Refractory Chronic Rhinosinusitis

Editors

ABTIN TABAEE
EDWARD D. MCCOUL

OTOLARYNGOLOGIC CLINICS OF NORTH AMERICA

www.oto.theclinics.com

Consulting Editor
SUJANA S. CHANDRASEKHAR

February 2017 • Volume 50 • Number 1

ELSEVIER

1600 John F. Kennedy Boulevard • Suite 1800 • Philadelphia, Pennsylvania, 19103-2899

http://www.oto.theclinics.com

OTOLARYNGOLOGIC CLINICS OF NORTH AMERICA Volume 50, Number 1
February 2017 ISSN 0030-6665, ISBN-13: 978-0-323-49669-8

Editor: Jessica McCool
Developmental Editor: Alison Swety

Otolaryngologic Clinics of North America (ISSN 0030-6665) is published bimonthly by Elsevier, Inc., 360 Park Avenue South, New York, NY 10010-1710. Months of issue are February, April, June, August, October, and December. Business and Editorial Offices: 1600 John F. Kennedy Blvd., Suite 1800, Philadelphia, PA 19103-2899. Customer Service Office: 6277 Sea Harbor Drive, Orlando, FL 32887-4800. Periodicals postage paid at New York, NY and additional mailing offices. Subscription prices are $381.00 per year (US individuals), $803.00 per year (US institutions), $100.00 per year (US student/resident), $500.00 per year (Canadian individuals), $1017.00 per year (Canadian institutions), $556.00 per year (international individuals), $1017.00 per year (international institutions), $270.00 per year (international & Canadian student/resident). Foreign air speed delivery is included in all *Clinics'* subscription prices. All prices are subject to change without notice. **POSTMASTER:** Send address changes to *Otolaryngologic Clinics of North America*, Elsevier Health Sciences Division, Subscription Customer Service, 3251 Riverport Lane, Maryland Heights, MO 63043. **Telephone: 1-800-654-2452 (U.S. and Canada); 314-447-8871 (outside U.S. and Canada). Fax: 314-447-8029. E-mail: journalscustomerservice-usa@elsevier.com (for print support); journalsonlinesupport-usa@elsevier.com (for online support).**

Reprints. For copies of 100 or more of articles in this publication, please contact the Commercial Reprints Department, Elsevier Inc., 360 Park Avenue South, New York, NY 10010-1710. Tel.: 212-633-3874; Fax: 212-633-3820; E-mail: reprints@elsevier.com.

Otolaryngologic Clinics of North America is also published in Spanish by McGraw-Hill Interamericana Editores S.A., P.O. Box 5-237, 06500 Mexico D.F., Mexico.

Otolaryngologic Clinics of North America is covered in *MEDLINE/PubMed (Index Medicus), Current Contents/Clinical Medicine, Excerpta Medica, BIOSIS, Science Citation Index,* and *ISI/BIOMED.*

PROGRAM OBJECTIVE
The goal of the *Otolaryngologic Clinics of North America* is to provide information on the latest trends in patient management, the newest advances; and provide a sound basis for choosing treatment options in the field of otolaryngology.

LEARNING OBJECTIVES
Upon completion of this activity, participants will be able to:
1. Review the classification and diagnosis of chronic rhinosinusitis.
2. Discuss treatments for chronic rhinosinusitis including topical therapies, office therapies, and sinus surgery.
3. Recognize comorbidities with chronic rhinosinusitis including nasal polyps and genetic and immune dysregulation, among others.

ACCREDITATION
The Elsevier Office of Continuing Medical Education (EOCME) is accredited by the Accreditation Council for Continuing Medical Education (ACCME) to provide continuing medical education for physicians.

The EOCME designates this enduring material for a maximum of 15 *AMA PRA Category 1 Credit*(s)™. Physicians should claim only the credit commensurate with the extent of their participation in the activity.

All other health care professionals requesting continuing education credit for this enduring material will be issued a certificate of participation.

DISCLOSURE OF CONFLICTS OF INTEREST
The EOCME assesses conflict of interest with its instructors, faculty, planners, and other individuals who are in a position to control the content of CME activities. All relevant conflicts of interest that are identified are thoroughly vetted by EOCME for fair balance, scientific objectivity, and patient care recommendations. EOCME is committed to providing its learners with CME activities that promote improvements or quality in healthcare and not a specific proprietary business or a commercial interest.

The planning committee, staff, authors and editors listed below have identified no financial relationships or relationships to products or devices they or their spouse/life partner have with commercial interest related to the content of this CME activity:
Adrianne Brigido; Roy R. Casiano, MD, FACS; Sujana S. Chandrasekhar, MD, FACS; Adam S. DeConde, MD; Jean Anderson Eloy, MD, FACS; Ashleigh Halderman, MD; Benjamin P. Hull, MD, MHA; Edward C. Kuan, MD, MBA; Andrew P. Lane, MD; Corinna G. Levine, MD, MPH; Emily Marchiano, MD; Jessica McCool; Edward D. McCoul, MD, MPH; Premkumar Nandhakumar; Gurston Nyquist, MD; Mindy Rabinowitz, MD; Marc Rosen, MD; Akshay Sanan, MD; Timothy L. Smith, MD, MPH; Jeffrey D. Suh, MD; Megan Suermann; Alison Swety; Andrew Thamboo, MD, MHSc, FRCSC; Alejandro Vázquez, MD; Thad W. Vickery, BA; Evan S. Walgama, MD; Yi Chen Zhao, MBBS, PhD, FRACS.

The planning committee, staff, authors and editors listed below have identified financial relationships or relationships to products or devices they or their spouse/life partner have with commercial interest related to the content of this CME activity:
Rakesh K. Chandra, MD is a consultant/advisor for, with research support from, Intersect ENT Inc.
Peter H. Hwang, MD is a consultant/advisor for Olympus America; Arinex Pty Ltd; 480 Biomedical; Sinnwave; and Intersect ENT Inc, and has stock ownership in Intersect ENT Inc.
Zara M. Patel, MD is on the speakers' bureau for Intersect ENT Inc, and is a consultant/advisor for Medtronic and Patara Pharma.
Vijay R. Ramakrishnan, MD is a consultant/advisor for Medtronic, and has research support from the National Institutes of Health, Flight Attendant Medical Research Institute; and the Cystic Fibrosis Foundation.
Abtin Tabaee, MD is a consultant/advisor for Spirox, Inc.
Peter-John Wormald, MD, FRACS, FRCS, MBChB is a consultant/advisor for NeilMed Pharmaceuticals Inc and ENT Technologies, and receives royalties/patents from Medtronic.

UNAPPROVED/OFF-LABEL USE DISCLOSURE
The EOCME requires CME faculty to disclose to the participants:
1. When products or procedures being discussed are off-label, unlabelled, experimental, and/or investigational (not US Food and Drug Administration [FDA] approved); and
2. Any limitations on the information presented, such as data that are preliminary or that represent ongoing research, interim analyses, and/or unsupported opinions. Faculty may discuss information about pharmaceutical agents that is outside of FDA-approved labelling. This information is intended solely for CME

and is not intended to promote off-label use of these medications. If you have any questions, contact the medical affairs department of the manufacturer for the most recent prescribing information.

TO ENROLL
To enroll in the *Otolaryngologic Clinics of North America* Continuing Medical Education program, call customer service at 1-800-654-2452 or sign up online at http://www.theclinics.com/home/cme. The CME program is available to subscribers for an additional annual fee of USD 260.

METHOD OF PARTICIPATION
In order to claim credit, participants must complete the following:
1. Complete enrolment as indicated above.
2. Read the activity.
3. Complete the CME Test and Evaluation. Participants must achieve a score of 70% on the test. All CME Tests and Evaluations must be completed online.

CME INQUIRIES/SPECIAL NEEDS
For all CME inquiries or special needs, please contact elsevierCME@elsevier.com.

Contributors

CONSULTING EDITOR

SUJANA S. CHANDRASEKHAR, MD, FACS
Clinical Professor of Otolaryngology-Head and Neck Surgery, Hofstra-Northwell School of Medicine, Clinical Associate Professor of Otolaryngology-Head and Neck Surgery, Icahn School of Medicine at Mount Sinai, Past President, American Academy of Otolaryngology-Head and Neck Surgery, Director, New York Otology, New York, New York

EDITORS

ABTIN TABAEE, MD
Associate Professor, Department of Otolaryngology, Weill Cornell Medicine–New York Presbyterian Hospital, New York, New York

EDWARD D. McCOUL, MD, MPH
Associate Professor, Department of Otorhinolaryngology, Ochsner Clinic, New Orleans, Louisiana

AUTHORS

ROY R. CASIANO, MD, FACS
Professor and Vice Chairman; Immediate Past President, American Rhinologic Society; Director, Rhinology and Endoscopic Skull Base Program, Department of Otolaryngology–Head & Neck Surgery, University of Miami, Miller School of Medicine, Miami, Florida

RAKESH K. CHANDRA, MD
Professor; Division Chief of Rhinology and Skull Base Surgery, Department of Otolaryngology, Vanderbilt University, Nashville, Tennessee

ADAM S. DeCONDE, MD
Division of Otolaryngology–Head & Neck Surgery, Department of Surgery, University of California San Diego, San Diego, California

JEAN ANDERSON ELOY, MD, FACS
Professor and Vice Chairman; Director, Rhinology and Sinus Surgery; Director, Otolaryngology Research; Co-Director, Endoscopic Skull Base Surgery Program, Department of Otolaryngology - Head and Neck Surgery, Center for Skull Base and Pituitary Surgery, Neurological Institute of New Jersey; Professor of Neurological Surgery, Professor of Ophthalmology and Visual Science, Departments of Neurological Surgery and Ophthalmology and Visual Science, Rutgers New Jersey Medical School, Newark, New Jersey

ASHLEIGH HALDERMAN, MD
Assistant Professor, Department of Otolaryngology–Head & Neck Surgery,
UT Southwestern Medical Center, Dallas, Texas

BENJAMIN P. HULL, MD, MHA
Clinical Instructor, Department of Otolaryngology, Vanderbilt University, Nashville,
Tennessee

PETER H. HWANG, MD
Professor, Department of Otolaryngology–Head & Neck Surgery, Stanford School of
Medicine, Stanford Sinus Center, Palo Alto, California

EDWARD C. KUAN, MD, MBA
Resident Physician, Department of Head and Neck Surgery, UCLA Medical Center,
Los Angeles, California

ANDREW P. LANE, MD
Professor, Department of Otolaryngology–Head & Neck Surgery, Johns Hopkins
Outpatient Center, Johns Hopkins School of Medicine, Baltimore, Maryland

CORINNA G. LEVINE, MD, MPH
Assistant Professor, Rhinology & Skull Base Surgery Fellow, Department of
Otolaryngology, University of Miami, Miller School of Medicine, Miami, Florida

EMILY MARCHIANO, MD
Department of Otolaryngology–Head & Neck Surgery, Neurological Institute of
New Jersey, Rutgers New Jersey Medical School, Newark, New Jersey

EDWARD D. McCOUL, MD, MPH
Associate Professor, Department of Otorhinolaryngology, Ochsner Clinic, New Orleans,
Louisiana

GURSTON NYQUIST, MD
Associate Professor, Department of Otolaryngology–Head & Neck Surgery, Thomas
Jefferson University Hospital, Philadelphia, Pennsylvania

ZARA M. PATEL, MD
Assistant Professor, Department of Otolaryngology–Head & Neck Surgery, Stanford
University School of Medicine, Stanford, California

MINDY RABINOWITZ, MD
Assistant Professor, Department of Otolaryngology–Head & Neck Surgery, Thomas
Jefferson University Hospital, Philadelphia, Pennsylvania

VIJAY R. RAMAKRISHNAN, MD
Department of Otolaryngology–Head & Neck Surgery, University of Colorado, Aurora,
Colorado

MARC ROSEN, MD
Professor, Department of Otolaryngology–Head & Neck Surgery, Thomas Jefferson
University Hospital, Philadelphia, Pennsylvania

AKSHAY SANAN, MD
Resident Physician, Department of Otolaryngology–Head & Neck Surgery, Thomas
Jefferson University Hospital, Philadelphia, Pennsylvania

TIMOTHY L. SMITH, MD, MPH
Division of Rhinology and Sinus/Skull Base Surgery, Department of Otolaryngology–Head & Neck Surgery, Oregon Sinus Center, Oregon Health and Science University, Portland, Oregon

JEFFREY D. SUH, MD
Associate Professor, Department of Head and Neck Surgery, UCLA Medical Center, Los Angeles, California

ABTIN TABAEE, MD
Associate Professor, Department of Otolaryngology, Weill Cornell Medicine–New York Presbyterian Hospital, New York, New York

ANDREW THAMBOO, MD, MHSc, FRCSC
Clinical Instructor, Department of Otolaryngology–Head & Neck Surgery, Stanford University School of Medicine, Stanford, California

ALEJANDRO VÁZQUEZ, MD
Fellow in Rhinology, Sinus, and Endoscopic Skull Base Surgery, Department of Otolaryngology–Head & Neck Surgery, Neurological Institute of New Jersey, Rutgers New Jersey Medical School, Newark, New Jersey

THAD W. VICKERY, BA
University of Colorado School of Medicine, Aurora, Colorado

EVAN S. WALGAMA, MD
Clinical Instructor, Department of Otolaryngology–Head & Neck Surgery, Stanford School of Medicine, Stanford Sinus Center, Palo Alto, California

PETER-JOHN WORMALD, MD, FRACS, FRCS, MBChB
Department of Surgery–Otolaryngology Head & Neck Surgery, The University of Adelaide, Adelaide, South Australia, Australia

YI CHEN ZHAO, MBBS, PhD, FRACS
Professor of Otolaryngology, Department of Surgery–Otolaryngology Head & Neck Surgery, The University of Adelaide, Adelaide, South Australia, Australia

Contents

An estimated 4.5% of total US health care dollars have been devoted to mitigating chronic rhinosinusitis. The most recalcitrant of these patients undergo surgery, which fails to improve symptoms in approximately 25% of patients. Recent advances in informational, microbiomic, and genomic analysis have introduced the first set of tools that patients, physicians, politicians, and payers can apply to better forecast which patients will respond favorably to endoscopic sinus surgery. This article summarizes the forces driving the application of personalized medicine to CRS and how new advances can be applied to clinical practice.

Chronic rhinosinusitis (CRS) is a prevalent condition that is heterogeneous in disease characteristics and multifactorial in cause. Although sinonasal mucosal inflammation in CRS is often either reversible or well-managed medically and surgically, a significant proportion of patients has a refractory form of CRS despite maximal therapy. Two of the several described factors thought to contribute to disease recalcitrance are genetic influences and dysfunction of the host immune system. Current evidence for a genetic basis of CRS is reviewed, as it pertains to putative abnormalities in innate and adaptive immune function. The role of systemic immunodeficiencies in refractory CRS is discussed.

Bacterial pathogens and microbiome alterations can contribute to the initiation and propagation of mucosal inflammation in chronic rhinosinusitis (CRS). In this article, the authors review the clinical and research implications of key pathogens, discuss the role of the microbiome, and connect bacteria to mechanisms of mucosal immunity relevant in CRS.

> Our understanding of chronic rhinosinusitis (CRS) show biofilm and osteitis play a role in the disease's pathogenesis and refractory. Studies point to its role in pathogenesis and poor prognosis. Outside the research laboratory, biofilm detection remains difficult and specific treatment remains elusive. It is believed that osteitis is a nidus of inflammation and occurs more commonly in patients with refractory CRS. However, osteitis may be exacerbated by surgery and a marker of refractory disease, not a causative agent. Surgery remains the mainstay treatment for biofilm and osteitis with mechanical disruption and removal of disease load providing the most effective treatment.

> Chronic rhinosinusitis with nasal polyposis (CRSwNP) represents a subset of chronic sinusitis with various causes. Some forms of the disease are driven by allergy, often in association with asthma. Refractory CRSwNP can be associated with cystic fibrosis and other clinical syndromes. More recent literature is presented regarding roles of innate immunity and superantigens. Effective treatment of CRSwNP requires careful endoscopic sinus surgery followed by an individualized treatment plan that often includes oral and topical steroids. Recidivism of polyps is common, and patients require long-term follow-up.

> Aspirin-exacerbated respiratory disease (AERD) is characterized by the triad of asthma, sinonasal polyposis, and aspirin intolerance. The hallmark of the disease is baseline overproduction of cysteinyl leukotrienes via the 5-lipoxygenase pathway, exacerbated by ingestion of aspirin. Patients with AERD have high rates of recidivistic polyposis following sinus surgery, although the improvement in quality of life following surgery is similar to aspirin-tolerant patients. The diagnosis is secured by a positive aspirin provocation test, usually administered by a medical allergist. Aspirin therapy is a unique treatment consideration for patients with AERD.

> Systemic and odontogenic etiologies of chronic rhinosinusitis, although rare, are an integral consideration in the comprehensive management of patients with sinonasal disease. Proper knowledge and timely recognition of each disease process, with referrals to appropriate consultants, will facilitate treatment, because many of these conditions require both local and systemic therapy. In some instances, medical therapy plays a pivotal role, with surgery being a supplemental treatment technique. We review the most commonly encountered systemic etiologies of chronic rhinosinusitis and odontogenic sinusitis, including clinical presentation, diagnosis, management, and treatment outcomes.

Office procedures in chronic rhinosinusitis (CRS) can be considered before and after medical management, as well as before and after surgical management. This article focuses specifically on refractory CRS, meaning those patients who have failed medical and surgical management already. The options available in the management of refractory CRS depend on the personnel, equipment, and instrumentation available in the office setting; surgeon experience; and patient suitability and tolerability. This article provides readers with possible procedural options that can be done in their clinics with indications, patient selection, potential complications, and postoperative considerations.

Topical therapy has become an important tool in the otolaryngologist's armamentarium for refractory chronic rhinosinusitis (CRS). Daily high-volume sinonasal saline irrigation and standard metered-dose topical nasal steroid therapy are supported by the most evidence. Nonstandard topical sinonasal steroid therapies are a potential option for refractory CRS. Current evidence recommends against the use of topical antifungal therapy and topical antibiotic therapy delivered using spray and nebulized techniques in routine cases of CRS. Stents are a new modality with preliminary data showing they are an option when traditional treatment has failed. Further research with long-term effects and outcomes studies for refractory CRS are needed.

Refractory chronic rhinosinusitis can be challenging to treat. Initial treatment focuses on medical and nonsurgical treatments. If these treatments fail, revision endoscopic sinus surgery is an option. A plan for revision surgery must address anatomic factors contributing to recurrence. Preoperative imaging and sinonasal endoscopy are systematically reviewed; areas of disease and "danger" zones are identified. Traditional anatomic landmarks are often obscured or absent; thus, a set of consistent landmarks (unchanged despite prior surgery) are used to navigate the revision endoscopic sinus surgery. Wide sinusotomies permit visualization and access to disease intraoperatively. Large sinus openings also facilitate postoperative debridements in clinic, endoscopic disease monitoring, and topical sinus therapy.

 Video content accompanies this article at http://www.oto.theclinics.com.

This review discusses extended endoscopic and open sinus surgery for refractory chronic rhinosinusitis. Extended maxillary sinus surgery including endoscopic maxillary mega-antrostomy, endoscopic modified medial maxillectomy, and inferior meatal antrostomy are described. Total/complete ethmoidectomy with mucosal stripping (nasalization) is discussed. Extended endoscopic sphenoid sinus procedures as well as their indications and potential risks are reviewed. Extended endoscopic frontal sinus procedures, such the modified Lothrop procedure, are described. Extended open sinus surgical procedures, such as the Caldwell-Luc approach, frontal sinus trephine procedure, external frontoethmoidectomy, frontal sinus osteoplastic flap with or without obliteration, and cranialization, are discussed.

Edward D. McCoul and Abtin Tabaee

Patients with refractory chronic rhinosinusitis, by definition, have persistent, poorly controlled symptoms and objective inflammatory findings despite prior medical and surgical therapy. These patients represent a diagnostic and treatment challenge given the complexity of the underlying disease factors and the limitations in available management options. This article presents a practical framework for clinical evaluation and treatment. Germane to discussion are emerging concepts in refractory chronic rhinosinusitis that will likely have important implications in the near future.

OTOLARYNGOLOGIC CLINICS
OF NORTH AMERICA

RELATED INTEREST

Immunology and Allergy Clinics of North America
August 2016 (Vol. 36, Issue 3)
Severe Asthma
Rohit K. Katial, *Editor*
Available at: http://www.immunology.theclinics.com

THE CLINICS ARE AVAILABLE ONLINE!
Access your subscription at:
www.theclinics.com

Foreword

Chronic Rhinosinusitis: A "Simple" Complex Condition

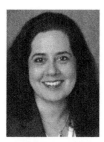

Sujana S. Chandrasekhar, MD, FACS
Consulting Editor

Often in medicine, what seems simple is actually very complex. That is the case with chronic rhinosinusitis (CRS). CRS is a common chronic illness in the United States and worldwide, affecting all age groups. In the United States, its prevalence is 146 per 1000 population; 12.3% of adults are diagnosed with CRS, according to Centers for Disease Control and Prevention data. In Europe, the incidence is 10.9%, as per GA2LEN data. In China, it may be as high as 13%. Self-diagnosis and treatment complicate our ability to understand the actual prevalence of this disorder.

There is a plethora of over-the-counter and herbal remedies for CRS, and this condition is managed by the following: the patient themselves in self-diagnosis, family physicians, internists, pediatricians, allergists, nurse practitioners, and otolaryngologists. But such a common and vexing condition is not simple, with layers of potential causes, findings, treatments, and reasons for treatment failures. In addition, the association of CRS with lower airways disease, including asthma, makes this more than just a stuffy nose problem. Genetic susceptibility, various viral and bacterial pathogens, existence of biofilms that make treatment very difficult, and mucosal and bony changes, including polyposis and osteitis, all lead to the complexity of this condition.

Drs Abtin Tabaee and Edward D. McCoul have compiled a comprehensive review of CRS in this issue of *Otolaryngologic Clinics of North America*. The reader will be left with a thorough understanding of the state-of-the-art and -science in diagnosing, determining cause, and offering targeted medical, office-based, and/or surgical therapies to the patient who presents with CRS. I congratulate the authors of each article

Otolaryngol Clin N Am 50 (2017) xv–xvi
http://dx.doi.org/10.1016/j.otc.2016.10.003
0030-6665/17/© 2016 Published by Elsevier Inc.

on their far-ranging exploration of each subject, and the guest editors on being able to pull the information together in a practical manner at the end.

Sujana S. Chandrasekhar, MD, FACS
New York Otology
Otolaryngology-Head and Neck Surgery
Hofstra-Northwell School of Medicine
1421 Third Avenue, 4th Floor
New York, NY 10028, USA

E-mail address:
ssc@nyotology.com

Preface

Refractory Chronic Rhinosinusitis

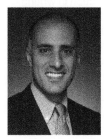
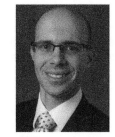

Abtin Tabaee, MD   Edward D. McCoul, MD, MPH
Editors

The past decade has witnessed a dramatic increase in the quality and volume of research into the basic science underpinnings and clinical experience associated with chronic rhinosinusitis (CRS). As the depth of knowledge regarding CRS has expanded, so too has our collective humility in the face of the complex challenges associated with diagnosis and treatment. No longer considered a single entity, CRS is now understood as a group of inflammatory disorders with distinct cofactors and pathophysiologic events. From a practical perspective, the endpoint of the clinical manifestations and our broad treatment options is similar for many of the different subtypes, but these will likely become more granular as subtle nuances in disease morphology become discernable with improved diagnostic tests and personalized treatment pathways.

No other aspect of rhinologic care for inflammatory disease represents a greater challenge to our field than refractory CRS, defined as persistent symptoms and objective inflammatory findings despite medical and surgical therapy. The negative quality-of-life impact, disease morbidity, and health care utilization for these patients are disproportionate and costly. Although our understanding of the underlying reasons for treatment failure has previously been limited, we are now approaching meaningful diagnostic and treatment pathways for many of these patients. The current issue of *Otolaryngologic Clinics of North America* explores refractory CRS from both pathophysiologic and clinical perspectives.

An esteemed list of authors has provided a series of complementary articles that both summate the latest advances in the field and provide a framework for approaching a patient with currently available modalities. The issue commences with a discussion of classification for the different CRS subtypes and how this may translate to a personalized approach to treatment. Subsequent articles discuss the various pathophysiologic factors that may exist in patients with refractory CRS, including dysregulated microbiome, genetic factors, biofilm, inflammatory injury, osteitis, and systemic

Otolaryngol Clin N Am 50 (2017) xvii–xviii
http://dx.doi.org/10.1016/j.otc.2016.11.001
0030-6665/17/© 2016 Published by Elsevier Inc.

disorders. The final portion of the issue explores different types of treatment modalities, including office-based, medical, and surgical options. Practical applications of these treatments as well as supporting clinical research studies are presented. Common to any discussion of an emerging field, there are as many questions in flux as there are well-defined principles.

We are immensely grateful to our publishing team for the opportunity to guest-edit this issue and to the contributing authors for their expertise and dedication in writing a series of deeply meaningful discussions and practical approaches to the care of patients with refractory CRS. Their collective wisdom is the core of this discussion. It is our hope that this issue will serve as a reference for clinical rhinology practice and as a reflection of both the current understanding and the future directions in the field.

Abtin Tabaee, MD
Department of Otolaryngology
Weill Cornell Medicine–New York Presbyterian Hospital
1305 York Avenue, 5th Floor
New York, NY 10021, USA

Edward D. McCoul, MD, MPH
Department of Otorhinolaryngology
Ochsner Clinic
1514 Jefferson Highway, CT-4
New Orleans, LA 70121, USA

E-mail addresses:
atabaee1@gmail.com (A. Tabaee)
emccoul@gmail.com (E.D. McCoul)

Classification of Chronic Rhinosinusitis—Working Toward Personalized Diagnosis

Adam S. DeConde, MD[a], Timothy L. Smith, MD, MPH[b],*

KEYWORDS

- Chronic rhinosinusitis • Precision medicine • Personalized medicine • Microbiome
- Cluster analysis • Phenotype • Endotype • Epidemiology

KEY POINTS

- The costs of chronic rhinosinusitis (CRS) are massive and increasing, with an estimated 4.5% of total US health care expenditures devoted to CRS care in 2011.
- Stratification of CRS by polyp status and baseline clinical history is not predictive of treatment outcomes.
- Baseline lost productivity, age, and the Sinonasal Outcome Test-22 score can effectively stratify patients into 5 distinct clusters with distinct responses to endoscopic sinus surgery.
- Genotypic data that can be discerned by an in-clinic taste test are associated with surgical outcomes in patients with CRS without nasal polyps.
- Baseline microbiomic data are associated with clinical phenotypes as well as surgical outcomes.

INTRODUCTION

Medicine as a whole is at the precipice of a revolution. The crucible of unprecedented advances in big data and financial and political pressure to provide increasingly efficient care are fueling these rapid changes. Management of CRS is particularly

Potential Conflicts of Interest: None.
Financial Disclosures: A.S. DeConde and T.L. Smith are consultants for IntersectENT, Incorporated (Menlo Park, California), which is not affiliated with this article. T.L. Smith is supported by a grant for this investigation from the National Institute on Deafness and Other Communication Disorders (NIDCD), one of the National Institutes of Health, Bethesda, Maryland (R01 DC005805; PI/PD: T.L. Smith).
[a] Division of Otolaryngology-Head & Neck Surgery, Department of Surgery, University of California San Diego, 200 W. Arbor, #8895, San Diego, CA 92103, USA; [b] Division of Rhinology and Sinus/Skull Base Surgery, Department of Otolaryngology – Head and Neck Surgery, Oregon Sinus Center, Oregon Health and Science University, 3181 South West Sam Jackson Park Road, PV-01, Portland, OR 97239, USA
* Corresponding author.
E-mail address: smithtim@ohsu.edu

Otolaryngol Clin N Am 50 (2017) 1–12
http://dx.doi.org/10.1016/j.otc.2016.08.003

susceptible to these changes for various reasons. Although CRS is a devastating disease, it is not life threatening, and in the modern era, the value of treatments has to be justified. It is also a hugely expensive disease, with some estimates placing the direct costs at 4.5% of the entire health care expenditure.[1] Given that patients with medically recalcitrant disease that undergo endoscopic sinus surgery (ESS) fail to make clinically significant improvements approximately one-fourth of the time,[2] there will be pressure on clinicians to refine these outcomes and justify the costs.

CRS is also now recognized as a complex multifactorial disease with a poorly understood interplay between anatomy, microbiome, and innate immunity that yields the common final pathway of 2 of 4 cardinal symptoms with characteristic endoscopic and radiographic findings.[3] New technological advances in all of these fields will help to refine outcomes, but will also require the clinician to be more facile in increasingly sophisticated technologies. Identification of patients who are good and bad surgical candidates will increasingly be demanded of the physician by patients, politicians, and payers.

This article covers the financial pressures that are driving the demand for a more efficient delivery of care, as well as the informatics and technical advances that are facilitating these refinements.

Epidemiology

A large range in prevalence of CRS is likely, due to variation of epidemiologic methods. Large questionnaire-based studies avoid the pitfalls of geographic variation and support US and European rates of CRS at approximately 10%. Confirmation of the veracity of the questionnaire-based methodology with clinical evaluations supports the accuracy of this methodology.

Understanding the true prevalence of a disease such as CRS is a critical yet challenging endeavor. Accurate prevalence estimates facilitate judicious application of research, as well as industry and health care resources in addressing CRS, and thus it behooves patients, the medical profession, and society to accurately document its prevalence. It is somewhat confusing to find that the literature on CRS reflects a wide range of prevalence, at 2% to 15%.[4,5] The range of prevalence is in part driven by the underlying methodology of the epidemiologic study: large-scale questionnaire evaluations and small-scale clinical evaluations.

Questionnaire-Based Evaluations

It has been a relatively recent development that broadly accepted diagnostic criteria for CRS have been adopted.[3,6] Epidemiologic studies, therefore, that predate modern definitions are limited by a lack of sensitivity and specificity and are not directly comparable. Although modern definitions of CRS require both subjective patient-reported symptoms along with physician-reported radiographic and/or endoscopic endpoints, there are practical limitations in obtaining large, population-level studies that include radiographic and endoscopic endpoints. Given these inherent limitations, a current examination of the literature places the true US prevalence of CRS at approximately 10%.[7]

Several national surveys support this number. The US National Health Interview Survey was carried out in 2012 and is the largest of these surveys.[7] It included 234,921 adults and 12.1% of subjects reported having been given the diagnosis of sinusitis by a health care provider in the preceding year. This likely is an overestimate of CRS rates, since the questionnaire did not clarify whether the diagnosis given was for acute or chronic disease. However, the 2008 Global Allergy and Asthma European Network questionnaire-based survey included 57,128 respondents based on the presence of at least 12 weeks of CRS patient-reported symptoms set forth in the European Position Paper on Rhinosinusitis and Nasal Polyps[4,8] and found a similar prevalence of 10.9%. The Canadian analog to these surveys found a prevalence of 5.2% in 73,364 respondents.[7] (**Table 1**).

Clinical Evaluations

Clinical evaluations are for the most part plagued by the inherent limitations of small sample size with a high likelihood of geographic and selection biases.[5] However, a follow-up study of the 2008 Global Allergy and Asthma European Network survey is worth reviewing. A subset of respondents to that survey was evaluated by an otolaryngologist.[9] Thirty-percent of the CRS diagnoses by survey were overturned; yet an additional 15% of respondents previously negative for CRS were classified as having CRS. This study helps confirm the relative veracity of the questionnaire-based approach, and suggests that not much value is added to the more expensive clinical evaluation.

SOCIETAL BURDEN OF CHRONIC RHINOSINUSITIS

Medically recalcitrant CRS is a massive burden for the individual patient. In fact, patients with CRS report more impairment of quality of life than patients with Parkinson disease, coronary disease requiring percutaneous intervention, and moderate chronic obstructive pulmonary disease (COPD). The estimated direct costs of CRS are increasing, with approximately $60 billion spent in 2011, representing 4.5% of overall health care expenditure for the year. Indirect costs of medically recalcitrant CRS can be massive, with mean costs of approximately 30% of annual income in patients who elect surgical therapy.

The high prevalence of CRS and the significant quality-of-life impact of CRS suggest that it weighs heavily on society. However, determining the societal burden of any disease state is, in a way, defining the value of resolving the disease state. This process is not trivial, and has only been possible recently for CRS. The value of controlling CRS is a function of the benefit obtained in controlling the disease divided by the cost to avoid it. In the case of CRS, the costs of the disease are captured by the direct costs of therapies and the indirect costs of uncontrolled disease.

Burden to the Individual

The benefit of avoiding CRS or resolving CRS is captured by a metric known as the health utility value. The utility value of any given health state is an effort to determine the preference of that health state over any other health state. Several mechanisms exist to determine the health utility of a given disease state, but 1 mechanism includes asking subjects to estimate how much time they would be willing to sacrifice to avoid a

Table 1
Questionnaire-based epidemiology of chronic rhinosinusitis

Author, Year	Survey	Location	Subjects	CRS Prevalence
Chen et al,[7] 2003	NPHS	Canada	73,364	5.2%
Hastan et al,[8] 2011	GA²LEN	Europe	57,128	10.9%
Blackwell et al,[6] 2014	NHIS	United States	234,921	12.10%

Abbreviations: GA²LEN, Global Allergy and Asthma European Network; NHIS, National Health Interview Survey; NPHS, National Population Health Survey.

certain poorer health sate. For example, asking a respondent to choose the number of years they would live disease-free compared with 10 years of life with CRS. Hypothetically, if the subject responded that 6.5 years of life without CRS is equivalent to 10 years with it, the utility value would be reflect the utility value of CRS, 0.65 (6.5 years divided by 10). At baseline, the mean utility value for patients with medically recalcitrant CRS was 0.65.[10] To give this number some context, CRS ranks lower than Parkinson disease,[11] coronary artery disease requiring percutaneous intervention,[12] and moderate COPD.[13] These findings were corroborated by Remenschneider and colleagues,[13] who found a diminished, but higher utility value of 0.81, which still places CRS in line with diseases such as asthma, COPD, and angina.

Burden to Society

The purely economic burden of CRS is truly staggering and consists of both the direct and indirect costs of the disease. The direct costs to society reflect the money spent on such things as medicines, doctor visits, surgeries, and tests, and the most recent analysis estimates the annual costs at $60.2 to $64.5 billion in 2011.[1] These estimates are in part a function of what prevalence estimate is used to extrapolate the costs. In this analysis, a conservative estimate of 3.5% was used; yet the costs represent 4.5% to 4.8% of the overall expenditures of US healthcare in 2011. The indirect costs represent the economic burden that results from decreased productivity of the population. Productivity loss is accounted for through absenteeism (missed work) and presenteeism (reduced work productivity). For an individual with medically refractory CRS (ie, uncontrolled disease), assuming mean income (in the US in 2013 approximately $31,000 annually), indirect costs result in $10,077 loss of income annually in patients who elect surgery and $3500 in patients who elect continued medical therapy.[14,15] Extrapolating these losses nationwide puts indirect costs for these patients at approximately $12.8 billion in 2013 (**Table 2**).

PRECISION MEDICINE

I want the country that eliminated polio and mapped the human genome to lead a new era of medicine—one that delivers the right treatment at the right time.
—President Barack Obama introducing the Precision Medicine Initiative in the 2015 State of the Union Address.

Given the high costs and suffering associated with CRS, optimization of therapeutic interventions is a valuable endeavor. Ideally, pretreatment stratification of patients would have clinically actionable characteristics. This level of precision would theoretically improve outcomes while decreasing unnecessary treatments for patients who are unlikely responders. An increase in health care efficiency is appealing to government officials in times of increasing austerity, and an increase in efficient targeting of interventions will be valuable for patients and health care providers also. Given

Table 2
Costs of chronic rhinosinusitis in 2014 US dollars

Author, Year	Methodology	Direct Costs	Indirect Costs
Ray et al,[16] 1999	Delphi technique	$5.8 billion	—
Bhattacharyya,[17] 2011	2007 Medical Expenditure Panel Survey	$9.8 billion	—
Smith et al,[18] 2015	Systematic review	$9.9 billion	$13 billion
Caulley et al,[1] 2015	2011 Medical Expenditure Panel Survey	$67.8 billion	—

that clinicians in many ways have been practicing personalized medicine since the profession's inception, the term precision medicine has been advocated to clarify the uniquely contemporary concept of application of big data to greatly increase the resolution with which an individual or disease process can be stratified.

Precision medicine is a tantalizing revolution that is thought to be imminent given the convergence of innovations in genetics, informatics, proteomics, microbiomics, metabolomics, and epigenetics.[19] The amount of information that can be obtained relatively inexpensively could allow for an unprecedented degree of stratification. Enthusiasm for this movement is reflected and fueled by the recent announcement of the Precision Medicine Initiative by President Barack Obama in his Jan. 20, 2015, State of the Union Address, supported by $215 million.[20] Such an investment is an important start to making precision medicine a reality and ensures that it will in part frame the direction of future research and care.

The implications for patients with CRS are important given the aforementioned costs of the disease, but also given the fact that CRS is a heterogeneous disease. CRS is likely a broad group of immune dysfunctional states that are united by the final common pathway of chronic symptoms. It seems reasonable to assume that to some degree individual idiosyncrasies would predispose one to success or failure of any given intervention. The following sections seek to summarize the current understanding of the classification and stratification of CRS and treatment implications.

CLASSIFICATION OF CHRONIC RHINOSINUSITIS

Classification of CRS is broadly categorized into phenotypes (clinical manifestation) and endotypes (biomarker and underlying pathogenesis). Classifications by phenotype (eg, phenotype, clinical history) historically have failed to stratify patients into actionable groups.

Clinically meaningful stratification of CRS has been pursued for many years. Classification schemes have historically been dominated by an effort to group CRS by the underlying pathophysiology or presence or absence of nasal polyps. Classification of CRS by its clinical manifestation is referred to as phenotyping, whereas classification by the underlying pathophysiologic mechanisms is termed endotyping. Clinical subtyping has reached the level of national guidelines, with stratification into CRS with nasal polyps (CRSwNP) and CRS without nasal polyps (CRSsNP).[3,4] Others argue that the presence and absence of eosinophils has also been implicated as an important branch point stratifying CRS[21,22] (**Table 3**). The challenge remains, however, that despite these efforts, the classification of CRS remains broad, with significant overlap between subtypes, and the stratification has not translated to clinically meaningful stratification.[2,23] This has led to efforts refining baseline phenotypic evaluation as well as the pursuit of novel endotypic biomarkers that would more accurately forecast treatment outcomes.

Phenotypic Classification of chronic rhinosinusitis

Cluster analysis of 103 clinical variables in a prospective, multicenter cohort has identified 3 easily obtainable baseline data points that stratify patients into distinct clusters. Clusters respond differentially to surgical intervention, with 3 of 5 patients making lasting, clinically meaningful improvement, while the other 2 patients fail to improve.

Part of the challenge of identifying clinical data that are actionable is in part due to the challenge in collecting a large number of baseline clinical variables in a high-quality way across a variety of geographies and institutions. Once the data are collected, the analysis required to sift through the massive amount of data is not trivial. Fortunately, a

Table 3			
Proposed classifications of chronic rhinosinusitis			
Classification Scheme	**Authors**	**Data Supporting**	**Correlates with Outcomes?**
Endoscopic (polyp vs nonpolyp)	EPOS,[4] Adult Sinusitis Guidelines,[3] Smith et al,[2] 2010	Expert opinion, pathomechanistic data, cohort data	No
Microscopic (high vs low eosinophilia)	Soler et al,[21] 2010, Czerny et al,[23] 2014, Kountakis et al,[22] 2004, Thompson et al,[24] 2016	Cohort data	Mixed
Clinical (without baseline PROMS)	Smith et al,[2] 2010	Cohort data	No
Clinical (with baseline PROMS)	Soler et al,[25] 2016	Cohort data	Yes
Microbiomic (biodiverse vs uniform)	Ramakrishnan et al,[26] 2015	Single-institution cohort data	Yes
Genomic (supertaster vs non-supertaster)	Adappa et al,[27] 2016	Single-institution cohort data	Yes

large, multicenter prospective cohort of medically recalcitrant patients electing either medical or surgical therapy has recently been accrued (Clinical Trial NCT01332136).[28]

A cluster analysis of these data incorporated 103 baseline clinical variables in a cohort of 482 patients who elected surgery.[28] Cluster analysis seeks to group sets of variables into groups with similar characteristics. Cluster analysis is unsupervised, in that it approaches the variables indifferently without any hypothesis. The advantage of this methodology is that the data are systematically grouped without bias to optimize clustering. A complete description of the characteristics of each cluster yielded in the analysis by Soler and colleagues[28] is beyond the scope of this article, and not as clinically relevant as discussing which clinical characteristics best predict cluster placement.

Only 3 clinical variables are required to effectively stratify patients into the correct clusters 90% of the time.[28] The first branch point in the sorting algorithm is missed productivity in the past 90 days, followed by age, and finally by SNOT-22 total (**Fig. 1**). Comparison of medication usage across clusters reveals that medication usage was significantly different. This is in contrast to a preliminary cluster analysis in which no patient-reported outcome measures were included in the cluster analysis. Without patient-reported outcome measures in the analysis, the patients stratify along more traditional lines (ie, polyp status or endoscopic and radiographic scores), yet the clusters no longer differ along clinically relevant measures such as patient-reported measures or medication usage.

Application of the clinical criteria that predicted clustering to the same cohort after recruitment of more patients (n = 690) was used to predict outcomes after surgical therapy.[25] The primary outcome was interval change of SNOT-22 at 6, 12, and 18 months. Indeed, the clusters responded differentially to surgical interventions, with cluster 1 and cluster 5 showing no significant advantage of surgery over continued medical therapy at 18-month follow-up and clusters 2 to 4 showing a clinically and statistically significant improvement at 18 months on the SNOT-22 (see

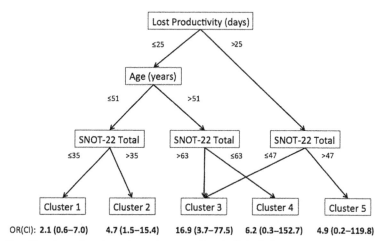

Fig. 1. Stratification of patients into clusters using 3 clinical characteristics with associated odds ratios (at bottom) of achieving improvement of at least a minimal clinically important difference after sinus surgery compared with medical management. 99.5% confidence interval, lost productivity, missed days of work in last 90 days, odds ratio, SNOT-22, Sinonasal Outcome Test-22.

Fig. 1). These findings are an important proof of concept that demonstrates that baseline characteristics can be used to not only stratify patients with CRS, but also to forecast response to surgical therapies when analyzed systematically.

Endotyping chronic rhinosinusitis

Contemporary enthusiasm for precision medicine is in large part fueled by advances in genomics and microbiomics. Application of these technologies to CRS is a recent phenomenon, yet there are already advances that can improve targeted therapies. Identifying biomarkers in CRS that forecast therapy outcomes is challenging and expensive. Frequently, studies are on groups of patients 1 order of magnitude less than the clinical investigations, and eventually these cohorts will have to grow. The following section highlights 2 efforts in endotyping of CRS that are associated with treatment outcomes.

Microbiomic classification of chronic rhinosinusitis

Microbiomics in CRS seek to apply ecological theories and measures to CRS. The sinus microbiome can be measured by the number of species (ie, richness) and the degree to which each species is represented (ie, complexity and evenness). Patients with increased richness, complexity, and evenness in the sinus microbiome at the time of surgery are less likely to have revision procedures and require postoperative systemic medical therapies.

A significant body of research has recently emerged on the impact of commensal gut bacteria on human health. Gut microbiota has been linked to early immunologic development, maintaining immune homeostasis, outcompeting pathogens, and modulating susceptibility to inflammatory and allergic diseases.[29–31] It has also become clear that healthy sinuses are in no way sterile environments.[32] It stands to reason (and data support the notion), that sinus microbiota plays an important role in modulating the inflammatory process of CRS.[33] Evidence from the lower airway also suggests that microbiota plays an important role in maintaining health and exacerbating disease.[34,35]

Part of the challenge for clinicians in consuming microbiome data is that the concept of the sinus as an ecosystem along with the analysis associated with such a paradigm is relatively novel. A full evaluation of the microbiota of the sinuses requires advanced molecular techniques. Broad-range 16S rRNA amplification and sequencing have increased sensitivity and allow for quantification of the bacterial species when compared with traditional clinical cultures that are currently routinely used.[36] Much more data, therefore, are generated by such analysis in contrast to clinical cultures.

Microbiome analysis is an application of ecological and biodiversity principles to a microscopic environment. As opposed to identifying a single pathogen, the analysis is geared at understanding the entire balance of the system. An infection can be thought of as an introduction of an invasive species into an environment, and surgery and antibiotics an exercise in repopulation after decimation of an ecosystem.[37] Although a deep understanding of these concepts and terminology is beyond the scope of this article, the reality is that moving forward clinicians will need to have at least a conversational understanding of the microbiomic concept with the associated vocabulary.

Species richness is simply a quantification of the number of species identified. Richness does not take into account the proportion of any given species, however. The complexity and evenness are indices that measure the degree to which the number of bacteria present is spread across the number of species present. For example, if the number of bacteria is evenly distributed (ie, the same number of bacteria of each species is represented) across species, then the evenness is 1, and as the distribution gets less even the score approaches zero.[38] In CRS, the literature has only just begun to go into press, and over the next 10 years, this data will become increasingly relevant.

With that foundation, examination of the early literature linking sinus microbiota with clinical outcomes is feasible. A relatively large cohort of patients (n = 56) undergoing endoscopic sinus surgery by a single surgeon for medically refractory CRS had an examination of microbiota at time of surgery.[26] These subjects were compared with controls, patients undergoing endoscopic approaches to intracranial skull base pathology or undergoing nasal airway surgery without CRS. At baseline, Ramakrishnan and colleagues sought to correlate microbiome characteristics with clinical phenotypes. Of 12 different clinical data points, only asthma and presence of purulence were significantly associated with sinus microbiota profiles. These variables remained significant when included in a 2-predictor model as well. Purulence on endoscopic examination was associated with increased *Bacteriodetes* and *Fusobacteria*, which are obligate anaerobes that may represent opportunistic pathogens when sinus ventilation is impaired.

The clinical endpoints employed by Ramakrishnan and colleagues[26] lacked patient-reported outcome measures, but did use hard clinical endpoints (medication usage and need for additional procedures) at a minimum of 6-month follow-up. An optimal outcome was defined as no further use of antibiotics, systemic steroids (beyond perioperative systemic therapies), or revision surgical therapy, with at least a 50% reduction in endoscopic scoring. Of the 27 subjects with CRS, approximately half had an optimal outcome. Optimal outcomes were associated with increased richness, evenness, and complexity. The association of increased richness, evenness, and complexity of sinus microbiota at baseline with optimal results makes intuitive biological sense. An increased baseline microbiome biodiversity might decrease the risk of postoperative infection through pathogen exclusion.

The true value of microbiome data in categorizing CRS has yet to be determined. The techniques required to accurately assess the sinus microbiome remain relegated to laboratories with a relatively high expense. The findings of Ramakrishnan and colleagues[26] need to be validated across larger cohorts with a greater number of clinical variables. Incorporation of patient-reported outcome measures is a valuable next step in determining the ability of the microbiome to predict baseline and post-treatment quality of life. Regardless, this early work holds great promise in refining the clinical model proposed by Soler and colleagues.[25]

Genomic classification of chronic rhinosinusitis

A bitter taste receptor, T2R38, has been recently identified in sinonasal ciliated epithelium. T2R38 plays an important role in sinonasal mucosa, sensing gram-negative bacteria, and modulating the innate immune system antimicrobial response. The T2R38 has a functional and nonfunctional form. Patients with CRSsNP homozygote for the functional form T2R38 have greatly long-term improved patient-reported outcomes after ESS. Functional T2R38 homozygosity can be accurately determined by a clinic-based test.

Until recently, no studies demonstrated any compelling genetic linkage to CRS treatment outcomes. The evaluation of the role of bitter taste receptors in innate immunity is a testament to the efficacy and rapidity of translational medicine. It has only been approximately 5 years since gustatory bitter taste receptors were even first identified in the lower airway,[39] and a compelling story of their role in innate immunity and the clinical consequences has since been elucidated.

Since the discovery of bitter taste receptors in the lower airways, presence of bitter taste signaling molecules were found to also be expressed within the nasal cavity.[40] One such bitter taste receptor, T2R38, was found to be expressed in ciliated human sinonasal epithelial cells.[41] A quorum-sensing molecule that is secreted by gram-negative organisms such as *Pseudomonas aeruginosa* in fact activates this receptor. T2R38 is thus an important means by which sinonasal mucosa recognizes presence of gram-negative bacteria. Further, activation of the T2R38 receptor creates a calcium-dependent increase in nitric oxide, which results in both antibacterial peptide secretion and increased ciliary beat frequency.[42]

The T2R38 protein has 2 common polypmorphisms that yield an active version and an inactive version. Any given individual gets 1 version from each parent, and thus 3 possible genotypes exist: homozygote functional T2R38, heterozygote T2R38, homozygote dysfunctional T2R38. These genotypes essentially follow Mendelian genetics, with a 20%, 50%, and 30% population distribution, respectively.[43] Conveniently, the genotypes correlate with an individual's taste sensitivity to the molecule phenlthiocarbamide, providing a convenient way to classify patients into supertasters (ie, homozygotes for functional T2R38), intermediate tasters (ie, heterozygote for functional T2R38), and nontasters (ie, homozygote for dysfunctional T2R38).[43]

Given the role that T2R38 plays in innate immunity, it would stand to reason that patients with nonfunctional T2R38 would be more susceptible to CRS. Study of a cohort of 207 patients who underwent endoscopic sinus surgery for medically refractory CRS demonstrated that the functional T2R38 homozygotes had long-term improved outcomes after ESS.[27] Interestingly, the improved outcomes after sinus surgery associated with functional T2R38 homozygosity only held true for CRSsNP. This supports the concept that CRSwNP and CRSsNP are distinct pathologic entities; yet it may be that the study was underpowered, as there was a difference in mean improvement on SNOT-22 (31+-25 vs 24+-22, $P = .13$), but it did not reach statistical significance. However, when the patients were stratified by polyp status, patients with CRSsNP and homozygosity for functional T2R38 reported significantly better outcomes, with mean improvement on SNOT-22 of 38+-21 versus 12+-22, $P = .006$.[27] Examination of the preoperative bitter taste test revealed that patients with high sensitivity to phenylthio-carbamide had a mean SNOT-22 improvement of 21 plus or minus 20 in CRSsNP compared with 4 plus or minus 21 in nontasters.

These findings are significant, as they represent the first stratification of CRS outcomes by genotype. They also highlight a significant endotypic difference between CRSwNP and CRSsNP, as the T2R38 receptor does not appear to impact clinical outcomes in CRSwNP. The study is limited by its sample size and lack of other potentially important data such as microbiome characteristics, which could potentially correlate with genotype of the innate immune system. Regardless, this work is a significant and exciting step toward delivering clinically meaningful precision medicine for CRS.

SUMMARY

Although in its earliest stages, the reality of precision medicine is here. The direct and indirect costs of CRS are staggering, estimated to be between $20 and $60 billion annually. Even modest improvements in efficiency of care would have a large societal benefit. Recent advances in clinical phenotyping, microbiomics, and genomics have already refined the ability to forecast patients who are likely to succeed with surgical management. Analysis of clinical phenotypes has revealed 5 distinct clusters of patients that can accurately be sorted through 3 easily accessible pieces of data (SNOT-22 score, lost productivity and age). Microbiomics and CRS, although novel, have already demonstrated that diverse and even microbiomic sinus ecosystems are associated with improved surgical outcomes. Application of this information will require wide distribution of diagnostic testing prior to broad application. Finally, genomics has identified a subgroup of patients with CRSsNP that can be distinguished in clinic with a taste test that predicts improved outcomes after ESS. These are only the earliest steps in an increasingly sophisticated and complicated approach to CRS.

REFERENCES

1. Caulley L, Thavorn K, Rudmik L, et al. Direct costs of adult chronic rhinosinusitis by using 4 methods of estimation: results of the US Medical Expenditure Panel Survey. J Allergy Clin Immunol 2015;136(6):1517–22.
2. Smith TL, Litvack JR, Hwang PH, et al. Determinants of outcomes of sinus surgery: a multi-institutional prospective cohort study. Otolaryngol Head Neck Surg 2010;142(1):55–63.
3. Rosenfeld RM, Piccirillo JF, Chandrasekhar SS, et al. Clinical practice guideline (update): adult sinusitis. Otolaryngol Head Neck Surg 2015;152(2 Suppl):S1–39.
4. Fokkens W, Lund V, Mullol J, European Position Paper on Rhinosinusitis and Nasal Polyps Group. European position paper on rhinosinusitis and nasal polyps 2007. Rhinol Suppl 2007;20:1–136.
5. Shashy RG, Moore EJ, Weaver A. Prevalence of the chronic sinusitis diagnosis in Olmsted County, Minnesota. Arch Otolaryngol Head Neck Surg 2004;130(3):320–3.
6. Blackwell DL, Lucas JW, Clarke TC. Summary health statistics for U.S. adults: national health interview survey, 2012. Vital Health Stat 10 2014;260:1–161.
7. Chen Y, Dales R, Lin M. The epidemiology of chronic rhinosinusitis in Canadians. Laryngoscope 2003;113(7):1199–205.
8. Hastan D, Fokkens WJ, Bachert C, et al. Chronic rhinosinusitis in Europe – an underestimated disease. A GA^2LEN study. Allergy 2011;66(9):1216–23.
9. Lange B, Thilsing T, Baelum J, et al. Diagnosing chronic rhinosinusitis: comparing questionnaire-based and clinical-based diagnosis. Rhinology 2013;51(2):128–36.

10. Brazier J, Roberts J, Deverill M. The estimation of a preference-based measure of health from the SF-36. J Health Econ 2002;21(2):271–92.
11. Hatoum HT, Brazier JE, Akhras KS. Comparison of the HUI3 with the SF-36 preference based SF-6D in a clinical trial setting. Value Health 2004;7(5):602–9.
12. Kontodimopoulos N, Argiriou M, Theakos N, et al. The impact of disease severity on EQ-5D and SF-6D utility discrepancies in chronic heart failure. Eur J Health Econ 2011;12(4):383–91.
13. Remenschneider AK, Scangas G, Meier JC, et al. EQ-5D-derived health utility values in patients undergoing surgery for chronic rhinosinusitis. Laryngoscope 2015;125(5):1056–61.
14. Rudmik L, Smith TL, Schlosser RJ, et al. Productivity costs in patients with refractory chronic rhinosinusitis. Laryngoscope 2014;124(9):2007–12.
15. Rudmik L, Soler ZM, Smith TL, et al. Effect of continued medical therapy on productivity costs for refractory chronic rhinosinusitis. JAMA Otolaryngol Head Neck Surg 2015;141(11):969–73.
16. Ray NF, Baraniuk JN, Thamer M, et al. Healthcare expenditures for sinusitis in 1996: contributions of asthma rhinitis, and other airway disorders. J Allergy Clin Immunol 1999;103:408–14.
17. Bhattacharyya N. Incremental health care utilization and expenditures for chronic rhinosinusitis in the United States. Ann Otol Rhinol Laryngol 2011;120(7):423–7.
18. Smith KA, Orlandi RR, Rudmik L. Cost of adult chronic rhinosinusitis: a systematic review. Laryngoscope 2015;125(7):1547–56.
19. Jameson JL, Longo DL. Precision medicine—personalized, problematic, and promising. N Engl J Med 2015;372(23):2229–34.
20. Collins FS, Varmus H. A new initiative on precision medicine. N Engl J Med 2015; 372(9):793–5.
21. Soler ZM, Sauer D, Mace J, et al. Impact of mucosal eosinophilia and nasal polyposis on quality-of-life outcomes after sinus surgery. Otolaryngol Head Neck Surg 2010;142(1):64–71.
22. Kountakis SE, Arango P, Bradley D, et al. Molecular and cellular staging for the severity of chronic rhinosinusitis. Laryngoscope 2004;114(11):1895–905.
23. Czerny MS, Namin A, Gratton MA, et al. Histopathological and clinical analysis of chronic rhinosinusitis by subtype. Int Forum Allergy Rhinol 2014;4(6):463–9.
24. Thompson CF, Price CPE, Huang JH, et al. A pilot study of symptom profiles from a polyp vs an eosinophilic-based classification of chronic rhinosinusitis. Int Forum Allergy Rhinol 2016;6:500–7.
25. Soler ZM, Hyer JM, Rudmik L, et al. Cluster analysis and prediction of treatment outcomes for chronic rhinosinusitis. J Allergy Clin Immunol 2016;137:1054–62. Available at: http://www.sciencedirect.com/science/article/pii/S0091674915031164. Accessed January 27, 2016.
26. Ramakrishnan VR, Hauser LJ, Feazel LM, et al. Sinus microbiota varies among chronic rhinosinusitis phenotypes and predicts surgical outcome. J Allergy Clin Immunol 2015;136(2):334–42.e1.
27. Adappa ND, Farquhar D, Palmer JN, et al. TAS2R38 genotype predicts surgical outcome in nonpolypoid chronic rhinosinusitis. Int Forum Allergy Rhinol 2016; 6(1):25–33.
28. Soler ZM, Hyer JM, Ramakrishnan V, et al. Identification of chronic rhinosinusitis phenotypes using cluster analysis. Int Forum Allergy Rhinol 2015;5(5):399–407.
29. McLoughlin RM, Mills KHG. Influence of gastrointestinal commensal bacteria on the immune responses that mediate allergy and asthma. J Allergy Clin Immunol 2011;127(5):1097–107 [quiz: 1108–9].

30. Tabas I, Glass CK. Anti-inflammatory therapy in chronic disease: challenges and opportunities. Science 2013;339(6116):166–72.
31. Frank DN, Pace NR. Gastrointestinal microbiology enters the metagenomics era. Curr Opin Gastroenterol 2008;24(1):4–10.
32. Ramakrishnan VR, Feazel LM, Gitomer SA, et al. The microbiome of the middle meatus in healthy adults. PLoS One 2013;8(12):e85507.
33. Abreu NA, Nagalingam NA, Song Y, et al. Sinus microbiome diversity depletion and Corynebacterium tuberculostearicum enrichment mediates rhinosinusitis. Sci Transl Med 2012;4(151):151ra124.
34. Sze MA, Dimitriu PA, Hayashi S, et al. The lung tissue microbiome in chronic obstructive pulmonary disease. Am J Respir Crit Care Med 2012;185(10): 1073–80.
35. Marri PR, Stern DA, Wright AL, et al. Asthma-associated differences in microbial composition of induced sputum. J Allergy Clin Immunol 2013;131(2): 346–52.e1–3.
36. Hauser LJ, Feazel LM, Ir D, et al. Sinus culture poorly predicts resident microbiota. Int Forum Allergy Rhinol 2015;5(1):3–9.
37. Costello EK, Stagaman K, Dethlefsen L, et al. The application of ecological theory toward an understanding of the human microbiome. Science 2012;336(6086): 1255–62.
38. Morgan XC, Huttenhower C. Chapter 12: human microbiome analysis. PLoS Comput Biol 2012;8(12):e1002808.
39. Shah AS, Ben-Shahar Y, Moninger TO, et al. Motile cilia of human airway epithelia are chemosensory. Science 2009;325(5944):1131–4.
40. Braun T, Mack B, Kramer MF. Solitary chemosensory cells in the respiratory and vomeronasal epithelium of the human nose: a pilot study. Rhinology 2011;49(5): 507–12.
41. Lee RJ, Xiong G, Kofonow JM, et al. T2R38 taste receptor polymorphisms underlie susceptibility to upper respiratory infection. J Clin Invest 2012;122(11): 4145–59.
42. Lee RJ, Kofonow JM, Rosen PL, et al. Bitter and sweet taste receptors regulate human upper respiratory innate immunity. J Clin Invest 2014;124(3):1393–405.
43. Kim U, Jorgenson E, Coon H, et al. Positional cloning of the human quantitative trait locus underlying taste sensitivity to phenylthiocarbamide. Science 2003; 299(5610):1221–5.

Genetic and Immune Dysregulation in Chronic Rhinosinusitis

 CrossMark

Ashleigh Halderman, MD[a], Andrew P. Lane, MD[b],*

KEYWORDS

- Chronic rhinosinusitis • Chronic rhinosinusitis with nasal polyps
- Chronic rhinosinusitis without nasal polyps • Genetics
- Single-nucleotide polymorphisms • Immune dysregulation
- Primary immunodeficiency

KEY POINTS

- Local defects in innate and adaptive immunity have been implicated in the pathogenesis of refractory chronic rhinosinusitis (CRS).
- A genetic basis in CRS is suggested by an association with well-defined heritable disorders as well as limited evidence of a familial inheritance pattern.
- More than 445 single-nucleotide polymorphisms have been associated with CRS, although these largely have not been replicated.
- Systemic immune dysregulation in refractory CRS may be demonstrated with laboratory testing of humoral and cell-mediated immunity.

INTRODUCTION

Chronic rhinosinusitis (CRS) is defined in adults as persistent symptoms of sinonasal inflammation for 12 or more weeks with confirmatory objective findings on nasal endoscopy or computed tomography (CT).[1,2] CRS is a multifactorial disease with proposed etiopathologies including occupational/environmental exposures, infection, immune dysfunction, and genetic predisposition. As understanding of the disease evolves, clinical phenotypes have emerged that allow subclassification within the entity once identified solely as CRS. The presence or absence of polyps is used as a primary distinction because of easily recognizable clinical features and underlying inflammatory profiles. CRS with nasal polyps (CRSwNP) is characterized by T helper (Th)-2 polarization, with eosinophilia, increased levels of interleukin-4 (IL-4), IL-5, and IL-13, as well as high local production of immunoglobulin E (IgE). CRS without nasal

a Department of Otolaryngology – Head and Neck Surgery, UT Southwestern Medical Center, 5323 Harry Hines Blvd, Dallas, TX 75390, USA; b Department of Otolaryngology – Head and Neck Surgery, Johns Hopkins Outpatient Center, Johns Hopkins School of Medicine, 6th Floor, 601 North Caroline Street, Baltimore, MD 21287-0910, USA
* Corresponding author.
E-mail address: alane3@jhmi.edu

Otolaryngol Clin N Am 50 (2017) 13–28
http://dx.doi.org/10.1016/j.otc.2016.08.009
0030-6665/17/© 2016 Elsevier Inc. All rights reserved.

oto.theclinics.com

polyps (CRSsNP) demonstrates a mixed cytokine profile that lacks Th2 polarization. High levels of interferon-γ (IFN-γ) and transforming growth factor-β have been reported in CRSsNP,[3] but the consistency of this feature continues to be under investigation.[4–6] Although Th2 polarization clearly characterizes CRSwNP in Western countries, evidence suggests that Th2 skewing may be absent in CRSwNP patients in China. This difference may be disappearing as the region undergoes modernization.[7] A third distinct phenotype of CRS is aspirin-exacerbated respiratory disease (AERD), which is fully discussed elsewhere in this issue.

Clinically, otolaryngologists encounter refractory forms of rhinosinusitis within each phenotype. No consensus statement defining recalcitrant CRS exists; however, broadly speaking, CRS is considered refractory when it responds poorly to medical and surgical therapy. Multiple theories and possible pathophysiologic mechanisms have been proposed to explain recalcitrance in CRS. In this review, the authors focus specifically on the contribution of genetics and immunologic dysregulation.

At the most basic level, support for an underlying genetic contribution to CRS stems from observations of familial inheritance patterns.[8–10] Most of these observations were made in patients with nasal polyps, and, therefore, conclusions about the familial inheritance pattern of CRSsNP cannot be drawn. In patients with nasal polyps, a heritability of 14% to 42% has been described.[9,10] Cohen and colleagues[10] subclassified CRSwNP patients into 3 groups: isolated polyps, polyps with asthma, and AERD. Interestingly, they found that AERD had the highest heritability (42%) followed by asthma and polyps (30%) and isolated polyps (15%). In addition, they demonstrated a correlation with the number of family members (frequency) with nasal polyposis and the severity of disease showing that severity is proportional to the penetrance of an underlying genetic component.

As a caveat, growing evidence suggests that multiple endotypes of CRS, yet to be fully elucidated, may be present beyond the CRSsNP/CRSwNP/AERD classification scheme. Recognition that CRS remains a complex and incompletely defined disease has important consequences for weighing the validity of genetic and immunologic studies. Without precise definitions of CRS subtypes, meaningful interpretation of research findings is difficult, particularly when detailed clinical information, including raw laboratory and radiographic findings, is not available. At present, differences among CRS subtypes are likely obscured by classifications based on an incomplete understanding, and current scoring systems used for clinical research do not capture CRS features with sufficient granularity. Because of the variety within CRS, more meticulous gathering of patient data with subclassification will almost certainly be necessary to detect true genetic and immunologic contributors. Even if precise categorization were possible, CRS fluctuates in severity and characteristics over time and can develop later in life, so flawed subtype assignments are possible, particularly in genetic studies. All of these challenges must be appreciated, and the existing CRS literature should be evaluated through this lens.

Innate Immunity and Epithelial Barrier Dysfunction in Chronic Rhinosinusitis

Among the mechanisms proposed to contribute to CRS pathogenesis and recalcitrance, many involve abnormalities of local mucosal immune defense. Sinonasal innate immune function begins with the physical epithelial barrier, mucus production, and mucociliary clearance, extending to involve secreted antimicrobial factors and phagocytic hematopoietic cells that combat infection in the airway lumen.[11] Multiple inflammatory mediators produced by epithelial cells and other nonlymphocytic cell populations interact with the adaptive immune system to drive antigen-specific antibody production. Although lymphocytes had long been assumed to be the principal drivers of chronic inflammation, it has become increasingly apparent that tissue-bound epithelial cells, fibroblasts, macrophages, dendritic cells, mast cells, and innate lymphoid cells (ILCs) also participate in perpetuating inflammation. These cell types lack the ability to generate antigen-specific receptors through gene recombination, but instead use germline-encoded pattern recognition receptors (PRR) that bind to microbial elements and to damage-associated molecules. Genetic aberration or dysregulation of any of these innate immune pathways has the potential to contribute to CRS recalcitrance, and there is a growing body of evidence to support this concept. Abnormal mucus viscoelasticity and diminished mucociliary clearance are linked to CRS, including in genetically based diseases such as cystic fibrosis (CF) and primary ciliary dyskinesia.[12,13] Alteration in expression of PRRs such as toll-like receptors (TLRs) and taste receptors may also be associated with refractory CRS.

Several antimicrobial products are present in mucus and the sinonasal mucosa and include:

- Acute phase proteins
- Neutralizing proteins
- Enzymes
- Opsonins
- Defensins
- Protease inhibitors
- Surfactants

Increased levels of surfactant protein A, lysozyme, C3, and C5 have been demonstrated in tissue specimens of CRSsNP compared with controls.[14–17] In CRSwNP, increased levels of lysozyme, C3, cathelicidin, and acidic mammalian chitinase have been demonstrated compared with controls.[15,17–19] Other studies have shown decreased levels of antimicrobial products in both CRSsNP and CRSwNP. Altogether, these findings indicate that abnormal functioning or regulation of the innate immune system is present in both CRSsNP and CRSwNP and may play a significant role in the persistent inflammation that is a hallmark of all CRS.

PRRs may be activated by pathogen-associated molecular patterns or damage-associated molecular patterns. These receptors are found on most cell types, including macrophages, lymphocytes, and epithelial cells. Interestingly, studies have shown that TLR2, TLR4, and TLR7 messenger RNA (mRNA) and protein levels are significantly lower in CRSsNP than controls.[20] Similar findings of altered expression of TLR2, TLR4, TLR7, and TLR9 have been demonstrated in sinonasal tissue from patients with CRSwNP.[21–24] Another class of PRRs, taste receptors, has been shown to be expressed by nasal solitary chemosensory cells and to modulate epithelial cell innate immune activity in vitro.[25,26] Dysregulation of taste receptors in CRS has been suggested but not demonstrated. Although some studies have shown downregulation of PRRs and others have shown upregulation of the same PRRs, these data in aggregate imply that dysfunction or dysregulation of innate immunity is present and potentially contributing to the pathogenesis of CRS.

One example of potential innate immune dysregulation in refractory CRS is decreased expression and function of the PRR TLR9.[23] TLR9 activation leads to the production and release of Th1 cytokines and may downregulate Th2 inflammation at the same time.[27–29] Interestingly, decreased expression of TLR9 has been demonstrated in sinonasal epithelial cells (SNEC) from patients with recalcitrant CRSwNP, which could indicate that a deficient Th1 response in these patients contributes to Th2 skewed inflammation in CRSwNP. Furthermore, IL-33, a mediator produced by SNEC that activates the production of pro-Th2 mediators from ILCs, has been shown to have 3 times higher levels of mRNA expression in treatment-resistant CRSwNP than treatment-responsive CRSwNP.[30] These studies support the concept that innate immune defects contribute to the more recalcitrant forms of CRSwNP and that the resistance to treatment may relate to dysregulated mucosal immunity.

Genetics of Innate Immunity in Chronic Rhinosinusitis

Single-nucleotide polymorphisms (SNPs) are single-nucleotide variations in the DNA sequence. When an SNP occurs in a coding region of DNA, variability in the amino acid sequence can be created.[31] There are many limitations to attempting to causally link SNPs with CRS pathogenesis. First, most genetic CRS studies have compared allele frequencies of SNPs between CRS patients and control subjects only in genes previously implicated in CRS pathogenesis. This comparison creates an inherent bias and simultaneously hinders identification of novel gene candidates. Pooling-based genome-wide association scans (GWAS) allow unbiased investigation of the human genome with analysis of hundreds of thousands of possible candidate SNPs at one time. Bosse and colleagues[32] identified nearly 600 SNPs from 445 genes potentially associated with CRS. Given the multifactorial nature of CRS, the effect size of genes relevant to CRS are likely to be small, necessitating large sample sizes to achieve sufficient statistical power. Most studies have been underpowered and may be confounded by genetically diverse patient populations. Even when an SNP is associated with CRS, this does not automatically imply direct causation through gene dysregulation. Some SNPs may represent unrelated markers genetically linked to an unknown causal genetic variation, whereas others may have indirect roles by affecting transcription of undetermined genes truly involved in CRS. In genome-wide comparisons, implementing statistical corrections for multiple testing is critical in order to avoid false positive associations. When associations are replicated in multiple studies, confidence grows that a true relationship exists.

Because genetic variation in innate immunity genes appears to be a promising target for studies in CRS, multiple investigations have been attempted, but to date, definitive relationships have not been demonstrated. Only a few associations have been replicated, most notably those mentioned above, and causal associations remain unproven. Other than the studies of patients with well-characterized defects of the bitter taste receptor TAS2R38 gene, functional assessments of identified genetic variations have not yet been reported. No association has been determined between TLRs or downstream signaling molecule SNPs and CRS, other than an unreplicated study of interleukin-1 receptor-associated kinase 4 (IRAK4) polymorphisms in Chinese patients. SNPs in the nitric oxide synthase (NOS) family of genes have also been investigated in CRS, again with few reports of unreplicated associations in limited studies. Other genes that have been implicated in individual studies include the met proto-oncogene, locus (hepatocyte growth factor receptor), and serpin peptidase inhibitor (SERPINA1), but confirmatory studies are needed.

Several SNPs for multiple innate immune genes putatively involved in CRS are summarized in **Table 1**. Replication studies have been performed for acyloxyacyl hydroxylase (AOAH), the bitter taste receptor T2R38, and the Cystic Fibrosis Transmembrane Regulator (CFTR locus), and these genes are discussed below.

Acyloxyacyl hydroxylase

Polymorphisms in the gene for AOAH were initially associated with asthma in a GWAS in 2006.[33] Diminished degradation of lipopolysaccharides in AOAH dysfunction leads to continuous stimulation of inflammation through a TLR-4-dependent

Table 1
Genes involved in innate immunity that have been associated with chronic rhinosinusitis

Gene	Variation	Phenotype	Study
AOAH	rs4504543	CRSsNP	Zhang et al,[37] 2012
CD14	rs2569190	CRSwNP	Bernstein et al,[78] 2009, Yazdani et al,[93] 2012
IRAK4	Multiple	CRSsNP, CRSwNP	Tewfik et al,[94] 2009
LTF	−140 A > G	CRSwNP	Zielinska-Blizniewska et al,[66] 2012
MET	Multiple	CRSwNP	Castano et al,[59] 2010
NOS1	Multiple	Mixed population	Zhang et al,[95] 2011
NOS1AP	rs4657164	Mixed population	Zhang et al,[95] 2011
NOS2A	Promoter VNTR	CRSwNP	Pascual et al,[96] 2008
SERPINA1	rs1243168	Mixed population	Kilty et al,[97] 2010
TLR2	Multiple	CRSwNP	Sachse et al,[98] 2010, Park et al,[99] 2011
TAS2R38	PAV/PAV, PAV/AVI, AVI/AVI	Mixed population	Adappa et al,[39] 2016

mechanism,[34–36] according to studies in AOAH knockout mice. Bosse and colleagues[32] identified an association with an AOAH SNP rs4504543 and CRS in their GWAS. Zhang and colleagues[37] replicated this finding and showed an association with rs4504543 and Chinese patients with CRSsNP.

Bitter taste receptors
Expression of type 2 receptor bitter taste receptors (T2Rs) has been demonstrated by cell types outside of the gustatory system, including ciliated epithelial cells and solitary chemosensory cells of the upper airway. In response to bitter stimuli, and notably quorum-sensing molecules of gram-negative bacteria, nasal epithelial cell T2R38 signaling activates release of antimicrobial peptides and nitric oxide in vitro while altering ciliary beat frequency.[26,38] Tas2R38 polymorphisms have also been associated with surgical outcomes in CRSsNP.[39]

Cystic Fibrosis Transmembrane Regulator Locus
A clear genetic link between mutations in the CFTR locus and CF, which in turn is strongly associated with CRSsNP and CRSwNP, suggests that CFTR mutations could contribute to CRS in the absence of CF. A GWAS for CRS genes by Pinto and colleagues[40] supported a relationship between CFTR and CRS. A large series published in the *Journal of the American Medical Association* in 2000 established that patients with CRS were significantly more likely to be CFTR carriers than were controls.[41] Of patients who underwent full sequencing of CFTR, 38% of patients with CRSsNP were found to have mutations. Other studies have shown much lower rates of CFTR mutations in patients with CRS; however, it is important to note that those studies only assessed the 23 most common CFTR mutations. It is thought that CFTR mutations can still affect mucociliary clearance, viscosity of mucus, and sinonasal inflammation in the carrier state.

Adaptive Immunity in Chronic Rhinosinusitis
Innate immunity plays complex roles in priming and modulating the adaptive immune response through stimulating cytokine production, driving further inflammatory

response and determining T-cell differentiation, among many other actions. Although the 2 arms of the immune system have been separated in this text, in reality, they are each highly dependent on the other and intricately linked. The major cell type of the adaptive immune system, lymphocytes, are activated by binding of antigen-specific receptors to release cytokines, chemokines, and/or immunoglobulins, which in turn recruit leukocytes and orchestrate inflammatory responses. Adaptive immune responses may be characterized by the dominantly expressed cytokines into Th1, Th2, and Th17 types. The inflammation in CRS is generally mixed, although Th2 skewing with local eosinophilia is a prominent feature of CRSwNP. The major Th2-associated cytokines are IL-4, IL-5, IL-9, and IL-13. CRSsNP is more heterogeneous and less defined by a specific cytokine profile, and both forms of CRS display activation of cytotoxic T-cells, macrophages, and neutrophils. Th17 inflammatory cytokines have also been described in CRS, particularly in noneosinophilic polyps, although the role of these mediators in CRS pathogenesis is uncertain.

A study by Jyonouchi and colleagues[42] evaluated sinonasal lavage from patients with treatment-resistant CRS (mixed types), and found elevated levels of IFN-γ, IL-5, IL-8, IL-10, and IL-18. These findings support the concept that Th1 and Th2 driven inflammation could be contributing to recalcitrant forms of CRS. Regulatory T-cell (Treg) dysfunction has also been described in CRS; however, their exact role is unclear, with conflicting reports of either Treg cell impairment[43] or increased numbers of Tregs in CRSwNP patients.[44] B-cells have also been implicated as contributing to CRSwNP, as evident by increased B-cell numbers as well as increased levels of chemotactic factors and cytokines that promote B-cell activation and proliferation in nasal polyps compared with tissue from CRSsNP and controls.[45–48] Levels of multiple immunoglobulins have been shown to be increased in nasal polyps without a concomitant increase in the peripheral blood, suggesting local rather than systemic activation of B-cell antibody production in polyps.

Genetics of Adaptive Immune Dysfunction in Chronic Rhinosinusitis

Asthma and atopy are characterized by a Th2 inflammatory cytokine profile and tissue eosinophilia similar to CRSwNP, which has led to a search for linked genetic variants in genes encoding Th2 inflammatory mediators in these diseases. In asthma and allergy, promoter polymorphisms in IL-4 (rs2243250)[49,50] and IL-13 (rs20541)[51,52] have been strongly and repeatedly implicated. A small number of less powerful studies of the IL4 promoter SNPs in CRSwNP have not demonstrated a relationship, although a single Chinese study identified a CRSwNP-associated SNP elsewhere in the IL-4 gene.[53,54] No association has been found between IL-13 polymorphisms and CRS.[55] The most intriguing Th2-associated cytokine may be IL-33, which is an important stimulus for type 2 ILCs. Genetic variation in IL-33 has been implicated in allergic diseases, and an association with asthma has been well replicated.[56] Currently, the one genetic study of IL-33 and CRS by Buysschaert and colleagues[57] looked at more than 700 well-phenotyped Belgian patients (284 patients with CRSwNP and 427 control subjects), finding that the SNP rs3939286 in the vicinity of the IL-33 start codon was significantly associated with CRSwNP, even when controlling for atopy. Whether this SNP directly impacts the expression or function of IL-33 remains to be determined. The IL-33 receptor, ST2, has also been a target of investigation, yielding inconsistent results among studies of Canadian, Belgian, and Chinese CRSwNP patients.[37,57–59] Other genes with unreplicated studies supporting association with CRSwNP include tumor necrosis factor-β (TNF-β),[60] A20 (modulator of nuclear factor kB activation),[61] IL-22 receptor a1,[62] and 2 inhibitory receptors of IL-1.[59,63] Finally, genes associated with arachidonic acid metabolism, including leukotriene C4 synthase,[64] prostaglandin D2 receptor,[65] and cyclooxygenase-2,[66] have been investigated in unreplicated studies with limited study power and phenotypically heterogeneous patients.

Of the several SNPs in genes for adaptive immunity, only a few have been replicated. Other SNPs implicated in CRS but not replicated are summarized in **Table 2**, and those that have been replicated are discussed in greater detail later.

IL1A

IL-1 is an inflammatory cytokine that activates T-cells and monocytes, induces the expression of inflammatory cytokines and proteins, and upregulates the expression of adhesion molecules. It is has been shown to be more highly expressed in nasal polyps.[67,68] IL-1 exists in 2 types, IL-1a and IL-1b, and the genes encoding both are located on chromosome 2.[69] A G-to-T base exchange SNP in exon 5 at +4845 of the IL1A gene results in an amino acid substitution of alanine to serine,[70] possibly modifying its functionality. This SNP (rs17561) has been associated with both nasal polyposis and CRS with and without polyps in separate studies. Erbek and colleagues demonstrated a significant association with both the 4845 GT and 4845 TT genotypes and nasal polyps in Turkish patients. The 4845 GG genotype was significantly more common in controls.[62] Mfuna Endam and colleagues[63] studied Canadian patients with CRS (both those with and without polyps were included), demonstrating an association with rs17561 polymorphism. Interestingly, a Finnish study of asthmatics demonstrated a significant association between the 4845 GG genotype (no polymorphism present) and need for surgical nasal polypectomy.[71] It is important to note that this study identified subjects with nasal polyps by self-report only, whereas Erbek and colleagues confirmed the presence of nasal polyps by both nasal endoscopy and CT. Mfunda Endam and colleagues identified subjects with CRS (both with and without polyps) according to the 2004 American Academy of Otolaryngology-Head and Neck Surgery Guidelines. All 3 studies were performed in geographically/ethnically (and therefore likely genetically) diverse patient populations. This factor along with differences in the identification of CRS and CRSwNP patients could explain the differing results and highlights the importance of strict definitions of CRS phenotypes. Regardless, the replication of an association with rs17561 and CRSsNP and CRSwNP is exciting and suggests the need for future study.

Table 2
Genes involved in adaptive immunity that have been associated with chronic rhinosinusitis

Gene	Variation	Phenotype	Study
CD8A	rs3810831	Mixed population	Alromaih et al,[100] 2013
IL10	rs1800629	CRSwNP	Bernstein et al,[78] 2009
IL1A	Multiple	CRSsNP, CRSwNP	Erbek et al,[77] 2007, Mfuna Endam et al,[62] 2010
IL1B	rs16944	Mixed population	Erbek et al,[77] 2007, Mfuna Endam et al,[62] 2010
IL1RL1	Multiple	CRSsNP, CRSwNP	Castano et al,[101] 2009
ILR1N	VNTR in intron 2	Mixed population	Cheng et al,[102] 2006
IL22RA1	Multiple	Mixed population	Endam et al,[103] 2009
IL33	rs3939286	CRSwNP	Buysschaert et al,[57] 2010
IL4	rs2243250	CRSsNP, CRSwNP	Yea et al,[53] 2006

Tumor necrosis factor-α

TNF-α acts synergistically in the process of chronic inflammation with IL-1 to regulate the extravasation of eosinophils into polyps by inducing upregulation of vascular adhesion molecules.[72] *TNFA*, the gene encoding TNF-α, is located on chromosome 6 within the class 3 region of the major histocompatibility complex.[73] Polymorphisms of the *TNFA* gene are associated with chronic inflammatory diseases including asthma, and the *TNFA* -308 G > A (rs1800629) polymorphism is seen relatively frequently in Caucasian populations.[69,74,75]

One SNP in the promoter region of *TNFA*, a G-to-A substitution at position -308, increases *TNFA* promoter activity because of preferential transcription factor binding to adenosine over guanine.[76] Two separate studies found the -308 GA genotype to be associated with CRSwNP in Turkish patients.[77] Bernstein and colleagues[78] also found that patients with the SNP rs1800629 show an increased susceptibility to CRSwNP over controls in a US study. A Hungarian study evaluated various subgroups of CRS patients including CRSsNP, CRSwNP, CRSwNP aspirin sensitive, and CRSwNP aspirin tolerant for an association with *TNFA* -308 G > A. Interestingly, they found that *TNFA* -380 G > A was positively associated with the CRSwNP aspirin-sensitive subgroup only.[75] All other subgroups, even those with nasal polyps who were aspirin tolerant, did not show a significant association with this polymorphism. Finally, in contradiction to the above studies, Mfunda Endam and colleagues[62] did not find an association between any of the *TNFA* polymorphisms that they investigated and the development of CRS. However, this study group included CRS patients both with and without polyposis and therefore is more heterogeneous than the other studies. Overall, multiple studies have suggested an association with the *TNFA* -308 G > A polymorphism with CRSwNP, which warrants further investigation and may suggest a potential therapeutic target.

Immunodeficiency in Chronic Rhinosinusitis

Primary immune deficiencies (PID) are inherited disorders of immunity resulting in either dysfunctional or nonfunctional portions of the immune system. More than 120 genes have been identified that contribute to primary immunodeficiency.[79] Any arm of the immune system (humoral, phagocytic, cellular or complement) can be affected. There are more than 200 genetic disorders affecting the immune system with an estimated prevalence of 1:2000 in the general population. Some of the more common PIDs with relevance in otolaryngology include

- Selective IgA deficiency
- IgG subclass deficiency
- Common variable immunodeficiency (CVID)
- Specific antibody deficiency
- Agammaglobulinemia

Common clinical manifestations of PID include recurrent infections (specifically, pneumonia, bronchiectasis, otitis media, and rhinosinusitis), unusually persistent or severe infections, and/or infections with rare organisms.[79,80] PID has been demonstrated as a risk factor in the development of CRS in multiple studies,[81–83] and patients with refractory CRS have higher rates of PID than the general population. In one study, an immune abnormality was identified in 55% of patients with recalcitrant CRS. CVID has been identified in 1.5% to 10% of patients with refractory CRS, whereas its incidence in the general population is thought to be around 1:50,000.[81,84,85] In addition, evidence for a humoral immunodeficiency on testing for functional antibody response has been demonstrated in 22% to 67% of patients with recalcitrant CRS.[81,82,86]

Finally, selective immunoglobulin deficiencies (IgA, IgM and IgG3 subclass) have been demonstrated at an increased rate in this patient population.[81,82,84,86]

In select patients who have failed standard medical and surgical therapy, it is reasonable to consider immunologic work. Given the complexity in interpreting test results and the possible need for management of PID, immunodeficiency workups should involve an immunologist. Screening tests for humoral immunodeficiency include complete blood count (CBC) with differential, serum levels of IgA, IgM, IgG, and IgG subclasses. If the above levels are abnormal, further investigation should be undertaken with IgG titers to specific antigens for diseases that a patient has either had or been immunized to (ie, mumps, tetanus, pneumococcus, and so forth). With the exception of IgA, confirmation of humoral immunodeficiencies requires demonstration of an impaired specific antibody response. An impaired response can be demonstrated by drawing prevaccine titers followed by vaccine administration and redrawing of titers 3 to 4 weeks later; this is often done with the Pneumovax vaccine. A 4-fold increase in any vaccinated serotype previously low on titer testing should be observed. Furthermore, greater than 50% of serotypes in children and greater than 70% in adults should respond.[79] If this testing is abnormal, then flow cytometry to count B cells or genetic testing may be indicated. **Fig. 1** is a flow chart for the laboratory workup for humoral immunodeficiencies.

Workup for cellular immunodeficiency similarly begins with a CBC and absolute lymphocyte counts. Cutaneous delayed hypersensitivity testing with intradermal tests

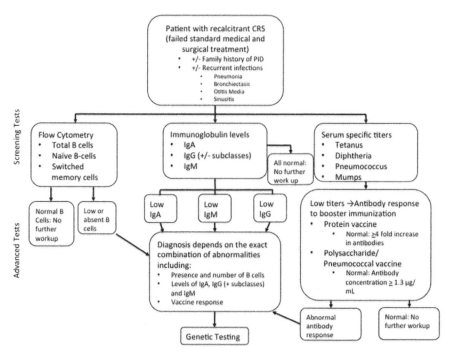

Fig. 1. Laboratory evaluation for suspected humoral deficiencies. Screening tests include immunoglobulin levels, serum-specific immunogolobulin titers, and B-lymphocyte flow cytometry. Low titers should be investigated further by testing for a specific antibody response to both protein and polysaccharide vaccines. Genetic testing should be considered in all patients diagnosed with a primary immunodeficiency.

is also recommended.[79] If either of these above tests indicates an abnormality, then further testing with T-cell flow cytometry or in vitro lymphocyte proliferation assays may be performed. Enzyme assays and a natural killer (NK) cytolysis assay complete the workup. Defects in granulocytes can be evaluated by an absolute neutrophil count and tests for neutrophil oxidative function. The workup for cellular and phagocytic immunodeficiencies is summarized in **Fig. 2**.

Complement function can be evaluated using 2 different assays. CH50 tests the classical complement activation pathway, whereas AH50 tests the alternative pathway. Any abnormal response can be worked up further with specific testing for components such as C3, C4, C1q, and C1 esterase inhibition. Again, at any step in the workup process, an abnormal result should prompt evaluation to an immunologist.

Recommended treatment of CRS in patients with PID includes both prophylactic antimicrobials and early culture-directed antibiotics.[87,88] In addition, endoscopic sinus surgery (ESS) in patients with CRS and underlying immunodeficiency has shown similar benefits as ESS in CRS patients with normal immunity.[89] Intravenous immunoglobulin G (IVIG) is a mechanism for inducing passive immunity in patients with immunodeficiencies. The literature regarding the impact of IVIG on sinusitis in patients with PID has been mixed. One study showed a short-term decrease in symptoms and frequency of sinopulmonary infections in patients on high-dose IVIG.[90] Other studies have shown an increased rate of CRS in patients on IVIG.[91,92] Besides an unclear benefit and possible detrimental effect on CRS symptoms in patients with PID, IVIG is associated with multiple side effects, including headache, nausea, tachycardia,

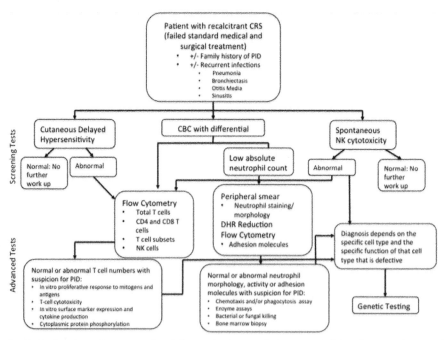

Fig. 2. Evaluation of suspected cellular and phagocytic immunodeficiencies. An abnormal absolute neutrophil count (ANC) on CBC should prompt further investigation into the morphology and function of neutrophils. Screening tests for cellular immune defects include flow cytometry, cutaneous delayed hypersensitivity, and an evaluation of NK cell cytotoxicity. DHR, Dihydrorhodamine.

shortness of breath, and anaphylaxis. Until more is understood about the impact of IVIG and CRS in patients with PID, comanagement of these patients with an immunologist and early detection and intervention of infections are appropriate.

SUMMARY

Refractory CRS is a highly heterogeneous disease process, complicating clear identification of causative factors. Abnormalities in the innate and adaptive immune functions of the sinonasal mucosa have been suggested by laboratory and clinical studies. Although CRS subtypes are incompletely defined, and the specific mechanisms through which immune dysfunction causes chronic inflammation remain to be elucidated, a general picture is emerging that local defects in mucosal immunity play a central role in driving and perpetuating the disease state. The study of the genetics of CRS is still in its infancy, and replication of genetic associations identified through GWAS is needed before detailed studies of involved pathogenic pathways and potential therapeutic targets can be contemplated. PIDs are inherited disorders that appear to be present at an increased prevalence in patients with recalcitrant CRS. The diagnosis of immunodeficiencies is complex and best done in coordination with an immunologist.

REFERENCES

1. Fokkens WJ, Lund VJ, Mullol J, et al. European position paper on rhinosinusitis and nasal polyps 2012. Rhinol Suppl 2012;23:3, p preceding table of contents, 1–298.
2. Benninger MS, Ferguson BJ, Hadley JA, et al. Adult chronic rhinosinusitis: definitions, diagnosis, epidemiology, and pathophysiology. Otolaryngol Head Neck Surg 2003;129(3 Suppl):S1–32.
3. Van Zele T, Claeys S, Gevaert P, et al. Differentiation of chronic sinus diseases by measurement of inflammatory mediators. Allergy 2006;61(11):1280–9.
4. Nagarkar DR, Poposki JA, Tan BK, et al. Thymic stromal lymphopoietin activity is increased in nasal polyps of patients with chronic rhinosinusitis. J Allergy Clin Immunol 2013;132(3):593–600.e12.
5. Stevens WW, Ocampo CJ, Berdnikovs S, et al. Cytokines in chronic rhinosinusitis. Role in eosinophilia and aspirin-exacerbated respiratory disease. Am J Respir Crit Care Med 2015;192(6):682–94.
6. Zhang N, Van Zele T, Perez-Novo C, et al. Different types of T-effector cells orchestrate mucosal inflammation in chronic sinus disease. J Allergy Clin Immunol 2008;122(5):961–8.
7. Van Crombruggen K, Zhang N, Gevaert P, et al. Pathogenesis of chronic rhinosinusitis: inflammation. J Allergy Clin Immunol 2011;128(4):728–32.
8. Lockey RF, Rucknagel DL, Vanselow NA. Familial occurrence of asthma, nasal polyps and aspirin intolerance. Ann Intern Med 1973;78(1):57–63.
9. Greisner WA 3rd, Settipane GA. Hereditary factor for nasal polyps. Allergy Asthma Proc 1996;17(5):283–6.
10. Cohen NA, Widelitz JS, Chiu AG, et al. Familial aggregation of sinonasal polyps correlates with severity of disease. Otolaryngol Head Neck Surg 2006;134(4):601–4.
11. Ramanathan M Jr, Lane AP. Innate immunity of the sinonasal cavity and its role in chronic rhinosinusitis. Otolaryngol Head Neck Surg 2007;136(3):348–56.
12. Majima Y, Hirata K, Matsubara T, et al. Viscoelastic properties of nasal mucus from patients with chronic sinusitis. Nihon Jibiinkoka Gakkai Kaiho 1983;86(6):644–51 [in Japanese].

13. Chen B, Antunes MB, Claire SE, et al. Reversal of chronic rhinosinusitis-associated sinonasal ciliary dysfunction. Am J Rhinol 2007;21(3):346–53.
14. Lee HM, Kang HJ, Woo JS, et al. Upregulation of surfactant protein A in chronic rhinosinusitis. Laryngoscope 2006;116(2):328–30.
15. Woods CM, Lee VS, Hussey DJ, et al. Lysozyme expression is increased in the sinus mucosa of patients with chronic rhinosinusitis. Rhinology 2012;50(2):147–56.
16. Schlosser RJ, Mulligan RM, Casey SE, et al. Alterations in gene expression of complement components in chronic rhinosinusitis. Am J Rhinol Allergy 2010;24(1):21–5.
17. Cui YH, Zhang F, Xiong ZG, et al. Increased serum complement component 3 and mannose-binding lectin levels in adult Chinese patients with chronic rhinosinusitis. Rhinology 2009;47(2):187–91.
18. Ramanathan M Jr, Lee WK, Lane AP. Increased expression of acidic mammalian chitinase in chronic rhinosinusitis with nasal polyps. Am J Rhinol 2006;20(3):330–5.
19. Park SK, Heo KW, Hur DY, et al. Chitinolytic activity in nasal polyps. Am J Rhinol Allergy 2011;25(1):12–4.
20. Detwiller KY, Smith TL, Alt JA, et al. Differential expression of innate immunity genes in chronic rhinosinusitis. Am J Rhinol Allergy 2014;28(5):374–7.
21. Zhao CY, Wang X, Liu M, et al. Microarray gene analysis of Toll-like receptor signaling elements in chronic rhinosinusitis with nasal polyps. Int Arch Allergy Immunol 2011;156(3):297–304.
22. Lane AP, Truong-Tran QA, Schleimer RP. Altered expression of genes associated with innate immunity and inflammation in recalcitrant rhinosinusitis with polyps. Am J Rhinol 2006;20(2):138–44.
23. Ramanathan M Jr, Lee WK, Dubin MG, et al. Sinonasal epithelial cell expression of toll-like receptor 9 is decreased in chronic rhinosinusitis with polyps. Am J Rhinol 2007;21(1):110–6.
24. Ramanathan M Jr, Lee WK, Spannhake EW, et al. Th2 cytokines associated with chronic rhinosinusitis with polyps down-regulate the antimicrobial immune function of human sinonasal epithelial cells. Am J Rhinol 2008;22(2):115–21.
25. Lee RJ, Cohen NA. Sinonasal solitary chemosensory cells "taste" the upper respiratory environment to regulate innate immunity. Am J Rhinol Allergy 2014;28(5):366–73.
26. Lee RJ, Kofonow JM, Rosen PL, et al. Bitter and sweet taste receptors regulate human upper respiratory innate immunity. J Clin Invest 2014;124(3):1393–405.
27. Serebrisky D, Teper AA, Huang CK, et al. CpG oligodeoxynucleotides can reverse Th2-associated allergic airway responses and alter the B7.1/B7.2 expression in a murine model of asthma. J Immunol 2000;165(10):5906–12.
28. Broide DH, Stachnick G, Castaneda D, et al. Immunostimulatory DNA mediates inhibition of eosinophilic inflammation and airway hyperreactivity independent of natural killer cells in vivo. J Allergy Clin Immunol 2001;108(5):759–63.
29. Farkas L, Kvale EO, Johansen FE, et al. Plasmacytoid dendritic cells activate allergen-specific TH2 memory cells: modulation by CpG oligodeoxynucleotides. J Allergy Clin Immunol 2004;114(2):436–43.
30. Reh DD, Wang Y, Ramanathan M Jr, et al. Treatment-recalcitrant chronic rhinosinusitis with polyps is associated with altered epithelial cell expression of interleukin-33. Am J Rhinol Allergy 2010;24(2):105–9.
31. Barreiro LB, Laval G, Quach H, et al. Natural selection has driven population differentiation in modern humans. Nat Genet 2008;40(3):340–5.

32. Bosse Y, Bacot F, Montpetit A, et al. Identification of susceptibility genes for complex diseases using pooling-based genome-wide association scans. Hum Genet 2009;125(3):305–18.
33. Barnes KC, Grant A, Gao P, et al. Polymorphisms in the novel gene acyloxyacyl hydroxylase (AOAH) are associated with asthma and associated phenotypes. J Allergy Clin Immunol 2006;118(1):70–7.
34. Shao B, Lu M, Katz SC, et al. A host lipase detoxifies bacterial lipopolysaccharides in the liver and spleen. J Biol Chem 2007;282(18):13726–35.
35. Ojogun N, Kuang TY, Shao B, et al. Overproduction of acyloxyacyl hydrolase by macrophages and dendritic cells prevents prolonged reactions to bacterial lipopolysaccharide in vivo. J Infect Dis 2009;200(11):1685–93.
36. Lu M, Varley AW, Ohta S, et al. Host inactivation of bacterial lipopolysaccharide prevents prolonged tolerance following gram-negative bacterial infection. Cell Host Microbe 2008;4(3):293–302.
37. Zhang Y, Endam LM, Filali-Mouhim A, et al. Polymorphisms in RYBP and AOAH genes are associated with chronic rhinosinusitis in a Chinese population: a replication study. PLoS One 2012;7(6):e39247.
38. Lee RJ, Xiong G, Kofonow JM, et al. T2R38 taste receptor polymorphisms underlie susceptibility to upper respiratory infection. J Clin Invest 2012;122(11):4145–59.
39. Adappa ND, Farquhar D, Palmer JN, et al. TAS2R38 genotype predicts surgical outcome in nonpolypoid chronic rhinosinusitis. Int Forum Allergy Rhinol 2016;6(1):25–33.
40. Pinto JM, Hayes MG, Schneider D, et al. A genomewide screen for chronic rhinosinusitis genes identifies a locus on chromosome 7q. Laryngoscope 2008;118(11):2067–72.
41. Wang X, Moylan B, Leopold DA, et al. Mutation in the gene responsible for cystic fibrosis and predisposition to chronic rhinosinusitis in the general population. JAMA 2000;284(14):1814–9.
42. Jyonouchi H, Sun S, Le H, et al. Evidence of dysregulated cytokine production by sinus lavage and peripheral blood mononuclear cells in patients with treatment-resistant chronic rhinosinusitis. Arch Otolaryngol Head Neck Surg 2001;127(12):1488–94.
43. Lan F, Zhang N, Zhang J, et al. Forkhead box protein 3 in human nasal polyp regulatory T cells is regulated by the protein suppressor of cytokine signaling 3. J Allergy Clin Immunol 2013;132(6):1314–21.
44. Pant H, Hughes A, Schembri M, et al. CD4(+) and CD8(+) regulatory T cells in chronic rhinosinusitis mucosa. Am J Rhinol Allergy 2014;28(2):e83–9.
45. Kato A, Peters A, Suh L, et al. Evidence of a role for B cell-activating factor of the TNF family in the pathogenesis of chronic rhinosinusitis with nasal polyps. J Allergy Clin Immunol 2008;121(6):1385–92, 1392.e1–2.
46. Hulse KE, Norton JE, Suh L, et al. Chronic rhinosinusitis with nasal polyps is characterized by B-cell inflammation and EBV-induced protein 2 expression. J Allergy Clin Immunol 2013;131(4):1075–83, 1083.e1–7.
47. Patadia M, Dixon J, Conley D, et al. Evaluation of the presence of B-cell attractant chemokines in chronic rhinosinusitis. Am J Rhinol Allergy 2010;24(1):11–6.
48. Peters AT, Kato A, Zhang N, et al. Evidence for altered activity of the IL-6 pathway in chronic rhinosinusitis with nasal polyps. J Allergy Clin Immunol 2010;125(2):397–403.e10.
49. Walley AJ, Cookson WO. Investigation of an interleukin-4 promoter polymorphism for associations with asthma and atopy. J Med Genet 1996;33(8):689–92.

50. Noguchi E, Shibasaki M, Arinami T, et al. Association of asthma and the interleukin-4 promoter gene in Japanese. Clin Exp Allergy 1998;28(4):449–53.
51. Hunninghake GM, Soto-Quiros ME, Avila L, et al. Polymorphisms in IL13, total IgE, eosinophilia, and asthma exacerbations in childhood. J Allergy Clin Immunol 2007;120(1):84–90.
52. Beghe B, Hall IP, Parker SG, et al. Polymorphisms in IL13 pathway genes in asthma and chronic obstructive pulmonary disease. Allergy 2010;65(4):474–81.
53. Yea SS, Yang YI, Park SK, et al. Interleukin-4 C-590T polymorphism is associated with protection against nasal polyps in a Korean population. Am J Rhinol 2006;20(5):550–3.
54. Zhang ML, Ni PH, Cai CP, et al. Association of susceptibility to chronic rhinosinusitis with genetic polymorphisms of IL-4 and IL-10. Zhonghua Er Bi Yan Hou Tou Jing Wai Ke Za Zhi 2012;47(3):212–7 [in Chinese].
55. Palikhe NS, Kim SH, Cho BY, et al. IL-13 gene polymorphisms are associated with rhinosinusitis and eosinophilic inflammation in aspirin intolerant asthma. Allergy Asthma Immunol Res 2010;2(2):134–40.
56. Ober C, Yao TC. The genetics of asthma and allergic disease: a 21st century perspective. Immunol Rev 2011;242(1):10–30.
57. Buysschaert ID, Grulois V, Eloy P, et al. Genetic evidence for a role of IL33 in nasal polyposis. Allergy 2010;65(5):616–22.
58. Plager DA, Kahl JC, Asmann YW, et al. Gene transcription changes in asthmatic chronic rhinosinusitis with nasal polyps and comparison to those in atopic dermatitis. PLoS One 2010;5(7):e11450.
59. Castano R, Bosse Y, Endam LM, et al. c-MET pathway involvement in chronic rhinosinusitis: a genetic association analysis. Otolaryngol Head Neck Surg 2010;142(5):665–71.e1-2.
60. Takeuchi K, Majima Y, Sakakura Y. Tumor necrosis factor gene polymorphism in chronic sinusitis. Laryngoscope 2000;110(10 Pt 1):1711–4.
61. Cormier C, Bosse Y, Mfuna L, et al. Polymorphisms in the tumour necrosis factor alpha-induced protein 3 (TNFAIP3) gene are associated with chronic rhinosinusitis. J Otolaryngol Head Neck Surg 2009;38(1):133–41.
62. Erbek SS, Yurtcu E, Erbek S, et al. Proinflammatory cytokine single nucleotide polymorphisms in nasal polyposis. Arch Otolaryngol Head Neck Surg 2007;133(7):705–9.
63. Mfuna Endam L, Cormier C, Bosse Y, et al. Association of IL1A, IL1B, and TNF gene polymorphisms with chronic rhinosinusitis with and without nasal polyposis: a replication study. Arch Otolaryngol Head Neck Surg 2010;136(2):187–92.
64. de Alarcon A, Steinke JW, Caughey R, et al. Expression of leukotriene C4 synthase and plasminogen activator inhibitor 1 gene promoter polymorphisms in sinusitis. Am J Rhinol 2006;20(5):545–9.
65. Benito Pescador D, Isidoro-Garcia M, Garcia-Solaesa V, et al. Genetic association study in nasal polyposis. J Investig Allergol Clin Immunol 2012;22(5):331–40.
66. Zielinska-Blizniewska H, Sitarek P, Milonski J, et al. Association of the -33C/G OSF-2 and the 140A/G LF gene polymorphisms with the risk of chronic rhinosinusitis with nasal polyps in a Polish population. Mol Biol Rep 2012;39(5):5449–57.
67. Kramer MF, Rasp G. Nasal polyposis: eosinophils and interleukin-5. Allergy 1999;54(7):669–80.
68. Hamaguchi Y, Suzumura H, Arima S, et al. Quantitation and immunocytological identification of interleukin-1 in nasal polyps from patients with chronic sinusitis. Int Arch Allergy Immunol 1994;104(2):155–9.

69. Haukim N, Bidwell JL, Smith AJ, et al. Cytokine gene polymorphism in human disease: on-line databases, supplement 2. Genes Immun 2002;3(6):313–30.
70. van den Velden PA, Reitsma PH. Amino acid dimorphism in IL1A is detectable by PCR amplification. Hum Mol Genet 1993;2(10):1753.
71. Karjalainen J, Joki-Erkkila VP, Hulkkonen J, et al. The IL1A genotype is associated with nasal polyposis in asthmatic adults. Allergy 2003;58(5):393–6.
72. Bernstein JM. Update on the molecular biology of nasal polyposis. Otolaryngol Clin North Am 2005;38(6):1243–55.
73. Carroll MC, Katzman P, Alicot EM, et al. Linkage map of the human major histocompatibility complex including the tumor necrosis factor genes. Proc Natl Acad Sci U S A 1987;84(23):8535–9.
74. Waldron-Lynch F, Adams C, Shanahan F, et al. Genetic analysis of the 3' untranslated region of the tumour necrosis factor shows a highly conserved region in rheumatoid arthritis affected and unaffected subjects. J Med Genet 1999; 36(3):214–6.
75. Szabo K, Kiricsi A, Revesz M, et al. The -308 G>A SNP of TNFA is a factor predisposing to chronic rhinosinusitis associated with nasal polyposis in aspirin-sensitive Hungarian individuals: conclusions of a genetic study with multiple stratifications. Int Immunol 2013;25(6):383–8.
76. Shiau MY, Wu CY, Huang CN, et al. TNF-alpha polymorphisms and type 2 diabetes mellitus in Taiwanese patients. Tissue Antigens 2003;61(5):393–7.
77. Batikhan H, Gokcan MK, Beder E, et al. Association of the tumor necrosis factor-alpha -308 G/A polymorphism with nasal polyposis. Eur Arch Otorhinolaryngol 2010;267(6):903–8.
78. Bernstein JM, Anon JB, Rontal M, et al. Genetic polymorphisms in chronic hyperplastic sinusitis with nasal polyposis. Laryngoscope 2009;119(7):1258–64.
79. Bonilla FA, Khan DA, Ballas ZK, et al. Practice parameter for the diagnosis and management of primary immunodeficiency. J Allergy Clin Immunol 2015;136(5): 1186–205.e1-78.
80. Yarmohammadi H, Estrella L, Doucette J, et al. Recognizing primary immune deficiency in clinical practice. Clin Vaccine Immunol 2006;13(3):329–32.
81. Alqudah M, Graham SM, Ballas ZK. High prevalence of humoral immunodeficiency patients with refractory chronic rhinosinusitis. Am J Rhinol Allergy 2010;24(6):409–12.
82. Vanlerberghe L, Joniau S, Jorissen M. The prevalence of humoral immunodeficiency in refractory rhinosinusitis: a retrospective analysis. B-ENT 2006;2(4): 161–6.
83. Sethi DS, Winkelstein JA, Lederman H, et al. Immunologic defects in patients with chronic recurrent sinusitis: diagnosis and management. Otolaryngol Head Neck Surg 1995;112(2):242–7.
84. Chee L, Graham SM, Carothers DG, et al. Immune dysfunction in refractory sinusitis in a tertiary care setting. Laryngoscope 2001;111(2):233–5.
85. Park MA, Li JT, Hagan JB, et al. Common variable immunodeficiency: a new look at an old disease. Lancet 2008;372(9637):489–502.
86. Tahkokallio O, Seppala IJ, Sarvas H, et al. Concentrations of serum immunoglobulins and antibodies to pneumococcal capsular polysaccharides in patients with recurrent or chronic sinusitis. Ann Otol Rhinol Laryngol 2001;110(7 Pt 1): 675–81.
87. Kuruvilla M, de la Morena MT. Antibiotic prophylaxis in primary immune deficiency disorders. J Allergy Clin Immunol Pract 2013;1(6):573–82.

88. Ocampo CJ, Peters AT. Antibody deficiency in chronic rhinosinusitis: epidemiology and burden of illness. Am J Rhinol Allergy 2013;27(1):34–8.
89. Khalid AN, Mace JC, Smith TL. Outcomes of sinus surgery in ambulatory patients with immune dysfunction. Am J Rhinol Allergy 2010;24(3):230–3.
90. Roifman CM, Gelfand EW. Replacement therapy with high dose intravenous gamma-globulin improves chronic sinopulmonary disease in patients with hypogammaglobulinemia. Pediatr Infect Dis J 1988;7(5 Suppl):S92–6.
91. Rose MA, Schubert R, Schmitt-Grohe S, et al. Immunoglobulins and inflammatory cytokines in nasal secretions in humoral immunodeficiencies. Laryngoscope 2006;116(2):239–44.
92. Quinti I, Soresina A, Spadaro G, et al. Long-term follow-up and outcome of a large cohort of patients with common variable immunodeficiency. J Clin Immunol 2007;27(3):308–16.
93. Yazdani N, Amoli MM, Naraghi M, et al. Association between the functional polymorphism C-159T in the CD14 promoter gene and nasal polyposis: potential role in asthma. J Investig Allergol Clin Immunol 2012;22(6):406–11.
94. Tewfik MA, Bosse Y, Lemire M, et al. Polymorphisms in interleukin-1 receptor-associated kinase 4 are associated with total serum IgE. Allergy 2009;64(5): 746–53.
95. Zhang Y, Endam LM, Filali-Mouhim A, et al. Polymorphisms in the nitric oxide synthase 1 gene are associated with severe chronic rhinosinusitis. Am J Rhinol Allergy 2011;25(2):e49–54.
96. Pascual M, Sanz C, Isidoro-Garcia M, et al. (CCTTT)n polymorphism of NOS2A in nasal polyposis and asthma: a case-control study. J Investig Allergol Clin Immunol 2008;18(4):239–44.
97. Kilty SJ, Bosse Y, Cormier C, et al. Polymorphisms in the SERPINA1 (Alpha-1-Antitrypsin) gene are associated with severe chronic rhinosinusitis unresponsive to medical therapy. Am J Rhinol Allergy 2010;24(1):e4–9.
98. Sachse F, Becker K, Rudack C. Incidence of staphylococcal colonization and of the 753Q Toll-like receptor 2 variant in nasal polyposis. Am J Rhinol Allergy 2010;24(1):e10–3.
99. Park CS, Cho JH, Park YJ. Toll-like receptor 2 gene polymorphisms in a Korean population: association with chronic rhinosinusitis. Otolaryngol Head Neck Surg 2011;144(1):96–100.
100. Alromaih S, Mfuna-Endam L, Bosse Y, et al. CD8A gene polymorphisms predict severity factors in chronic rhinosinusitis. Int Forum Allergy Rhinol 2013;3(8): 605–11.
101. Castano R, Bosse Y, Endam LM, et al. Evidence of association of interleukin-1 receptor-like 1 gene polymorphisms with chronic rhinosinusitis. Am J Rhinol Allergy 2009;23(4):377–84.
102. Cheng YK, Lin CD, Chang WC, et al. Increased prevalence of interleukin-1 receptor antagonist gene polymorphism in patients with chronic rhinosinusitis. Arch Otolaryngol Head Neck Surg 2006;132(3):285–90.
103. Endam LM, Bosse Y, Filali-Mouhim A, et al. Polymorphisms in the interleukin-22 receptor alpha-1 gene are associated with severe chronic rhinosinusitis. Otolaryngol Head Neck Surg 2009;140(5):741–7.

Bacterial Pathogens and the Microbiome

Thad W. Vickery, BA[a], Vijay R. Ramakrishnan, MD[b],*

KEYWORDS

- Bacteria • Chronic rhinosinusitis • Microbiome • Culture-independent microbiology
- Sinusitis

KEY POINTS

- The sinuses are not sterile. A population of bacteria is present in both health and disease, roughly in the same overall abundance, but qualitatively different in its makeup.
- As of yet, no single bacterial species or set of species has been definitively shown to be protective or causative in chronic rhinosinusitis (CRS).
- The overall function of the bacterial community may be most important, rather than the presence or absence of a single pathogen.
- Therapies used to treat CRS may induce microbiome alterations.
- Further research is indicated and required in this exciting field.

INTRODUCTION

Chronic rhinosinusitis (CRS) continues to be one of the most prevalent health care problems in the United States. Despite the significant morbidity, loss of productivity, and health care costs associated with CRS, the underlying processes that lead to disease remain poorly understood. The nonspecific clinical symptoms of nasal obstruction, rhinorrhea, facial pain, and anosmia may represent a common end point for various inflammatory mechanisms occurring in different anatomic areas. CRS is increasingly being appreciated as a clinical syndrome with a wide spectrum of overlapping disease physiology. For instance, CRS with nasal polyps (CRSwNP) often is

Disclosure Statement: The authors have no financial conflicts of interest to disclose. Research reported in this publication was supported by the National Institute On Deafness And Other Communication Disorders of the National Institutes of Health under award numbers K23DC014747 (V.R. Ramakrishnan) and T32DC01228003 (T.W. Vickery). The content is solely the responsibility of the authors and does not necessarily represent the official views of the National Institutes of Health.
[a] University of Colorado School of Medicine, 13001 East 17th Place, Aurora, CO 80045, USA;
[b] Department of Otolaryngology, Head and Neck Surgery, University of Colorado, 12631 East 17th Avenue, B205, Aurora, CO 80045, USA
* Corresponding author.
E-mail address: Vijay.Ramakrishnan@UCDenver.edu

Otolaryngol Clin N Am 50 (2017) 29–47
http://dx.doi.org/10.1016/j.otc.2016.08.004
oto.theclinics.com

characterized by eosinophilic inflammation and increased production of histamine, IL-5 and IL-13,[1] whereas CRS without nasal polyps (CRSsNP) is often considered a predominantly neutrophilic disease characterized by high levels of interleukin (IL)-1, IL-6, and tumor necrosis factor (TNF) α.[2] In practice, however, there are patients with CRSsNP with high levels of eosinophils and patients with CRSwNP who exhibit robust neutrophilic infiltration within the sinonasal epithelium. Thus, our classification of CRS in clinical practice is often not as simple as we would prefer.

Chronic Rhinosinusitis Pathophysiology and Immune Homeostasis

CRS is characterized by persistent inflammation, a dysregulated immune response, and host-microbial interactions that together result in disruption of epithelial barrier function, poor wound healing, tissue remodeling, and clinical symptoms. Historically the significance of bacteria in acute and CRS has focused on the interactions between a single bacterial pathogen and its host. However, developing concepts in microbial ecology, laboratory methods in culture-independent microbiology, and bioinformatics are furthering our capacity to study complex microbial communities as an entire functional unit. The nasal cavity and paranasal sinuses are the first tissues exposed to airborne environmental challenges, including pathogenic and nonpathogenic bacteria, viruses, fungi, allergens, and toxins. The mucosal surface uses several immune mechanisms to promote homeostasis, which can be broadly divided into innate and adaptive immunity. Many host factors impact the functionality of the immune response that is thought to predispose individuals to the development of CRS.[3]

Innate versus adaptive immunity

Innate immunity classically refers to the nonspecific defense mechanisms that are rapidly activated following exposure to antigenic material and confer immediate protection. Within the upper respiratory tract, this includes the physical barrier provided by the ciliated pseudostratified columnar respiratory epithelium that lines the sinonasal cavity. This resilient barrier contains interspersed goblet cells that secrete a viscoelastic mucous layer atop the epithelial surface composed of high-molecular-weight glycoprotein mucins and heavily glycosylated molecules. In conjunction with beating cilia, the enriched mucous layer promotes nonspecific mucociliary clearance of microbes and irritant particles.[4] Barrier dysfunction can contribute to CRS; when coupled with defects in mucociliary clearance that promote bacterial colonization, bacterial invasion and further barrier disruption may occur.[3,5] Classic genetic defects in ciliary function, such as cystic fibrosis and primary ciliary dyskinesia, are often used as examples; but acquired ciliary dysfunction occurs in CRS as well.[6] Poor barrier function and dysfunctional mucociliary clearance are host defects that predispose individuals to pathogen colonization and the development of recurrent infection.[7–9]

Sinonasal epithelial cells secrete enzymes, opsonins, defensins, permeabolizing proteins, and other endogenous antimicrobial products into the apical mucous layer. These host defense molecules are important for directly neutralizing microbes and recruiting inflammatory cells that modulate the immune response. Specifically, epithelial cells secrete enzymes, such as lysozyme, peroxidases, and chitinases, and the small cationic permeabolizing proteins, such as the defensins and cathelicidins. Additionally, proteins, such as lactoferrin, mucins, C-reactive protein, and secretory leukocyte proteinase inhibitor, collectively provide protection from bacteria, fungi, and viruses at the apical surface.[9–11]

When pathogens do invade the sinonasal epithelium, circulating professional phagocytes, possessing pattern recognition receptors (PRRs) on their cell surface, recognize pathogen-associated molecular patterns and damage-associated molecular patterns. When host epithelial cell PRRs bind pathogenic or damaged cell proteins, the acute inflammatory pathways are activated and the tissue becomes primed for the adaptive immune response.[10,12] Toll-like receptors (TLRs) are a subset of PRRs that allow phagocytes to recognize bacterial motifs, such as lipopolysaccharide (via TLR-4) and CpG repeats (via TLR-9) associated with gram-negative bacteria and bacterial DNA respectively.

Current literature suggests that variable gene expression of TLRs and other cytokines may predispose some individuals to develop CRS.[13] For example, patients with CRS demonstrate variable expression of TLR2 mRNA.[14,15] TLR2 is expressed on sinonasal epithelial cells and recognizes several bacterial, fungal, and viral proteins. Binding of a ligand to TLR2 activates the acute inflammatory response and also primes the adaptive immune response by increasing expression of major histocompatibility complex II (MHC-II) costimulatory molecules required to present antigens to T-follicular helper cells. The resulting Th1 response is necessary for clearance of *Streptococcus pneumoniae* infection, for example.[16,17] Another study identified decreased TLR9 mRNA expression in CRSsNP[18]; however, in-depth study of TLR-mediated disease in CRS is lacking.

In concert with the acute inflammatory response, cytotoxic natural killer (NK) cells are important to mounting an appropriate innate immune response. Although NK cells are often understood to induce apoptosis in viral-infected cells and tumor cells, they are becoming increasingly of interest in CRS. Patients with CRS have dysfunctional NK cells that demonstrate impaired degranulation and diminished release of TNF α and interferon (IFN) γ.[19]

The *adaptive immune system* is stimulated when PMNs and macrophages are recruited to the site of infection to fully eradicate bacterial infection and establish long-lasting cell-mediated immunity.[20] Antigen-presenting cells, such as monocytes, macrophages, B-lymphocytes, and dendritic cells, process complex protein antigens and present antigenic peptides on their surface that are then presented to T helper cells on the appropriate MHC. Binding of the antigen-MHC complex to the T-cell receptor activates the adaptive immune system and leads to longer-lasting T-effector cells and antibody-producing plasma cells.[21]

Although much attention is given to defective innate immunity in the development of CRS, the adaptive immune system is crucial for developing an appropriate T-cell response; much of the CRS literature supports polarized populations of T-follicular helper cells (either Th1 or Th2) in subsets of CRS. Th1 cells produce IFN γ, IL-2, and TNF α, which ultimately lead to a robust cell-mediated response and phagocyte-mediated inflammation. Th2 cells produce IL-4, IL-5, and IL-13 that promote a strong antibody response and the accumulation of eosinophils while inhibiting the phagocytes and the resulting potent inflammatory response.[22] Furthermore, the T-follicular helper cell environment influences macrophage differentiation into M1 macrophages that are necessary for mounting a vigorous inflammatory response against intracellular pathogens or M2 macrophages that are associated with eosinophilic states.[23] M2 macrophages are predominant in CRSwNP and may play a role in exacerbating polyposis because they are unable to phagocytose *Staphylococcus aureus*.[24] The inappropriate persistence of Th1 inflammation in CRSsNP and the ongoing recruitment of eosinophils and Th2 cells in CRSwNP are hallmarks of adaptive immune dysfunction characteristic in CRS.

Surface mucosal niche

Once thought to be a sterile environment in the healthy state, the paranasal sinuses are now widely appreciated to harbor rich and diverse populations of commensal bacteria. Commensals are most often defined as the community of microorganisms that colonize epithelial surfaces without causing harm to the host. Our understanding of commensal bacteria is evolving to recognize the shifting selective pressures in the microbial community that likely include other forms of symbiosis between host cells and neighboring bacteria including parasitism, mutualism and amensalism. Host defense mechanisms contribute to a unique mucosal environment that constantly applies selective pressure on epithelial microbes resulting in a surface mucosal niche. This niche varies between individuals and between different anatomic compartments.[25,26] There may be drivers of this niche beyond host mucosal immune function, including environmental exposures (eg, smoking) or medication usage (eg, antibiotics) **(Fig. 1)**. Bacteria, either live or their by-products, such as DNA, quorum-sensing molecules, or metabolized waste, interact with the immune system and can influence inflammatory processes.

Role of Bacteria in Initiation and Sustenance of Inflammation

Historically, many described CRS as a disease that resulted from a persistent or incompletely treated acute infection. Current understanding is that CRS is an *inflammatory* process rather than *infectious* but that inflammatory mechanisms modulated by commensal and pathogenic bacteria contribute to disease formation, beyond the simplistic notion of a single microbial pathogen interacting with a host and causing

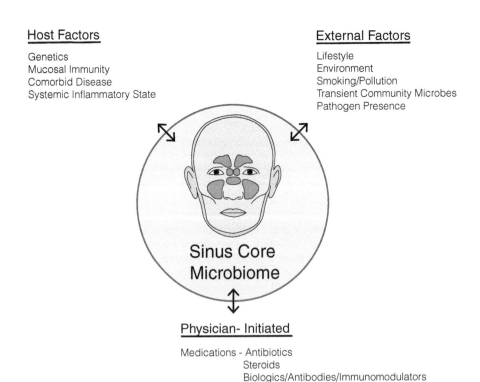

Host Factors

Genetics
Mucosal Immunity
Comorbid Disease
Systemic Inflammatory State

External Factors

Lifestyle
Environment
Smoking/Pollution
Transient Community Microbes
Pathogen Presence

Sinus Core
Microbiome

Physician- Initiated

Medications - Antibiotics
Steroids
Biologics/Antibodies/Immunomodulators
Surgery - Irrigation

Fig. 1. Potential factors influencing the sinus microbiome. (*Adapted from* Turnbaugh PJ, Ley RE, Hamady M, et al. The Human Microbiome Project. Nature 2007;449(7164):804–10.)

disease. Certainly, chronic inflammatory diseases can result from direct bacterial invasion at mucosal surfaces, resulting in compromised barrier function, a coordinated innate and adaptive immune response, and an acute inflammatory response, which may evolve into prolonged inflammation leading to tissue damage, remodeling, and fibrosis.[27] It is possible that in some patients, bacterial infection initiates the inflammatory process that never resolves; yet, in others it may be the case that a noninfectious inciting event initiates an inflammatory response that alters the native mucosal surface bacterial niche, which then propagates the disease once the original disease-causing event has concluded (**Fig. 2**).[28] Earlier studies of sinonasal microbiota used culture-based microbiology techniques, which have recently been usurped by nucleic acid–based molecular techniques that allow for more sensitive and less biased detection of microbes as well as the ability to characterize entire communities of microbes within the same sample.[29,30] Without evidence to support a definitive role for bacterial infection as the cause for CRS, future studies are needed to better understand the role of bacteria in host susceptibility to disease development.

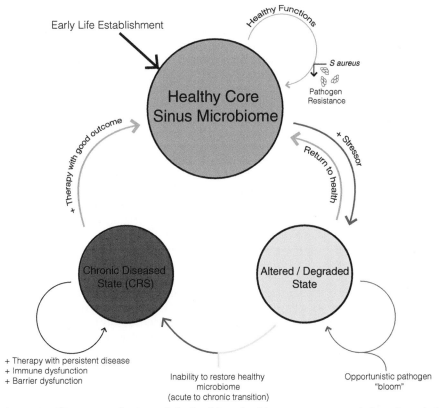

Fig. 2. Significant perturbations of the healthy microbiome state can result in a degraded state that is susceptible to disease. Once degraded and/or diseased, a goal may be to restore the rich and diverse healthy state. (*Adapted from* Lozupone CA, Stombaugh JI, Gordon JI, et al. Diversity, stability and resilience of the human gut microbiota. Nature 2012;489(7415):220–30.)

THE PARANASAL SINUS BIOME IN HEALTH AND DISEASE
The Microbiome

Host-microbe interactions are an established contributing factor in the formation of CRS, but evidence for the presence or absence of a single microbe resulting in disease is lacking. The shifting paradigm focuses on the unique composition of the entire bacterial community that colonizes the sinonasal mucosa also known as the microbiome. The microbiome is a potentially diverse community of microbiota existing in a delicate symbiotic relationship within a human microenvironment. These organisms possess great genetic potential to act as disease modifiers and contribute to the maintenance of health and formation of disease on all epithelial surfaces, including upper and lower airway.[31–33] In intestinal epithelia, early microbial colonization is essential for normal immunologic development and influences susceptibility to inflammatory and allergic diseases later in life.[34] In neonates, for example, early lower airway colonization with pathogens, such as *S pneumonia, Haemophilus influenzae*, and *Moraxella catarrhalis*, increases the risk of recurrent wheezing and asthma.[35] Additionally, several groups have demonstrated the importance of the microbiome on the host adaptive immune system through modulation of dendritic cells, Th17, and T-regulatory (Treg) cells.[36–39] Although much of bacterial microbiome research is still emerging, it is one of the most intriguing current topics of CRS research.

There remains a paucity of microbiome research on fungi, viruses, and bacteriophages in CRS, although growing evidence suggests that these microbes may contribute to a larger meta-organism in which interactions between and among all microbes and their host shape human health. Early efforts to describe microbial roles in CRS resulted in the fungal hypothesis, which suggested that CRS resulted from an overexuberant host response to *Alternaria* fungi.[40] Although this theory does not explain many of the defects observed in CRS, and current guidelines recommend against antifungal therapy for patients with CRS, there is continued research interest in the fungal microbiome.[41] Recent studies using sequencing of the fungal 18S ribosomal RNA gene demonstrate a rich and diverse population of commensal fungal taxa in middle meatal lavages from healthy patients and patients with CRS. Patients with CRS were found to have quantitative increases in the total amount of fungal 18S ribosomal RNA when compared with controls.[42] A 2014 prospective study by Cleland and colleagues[43] identified 207 unique fungal genera in 23 patients with CRS and 11 controls. Interestingly, fungal genera traditionally associated with CRS, such as *Alternaria* and *Aspergillus*, were found in very low abundance. This study also assessed postoperative changes in the fungal microbiome and found decreased richness at 6 and 12 weeks after surgery.[43] No studies to date have thoroughly profiled viral or bacteriophage populations within the paranasal sinuses, although there is certainly interest. For instance, recent evidence suggests that upper airway rhinovirus infection can alter the nasopharyngeal microbiome.[44] Further studies directed at characterizing the entire microbiome population in health are necessary in order to develop a more robust understanding of the role microbial diversity plays in sinonasal health as well as the generation of disease.

Bacteria in Health

Since the advent of culture-independent molecular techniques, several groups have used various techniques to characterize the sinonasal bacterial community in healthy individuals. Efforts to identify a distinct microbial profile in health are inconclusive, and there is currently no consensus on which bacteria predominate in or define the healthy state. Although several studies have characterized the bacterial communities in the upper airway, cross-study comparisons are difficult because of several variations in sampling methods, bacterial primer selection, sequencing methods, and data analysis pipelines.[45] Even so, there are several patterns that frequently emerge. These patterns include an abundance of *Propionibacterium acnes, Staphylococcus epidermidis, S aureus, and Corynebacterium* spp in health.[26,33,46,47] Of note, *Staphylococcus* spp, including *S aureus* and coagulase negative staphylococci, are present in healthy subjects and can behave in either pathogenic or commensal fashion based on particular strain, bacterial gene expression, and surrounding microbial interactions. Although native bacteria act to promote homeostasis within the sinonasal epithelia, disruption of this balance, known as *dysbiosis*, may allow commensal organisms to act as opportunistic pathogens in disease states.[48]

The Human Microbiome Project (HMP) consortium compiled 16S rRNA gene sequences collected from 18 different sites across the body in order to better associate the microbiome with human health.[49,50] Further analysis of the HMP data demonstrates that different human subjects possess unique native bacterial communities with highly variable taxonomic composition at the same body sites. These bacterial community profiles strongly associated with life-history characteristics, such as history of being breastfed as an infant, sex, and level of education. Interestingly, despite profound interperson and intraperson variability in the bacterial microbiome, community function remains constant; the community types from one body site are predictive of community types at other body sites within the same individual.[50,51] The association of bacterial community composition with life history factors, such as presence or absence of breastfeeding, raises questions about the source of commensal microbes. In the gastrointestinal literature, there are several studies that demonstrate that diet shapes the microbiome composition and different microbial profiles are associated with diseases, such as inflammatory bowel disease (IBD).[52] In addition to dietary factors, the upper airway microbiota are a known source of microbes that colonize the lung and stomach.[53] Ultimately, the aggregate of bacterial taxa in the sinus niche need to be better studied at a metagenome level to begin deciphering community function and how specific bacterial ecosystems are established.

Microbiome Changes in Disease

Several statistical indices are use to describe species diversity within a microbial community. *Alpha diversity* is the intracommunity diversity as measured by the total number and composition of species. *Beta diversity* is an estimate of the diversity (number and composition) comparison between different habitats. *Abundance* refers to the total amount of bacterial DNA that corresponds to specific bacterial taxa found within a sample. *Richness* describes the total number of species identified within a sample, that is, greater numbers of distinct species means higher richness. *Evenness* is a measure of how similar in number each species within a bacterial community is. Several studies have identified perturbations in the microbiome during CRS. In general, *S aureus* and anaerobes, including *Prevotella, Fusobacterium, Bacteroides* spp, and *Peptostreptococcus* spp, are consistently more abundant in CRS versus healthy controls.[26,41,46,47,54] Interestingly, although the abundance of pathogenic bacteria is increased in patients with CRS, the overall total quantity of bacteria does not seem to change compared with healthy individuals. This finding indicates that the sinus niche is filled by a given amount of bacteria, and a relative dominance of the niche by pathogens is associated with disease. In these studies, despite having a similar overall bacterial burden, microbial richness, evenness, and diversity of bacterial colonies were greatly diminished in CRS.[26,33,54] This observation supports the hypothesis that disturbances in the microbial community are a part of CRS. Just as ecologists associate the macroscopic biodiversity and biomass of rainforests and coral reef habitats with the overall health of the ecosystem, the microscopic biodiversity of bacteria within a host mucosal niche is considered a hallmark of health.

The frequent observation that CRS is associated with decreased microbial diversity parallels many other disease states. For example, decreased diversity in the gut microbiome is associated with obesity, active IBD, and psoriatic arthritis.[55–57] Although data are lacking to suggest that promoting bacterial diversity within the sinonasal niche would prevent or improve CRS, this may be a relevant consideration moving forward because the mainstays of CRS therapy are long-term broad-spectrum antibiotics and corticosteroids, which carry the potential to alter the microbiome composition.[58,59]

Are Microbiome Alterations a Cause or By-product of Disease?

Recent cross-sectional population studies have detected differences in the microbiome between patients with CRS and healthy individuals, but what does this really mean? One possibility is that community alterations in the microbiome lead to epithelial barrier and immune dysfunction resulting in disease. Alternatively, persistent inflammation at the mucosal surface may result in a prolonged immune response and/or alterations in the local microenvironment that shift the microbial community. Moreover, therapies administered for the disease (eg, antibiotic therapy and steroids) likely impact the microbiome and may confound these observations. The multitude of variables present that impact the mucosal niche makes establishing this causation difficult in the absence of animal models. In reality, any or all of these possibilities may occur (see **Fig. 1**).

The concept of perturbations in the microbial community resulting in disease, that is, *dysbiosis*, has been explored in the gastrointestinal tract. The normal gut flora plays an essential role in maintaining immune homeostasis, and disruptions in these mutualistic relationships are thought to lead to several conditions ranging from antibiotic-associated diarrhea and IBD to necrotizing enterocolitis and colorectal cancer.[48] Although disease-associated shifts in the bacterial microbiome have been observed in CRS, it remains unclear if this is an inciting factor in the development or propagation of disease or merely a consequence. Emerging data from cross-sectional analysis of specific patient populations suggest that host factors, such as a history of tobacco use, presence of asthma, or recent antibiotic use, can impact the microbiota.[30,46,60]

Given the panoply of disease mechanisms involved, the prolonged utilization of medical therapies, and the lack of a universal mouse model for the disease, human studies of CRS will require large-scale, multilevel, longitudinal design in order to delineate patterns of microbial perturbations and their significance. Such studies are critical to determining the role of the microbiome in disease formation, chronicity, severity and prognosis, and response to therapies.

CLINICAL IMPLICATIONS AND TREATMENT CONSIDERATIONS OF BACTERIAL PATHOGENS
Pathogens Often Implicated in Chronic Rhinosinusitis

Traditional culture-based study versus molecular techniques
Many culture-based studies of sinus specimens from patients with CRS identify the most common pathogens associated with CRS as *S aureus, Pseudomonas aeruginosa*, and, with specialized culture techniques, several species of anaerobes.[61–64] The bacterial pathogens implicated in CRS are distinct from those most often identified in acute bacterial rhinosinusitis (ABRS). Just as CRS is thought to be multifactorial, the incidence of ABRS may be higher in the setting of particular environmental

exposures, allergies, smoking, ciliary impairment, sinonasal anatomic variations, and transient bacterial infections.[65–67] However, the most often identified bacteria cultured in patients with ABRS are *Streptococcus pneumoniae, H influenzae, S pyrogenes, M catarrhalis*, and *S aureus.*[68]

Patients with refractory CRS often demonstrate both cellular and humoral immune dysfunction, as described earlier[69]; in these cases the most commonly isolated pathogens are *S aureus* and *P aeruginosa.*[63,64] Patients with CRS have a higher incidence of antibiotic resistance; this observation is especially notable in patients undergoing revision endoscopic sinus surgery (ESS) when compared with patients undergoing surgery for the first time.[70] True (ie, physiologic) antibiotic resistance in a dysbiotic community is difficult to assess but may be even higher than that documented in culture studies of antibiotic susceptibility.[71]

In the wake of emerging molecular and imaging techniques, several groups have interrogated the functional role of biofilms in CRS.[72–74] As the field embraces molecular identification techniques, it has become apparent that conventional culture methods are not on par with newer culture-independent techniques. Current data suggest that molecular techniques, such as 16S gene sequencing, demonstrate greater biodiversity, increased sensitivity, and the ability to identify anaerobic groups with greater specificity when compared with culture.[46,47] In practice, Hauser and colleagues[75] found clinical laboratory cultures to identify the dominant bacteria only 60% of the time. Presumably, identification of the dominant bacteria is the information sought by the clinician, as dysbiosis and decreased diversity in disease points to a single or few dominant organisms out of community balance as the cause of the condition. Culture-directed antibiotics are thought to be beneficial if there are signs of active infection, such as purulence, or if many antibiotics have already been administered; but the role of cultures is less clear in the absence of this history. As our understanding of the cause of CRS evolves, and our capacity to examine the entire microbial community increases, the utility of cultures in CRS requires further evaluation.

Staphylococcus aureus and Superantigens

S aureus and coagulase negative staphylococcus are the most common putative pathogens identified in CRS in North America.[68,76] Toxigenic strains of *S aureus* are known to be potent disease modifiers capable of disrupting barrier function, invading epithelial cells, modulating immune cells, and promoting polyp formation.[77] Staphylococcal superantigenic toxins (SAgs) are small molecules secreted during toxigenic *S aureus* infection that crosslink antigen-presenting cells and T cells by simultaneously binding MHC-II and the T-cell receptor. In contrast to conventional antigens, this direct activation of CD4+ and CD8+ T cells leads to a profound polyclonal immune response and generation of a Th2 cytokine environment. The Th2-skewing promotes eosinophil recruitment, the generation of polyclonal immunoglobulin E, Treg inhibition, mast cell degranulation, and the activation of M2 macrophages, which collectively result in generation of nasal polyps.[78–80]

The incidence and awareness of methicillin-resistant *S aureus* carriage in the anterior nares has increased in recent time and is known to contribute to surgical site infection and biofilm creation, slow mucosal healing after endoscopic sinus surgery, and result in greater overall morbidity.[72] Although *S aureus* is a major pathogen in CRS, most species remain methicillin-sensitive.[46,81,82] Because the colonization of healthy individuals with toxigenic strains of *Staphylococcus* is surprisingly common, multiple host and microenvironment factors likely contribute to *Staphylococcus*-implicated effects in CRS.

S aureus, P aeruginosa, H influenza, S pneumonia, M catarrhalis, and *Stenotrophomonas* are known to establish biofilms on the mucosal surface. *S aureus* biofilms in particular have been suggested to promote Th2 cytokines independently of SAgs.[83] Biofilm formation with any pathogen occurs in response to selective pressures within the mucosal niche, including antibiotic use, tobacco exposure, and loss of integrity of host epithelial immune barrier. The presence of biofilms is associated with increased disease severity and recalcitrance because antibiotics and host defenses do not efficiently penetrate the dense, 3-dimensional polysaccharide matrix. Once biofilms are established, they are difficult to clear and serve as a protected reservoir for pathogens to evolve virulence factors and shed planktonic bacteria that can incite acute exacerbations of disease.[84]

Pseudomonas aeruginosa

P aeruginosa infection of the paranasal sinuses is most frequently discovered in immune-compromised individuals, patients undergoing revision sinus surgery, or in the setting of ciliary dysfunction, such as in cystic fibrosis.[85–87] *P aeruginosa* secretes several virulence factors, including adhesins, secreted toxins (eg, exoenzyme S and exotoxin A), proteases, effector proteins (eg, elastase and alkaline protease), and pigments (eg, pyocyanin), which act to evade the immune system and disable host cells. Additionally, *P aeruginosa* uses active quorum sensing to organize tenacious biofilms at the epithelial surface and further evade host defenses.[88]

Anaerobes

Although advances in molecular sequencing have highlighted the preponderance of anaerobes in the CRS microbiome, in clinical practice, the identification of specific anaerobes is often complicated by limitations of culture techniques. The expansion of anaerobes in subsets of CRS may also result from alterations in the microbial community and local microenvironment.[30,89–91] Currently, anaerobes pose several challenges to the effective management of CRS. When identified by culture, this often influences antibiotic selection to include anaerobe coverage. In the case of anaerobes, such as Bacteroidetes and Fusobacteria, these pathogens are known to share mobile genetic elements that confer antibiotic resistance and increased virulence with other bacteria in the community.[92,93] Thus, these anaerobes, when expanded in CRS, may work synergistically with other opportunistic pathogens throughout a bacterial community leading to a pathogenic niche.

Antibiotic Resistance Associated with Pathogens in Chronic Rhinosinusitis Study

Antibiotic resistance is a natural phenomenon and is increasingly common in patients with refractory CRS.[70] Bacteria may acquire antibiotic resistance through random mutation or through exchange of genetic material. As discussed previously, the sinonasal bacterial niche experiences constant selective pressure from neighboring microbes and the host immune defenses. When this bacterial community proliferates in the presence of antibiotics, there is additional selective pressure that culls species with the defense mechanisms to withstand antimicrobials in the environment. There are several mobile genetic elements or *r* genes that confer resistance to particular antibiotics and may be passed vertically through generations of bacteria or horizontally from one bacterium to a neighboring bacterium.[94] Because antibiotics used to treat refractory CRS selectively eliminate the most susceptible members of the community, the potential of the microbiome to remain diverse and facilitate pathogen exclusion is reduced, theoretically allowing resistant bacteria to flourish and dominate. Innovative new strategies are needed to combat the increase of resistant superinfections in refractory CRS; perhaps an approach that includes promoting a diverse and healthy microbial community to exclude multiresistant pathogens will be explored in the future.

EMERGING RESEARCH CONCEPTS IN THE MICROBIOME
Role in Mucosal Immune Function

Although progress has been made to characterize the bacterial microbiome in health and disease, studies of host-microbe and microbe-microbe interactions occurring within the mucosal niche have only begun. The concept of pathogen exclusion refers to the ability of a microbial community to selectively inhibit the dominance of a single pathogen, which can occur actively through direct inhibition of pathogens by commensals within the niche. For example, S aureus may be inhibited by neighboring microbes, including S epidermidis, Corynebacterium spp, P aeruginosa, and fungal species.[25,95] Although the host innate immune defense uses several antimicrobial strategies to modulate surface microbes, the bacterial community itself possesses a much more dynamic capacity to shape microbes within the niche through the use of small molecule signals (quorum sensing), utilization of alternative nutrient sources, secreted antimicrobials, and transfer of mobile genetic elements over many generations. Expansion of pathogens may also be limited by passive mechanisms, such as competition for limited nutrients and the accumulation of metabolic waste products from indigenous microbes that inhibit pathogenic strains. For example, in the mouse intestine, enterohemorrhagic strains of Escherichia coli are known to compete with nonpathogenic strains for amino acids and other nutrients.[96,97]

Dysbiosis and Community Dynamics

Dysbiosis is the concept that disruption of mutualistic relationships in the microbiome may compromise health and contribute to human disease. If the healthy microbiome exists to serve a function or multiple functions, exogenous stressors that induce a dysbiosis may then influence the functional ability of the core microbiome, creating a temporary susceptibility for transitioning to a diseased state (see **Fig. 2**). It remains unclear whether dysbiosis is a primary trigger that leads to disease pathogenesis and if these community imbalances may be involved in determining severity or duration of disease.[48] But this is certainly an area of interest, as stability and resilience of the microbiome has a degree of interpersonal variance.[50,98]

Determinants of the Human Microbiome

The microbiome seems to be established early in infancy and is necessary for the development of normal mucosal immunity. Several gestational and postpartum environmental factors are known to contribute to the development of a healthy intestinal microbiome, including route of birth, gestational age at birth, breastfeeding, exposure to cigarette smoke or antibiotics, household milieu, and socioeconomic status.[99] In addition to environmental factors, there is intriguing evidence from twin studies to suggest that microbiome determinants are heritable but that genetics may play only a partial role in microbiome composition. These studies demonstrate that individuals have significant covariability in the species represented within their gut microbiome but that specific alleles held between monozygotic and dizygotic twins underlie the heritability of certain bacterial phyla.[55,100]

Stability refers to the degree of random change with time, and the resilience of a microbial community is defined by its ability to return to baseline following a perturbation in the community. Studies examining the stability and resilience of the sinonasal microbiome are limited, but emerging evidence suggests that the healthy adult microbiome is relatively stable over time.[25] Hauser and colleagues[98] determined that patients undergoing ESS and receiving postoperative oral antibiotics demonstrated a significant shift in the microbial composition 2 weeks postoperatively but that after 6 weeks the bacterial composition returned to the preintervention baseline in many patients. The significance of stability and resilience of the sinonasal microbiome is unclear at this point but may be identified as an important factor in disease susceptibility or response to therapy. For instance, the clinical scenario of a patient with an upper respiratory infection that subsequently develops into chronic sinus disease is quite common. If the native microbiota are not a stable and resilient population to begin with, then this perturbation could lead to prolonged shifts in the microbiome that then predispose to the formation of sinus disease, akin to the 2-hit hypothesis of carcinogenesis.[101]

Restoring a Healthy Microbiome: Prebiotics and Probiotics

With increasing evidence suggesting that dysbiosis participates in the onset or propagation of CRS, and data supporting the concept that microbial richness and diversity contribute to health, much interest has been devoted toward restoration of healthy microbial community function. The most obvious example of these efforts is with the use of probiotics and prebiotics. Probiotics are live bacteria or yeast that are introduced to a microbial community actively functioning to restore balance and/or functionality to the niche. Although significant research has been devoted to oral probiotics for the restoration of gastrointestinal microbes, similar trials investigating oral or topical probiotics in CRS are lacking. To date there has been one randomized controlled trial examining the utility of probiotics in CRS, which did not find any benefit.[102] Murine models have demonstrated proof of concept for the utility of introducing competing bacteria into the sinonasal milieu of infectious CRS using *Staphylococcus epidermidis* as a probiotic niche-occupier in *S aureus*–induced CRS in mice.[103] Prebiotics are non-nutritive fibers that, when delivered into a bacterial community, serve as substrates for bacteria and are thought to support the growth of desirable microbes within the community. The uses of prebiotics for nasal health are widely marketed by nutraceutical companies. However, there have not been any randomized controlled data that supports the use of prebiotics in the treatment of CRS.

Lastly, many of our antibiotics carry broad-spectrum activity and eradicate many species in addition to the target pathogen (ie, collateral damage), which may actually be unfavorable (**Fig. 3**). The development of narrow-spectrum antibiotics to selectively eliminate individual taxa from a microbial niche is appealing. In order to rationally move probiotics, prebiotics, and narrow-spectrum antibiotics into the rhinology clinic, we must develop a detailed description of the core microbiome or the core microbial components necessary for an individual to maintain sinonasal health. Restoring community function in the healthy state is a primary microbiome goal, just as restoring mucociliary function has been a functional goal in the management of CRS.[6]

A GENERAL APPROACH TO ANTIBIOTIC THERAPY FOR REFRACTORY CHRONIC RHINOSINUSITIS

Current Guidelines for Antibiotics in Chronic Rhinosinusitis

Although sinonasal saline irrigation and topical corticosteroids are the mainstays of medical therapy for CRS, current clinical practice guidelines do recommend the routine use of antibiotics.[104,105] If purulence is present on examination in patients with CRS, short-term culture-directed therapy has been recommended.[106–108] In

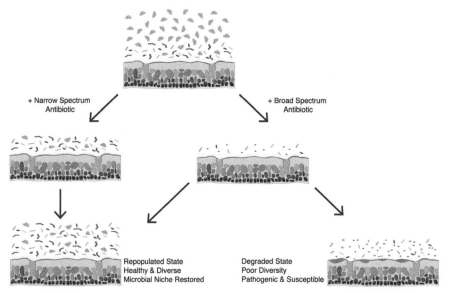

Fig. 3. Antibiotic use, coupled with subject-specific resilience, may potentially result in a degraded microbiome.

patients with CRSwNP who experience an acute exacerbation or persistent symptoms of CRS, a short course of systemic corticosteroid therapy remains the standard of care with the best early and long-term improvement in polyp scores,[109] although doxycycline may have a role in the patients as well.[110] Current clinical practice guidelines recommend consideration of long-term macrolide therapy, such as clarithromycin 250 to 500 mg daily, roxithromycin 150 mg daily, or azithromycin 500 mg weekly for 3 months in patients with CRSsNP only, as patients with nasal polyps did not benefit from long-term macrolide therapy when compared with placebo.[104,111,112] The *routine* use of antibiotics in CRS when acute infection is not present has been recently called into question, given the cost and potential harms of antibiotic use when the effectiveness of this therapy is not clear.[113]

Bacteria: Good, Bad, or Just There?

Increasing data suggest that diverse bacterial communities are important for maintaining human health, although much of our current CRS therapy is nonspecific and potentially eradicates large groups of both commensal and pathogenic bacteria. A recent culture-independent study has demonstrated that bacteria are present in roughly similar quantities in both healthy and diseased states.[29] Certainly, it is apparent that bacteria may function in a beneficial or detrimental manner to the host. However, it seems that much of the bacteria present are simply there, without a known role or function. It has also been noted that pathogens may be present in the healthy state, although in low abundance and housed within a richer and diverse population of other microbes.[26] It is currently challenging to determine if bacteria detected in disease always necessitates a therapeutic strategy for its eradication. Differences in microbial communities identified in recent CRS studies very well may be associations discovered because of confounding factors, such as the extensive and prolonged therapies used for the disease, namely, antibiotics. As a result, a more rational approach to judicious use of antibiotic therapy is needed in CRS.

REFERENCES

1. Bachert C, Gevaert P, Holtappels G, et al. Total and specific IgE in nasal polyps is related to local eosinophilic inflammation. J Allergy Clin Immunol 2001;107(4): 607–14.
2. Pawankar R, Nonaka M. Inflammatory mechanisms and remodeling in chronic rhinosinusitis and nasal polyps. Curr Allergy Asthma Rep 2007;7(3):202–8.
3. Kern RC, Conley DB, Walsh W, et al. Perspectives on the etiology of chronic rhinosinusitis: an immune barrier hypothesis. Am J Rhinol 2008;22(6):549–59.
4. Knowles MR, Boucher RC. Mucus clearance as a primary innate defense mechanism for mammalian airways. J Clin Invest 2002;109(5):571–7.
5. Peters AT, Kato A, Zhang N, et al. Evidence for altered activity of the IL-6 pathway in chronic rhinosinusitis with nasal polyps. J Allergy Clin Immunol 2010;125(2):397–403.e10.
6. Gudis D, Zhao KQ, Cohen NA. Acquired cilia dysfunction in chronic rhinosinusitis. Am J Rhinol Allergy 2012;26(1):1–6.
7. Hadfield PJ, Rowe-Jones JM, Mackay IS. The prevalence of nasal polyps in adults with cystic fibrosis. Clin Otolaryngol Allied Sci 2000;25(1):19–22.
8. Bush A, Chodhari R, Collins N, et al. Primary ciliary dyskinesia: current state of the art. Arch Dis Child 2007;92(12):1136–40.
9. Ooi EH, Psaltis AJ, Witterick IJ, et al. Innate immunity. Otolaryngol Clin North Am 2010;43(3):473–87, vii.
10. Claeys S, De Belder T, Holtappels G, et al. Human beta-defensins and toll-like receptors in the upper airway. Allergy 2003;58(8):748–53.
11. Ramanathan M, Lee WK, Spannhake EW, et al. Th2 cytokines associated with chronic rhinosinusitis with polyps down-regulate the antimicrobial immune function of human sinonasal epithelial cells. Am J Rhinol 2008;22(2):115–21.
12. Vandermeer J, Sha Q, Lane AP, et al. Innate immunity of the sinonasal cavity: expression of messenger RNA for complement cascade components and toll-like receptors. Arch Otolaryngol Head Neck Surg 2004;130(12):1374–80.
13. Kato A, Schleimer RP. Beyond inflammation: airway epithelial cells are at the interface of innate and adaptive immunity. Curr Opin Immunol 2007;19(6): 711–20.
14. Dong Z, Yang Z, Wang C. Expression of TLR2 and TLR4 messenger RNA in the epithelial cells of the nasal airway. Am J Rhinol 2005;19(3):236–9.
15. Detwiller KY, Smith TL, Alt JA, et al. Differential expression of innate immunity genes in chronic rhinosinusitis. Am J Rhinol Allergy 2014;28(5):374–7.
16. Hertz CJ, Kiertscher SM, Godowski PJ, et al. Microbial lipopeptides stimulate dendritic cell maturation via toll-like receptor 2. J Immunol 2001;166(4):2444–50.
17. Schwandner R, Dziarski R, Wesche H, et al. Peptidoglycan- and lipoteichoic acid-induced cell activation is mediated by toll-like receptor 2. J Biol Chem 1999;274(25):17406–9.
18. Ramanathan M, Lee WK, Dubin MG, et al. Sinonasal epithelial cell expression of toll-like receptor 9 is decreased in chronic rhinosinusitis with polyps. Am J Rhinol 2007;21(1):110–6.
19. Kim JH, Kim GE, Cho GS, et al. Natural killer cells from patients with chronic rhinosinusitis have impaired effector functions. PLoS One 2013;8(10):e77177.
20. Blair C, Naclerio RM, Yu X, et al. Role of type 1 T helper cells in the resolution of acute Streptococcus pneumoniae sinusitis: a mouse model. J Infect Dis 2005; 192(7):1237–44.
21. Hamilos DL. Antigen presenting cells. Immunol Res 1989;8(2):98–117.

22. Broere F, Apasov SG, Sitkovsky MV, et al. A2 T cell subsets and T cell-mediated immunity. In: Nijkamp FP, Parnham JM, editors. Principles of immunopharmacology: 3rd revised and extended edition. Basel (Switzerland): Birkhäuser Basel; 2011. p. 15–27.
23. Martinez FO, Helming L, Gordon S. Alternative activation of macrophages: an immunologic functional perspective. Annu Rev Immunol 2009;27:451–83.
24. Krysko O, Holtappels G, Zhang N, et al. Alternatively activated macrophages and impaired phagocytosis of S. aureus in chronic rhinosinusitis. Allergy 2011;66(3):396–403.
25. Yan M, Pamp SJ, Fukuyama J, et al. Nasal microenvironments and interspecific interactions influence nasal microbiota complexity and S. aureus carriage. Cell Host Microbe 2013;14(6):631–40.
26. Ramakrishnan VR, Feazel LM, Gitomer SA, et al. The microbiome of the middle meatus in healthy adults. PLoS One 2013;8(12):e85507.
27. Tabas I, Glass CK. Anti-inflammatory therapy in chronic disease: challenges and opportunities. Science 2013;339(6116):166–72.
28. Lozupone CA, Stombaugh JI, Gordon JI, et al. Diversity, stability and resilience of the human gut microbiota. Nature 2012;489(7415):220–30.
29. Ramakrishnan VR, Feazel LM, Abrass LJ, et al. Prevalence and abundance of Staphylococcus aureus in the middle meatus of patients with chronic rhinosinusitis, nasal polyps, and asthma. Int Forum Allergy Rhinol 2013;3(4):267–71.
30. Ramakrishnan VR, Hauser LJ, Feazel LM, et al. Sinus microbiota varies among chronic rhinosinusitis phenotypes and predicts surgical outcome. J Allergy Clin Immunol 2015;136(2):334–42.e1.
31. Turnbaugh PJ, Ley RE, Hamady M, et al. The human microbiome project. Nature 2007;449(7164):804–10.
32. Erb-Downward JR, Thompson DL, Han MK, et al. Analysis of the lung microbiome in the "healthy" smoker and in COPD. PLoS One 2011;6(2):e16384.
33. Abreu NA, Nagalingam NA, Song Y, et al. Sinus microbiome diversity depletion and Corynebacterium tuberculostearicum enrichment mediates rhinosinusitis. Sci Transl Med 2012;4(151):151ra124.
34. McLoughlin RM, Mills KHG. Influence of gastrointestinal commensal bacteria on the immune responses that mediate allergy and asthma. J Allergy Clin Immunol 2011;127(5):1097–107 [quiz: 1108–9].
35. Bisgaard H, Hermansen MN, Buchvald F, et al. Childhood asthma after bacterial colonization of the airway in neonates. N Engl J Med 2007;357(15):1487–95.
36. Ivanov II, Atarashi K, Manel N, et al. Induction of intestinal Th17 cells by segmented filamentous bacteria. Cell 2009;139(3):485–98.
37. Ivanov II, Frutos Rde L, Manel N, et al. Specific microbiota direct the differentiation of IL-17-producing T-helper cells in the mucosa of the small intestine. Cell Host Microbe 2008;4(4):337–49.
38. Worbs T, Bode U, Yan S, et al. Oral tolerance originates in the intestinal immune system and relies on antigen carriage by dendritic cells. J Exp Med 2006; 203(3):519–27.
39. Atarashi K, Tanoue T, Shima T, et al. Induction of colonic regulatory T cells by indigenous Clostridium species. Science 2011;331(6015):337–41.
40. Sasama J, Sherris DA, Shin SH, et al. New paradigm for the roles of fungi and eosinophils in chronic rhinosinusitis. Curr Opin Otolaryngol Head Neck Surg 2005;13(1):2–8.

41. Boase S, Foreman A, Cleland E, et al. The microbiome of chronic rhinosinusitis: culture, molecular diagnostics and biofilm detection. BMC Infect Dis 2013;13: 210.
42. Aurora R, Chatterjee D, Hentzleman J, et al. Contrasting the microbiomes from healthy volunteers and patients with chronic rhinosinusitis. JAMA Otolaryngol Head Neck Surg 2013;139(12):1328–38.
43. Cleland EJ, Bassiouni A, Bassioni A, et al. The fungal microbiome in chronic rhinosinusitis: richness, diversity, postoperative changes and patient outcomes. Int Forum Allergy Rhinol 2014;4(4):259–65.
44. Allen EK, Koeppel AF, Hendley JO, et al. Characterization of the nasopharyngeal microbiota in health and during rhinovirus challenge. Microbiome 2014;2: 22.
45. Wilson MT, Hamilos DL. The nasal and sinus microbiome in health and disease. Curr Allergy Asthma Rep 2014;14(12):485.
46. Feazel LM, Robertson CE, Ramakrishnan VR, et al. Microbiome complexity and Staphylococcus aureus in chronic rhinosinusitis. Laryngoscope 2012;122(2): 467–72.
47. Stephenson MF, Mfuna L, Dowd SE, et al. Molecular characterization of the polymicrobial flora in chronic rhinosinusitis. J Otolaryngol Head Neck Surg 2010; 39(2):182–7.
48. Frank DN, Zhu W, Sartor RB, et al. Investigating the biological and clinical significance of human dysbioses. Trends Microbiol 2011;19(9):427–34.
49. Human Microbiome Project Consortium. A framework for human microbiome research. Nature 2012;486(7402):215–21.
50. Human Microbiome Project Consortium. Structure, function and diversity of the healthy human microbiome. Nature 2012;486(7402):207–14.
51. Ding T, Schloss PD. Dynamics and associations of microbial community types across the human body. Nature 2014;509(7500):357–60.
52. Reshef L, Kovacs A, Ofer A, et al. Pouch inflammation is associated with a decrease in specific bacterial taxa. Gastroenterology 2015;149(3):718–27.
53. Bassis CM, Erb-Downward JR, Dickson RP, et al. Analysis of the upper respiratory tract microbiotas as the source of the lung and gastric microbiotas in healthy individuals. MBio 2015;6(2):e00037.
54. Choi EB, Hong SW, Kim DK, et al. Decreased diversity of nasal microbiota and their secreted extracellular vesicles in patients with chronic rhinosinusitis based on a metagenomic analysis. Allergy 2014;69(4):517–26.
55. Turnbaugh PJ, Hamady M, Yatsunenko T, et al. A core gut microbiome in obese and lean twins. Nature 2009;457(7228):480–4.
56. Ott SJ, Musfeldt M, Wenderoth DF, et al. Reduction in diversity of the colonic mucosa associated bacterial microflora in patients with active inflammatory bowel disease. Gut 2004;53(5):685–93.
57. Scher JU, Ubeda C, Artacho A, et al. Decreased bacterial diversity characterizes the altered gut microbiota in patients with psoriatic arthritis, resembling dysbiosis in inflammatory bowel disease. Arthritis Rheumatol 2015;67(1): 128–39.
58. Huang EY, Inoue T, Leone VA, et al. Using corticosteroids to reshape the gut microbiome: implications for inflammatory bowel diseases. Inflamm Bowel Dis 2015;21(5):963–72.
59. Modi SR, Collins JJ, Relman DA. Antibiotics and the gut microbiota. J Clin Invest 2014;124(10):4212–8.

60. Ramakrishnan VR, Frank DN. Impact of cigarette smoking on the middle meatus microbiome in health and chronic rhinosinusitis. Int Forum Allergy Rhinol 2015; 5(11):981–9.

61. Brook I, Frazier EH. Correlation between microbiology and previous sinus surgery in patients with chronic maxillary sinusitis. Ann Otol Rhinol Laryngol 2001;110(2):148–51.

62. Finegold SM, Flynn MJ, Rose FV, et al. Bacteriologic findings associated with chronic bacterial maxillary sinusitis in adults. Clin Infect Dis 2002;35(4):428–33.

63. Nadel DM, Lanza DC, Kennedy DW. Endoscopically guided cultures in chronic sinusitis. Am J Rhinol 1998;12(4):233–41.

64. Cleland EJ, Bassiouni A, Wormald PJ. The bacteriology of chronic rhinosinusitis and the pre-eminence of Staphylococcus aureus in revision patients. Int Forum Allergy Rhinol 2013;3(8):642–6.

65. Sande MA, Gwaltney JM. Acute community-acquired bacterial sinusitis: continuing challenges and current management. Clin Infect Dis 2004; 39(Suppl 3):S151–8.

66. Skoner DP. Complications of allergic rhinitis. J Allergy Clin Immunol 2000;105(6 Pt 2):S605–9.

67. Alho OP. Nasal airflow, mucociliary clearance, and sinus functioning during viral colds: effects of allergic rhinitis and susceptibility to recurrent sinusitis. Am J Rhinol 2004;18(6):349–55.

68. Fokkens WJ, Lund VJ, Mullol J, et al. European position paper on rhinosinusitis and nasal polyps 2012. Rhinol Suppl 2012;23:1–298.

69. Chee L, Graham SM, Carothers DG, et al. Immune dysfunction in refractory sinusitis in a tertiary care setting. Laryngoscope 2001;111(2):233–5.

70. Kingdom TT, Swain RE. The microbiology and antimicrobial resistance patterns in chronic rhinosinusitis. Am J Otolaryngol 2004;25(5):323–8.

71. Estrela S, Whiteley M, Brown SP. The demographic determinants of human microbiome health. Trends Microbiol 2015;23(3):134–41.

72. Suh JD, Ramakrishnan V, Palmer JN. Biofilms. Otolaryngol Clin North Am 2010; 43(3):521–30, viii.

73. Psaltis AJ, Ha KR, Beule AG, et al. Confocal scanning laser microscopy evidence of biofilms in patients with chronic rhinosinusitis. Laryngoscope 2007; 117(7):1302–6.

74. Oncel S, Pinar E, Sener G, et al. Evaluation of bacterial biofilms in chronic rhinosinusitis. J Otolaryngol Head Neck Surg 2010;39(1):52–5.

75. Hauser LJ, Feazel LM, Ir D, et al. Sinus culture poorly predicts resident microbiota. Int Forum Allergy Rhinol 2015;5(1):3–9.

76. Larson DA, Han JK. Microbiology of sinusitis: does allergy or endoscopic sinus surgery affect the microbiologic flora? Curr Opin Otolaryngol Head Neck Surg 2011;19(3):199–203.

77. Bachert C, Zhang N, Patou J, et al. Role of staphylococcal superantigens in upper airway disease. Curr Opin Allergy Clin Immunol 2008;8(1):34–8.

78. Pezato R, Świerczyńska-Krępa M, Niżankowska-Mogilnicka E, et al. Role of imbalance of eicosanoid pathways and staphylococcal superantigens in chronic rhinosinusitis. Allergy 2012;67(11):1347–56.

79. Pérez Novo CA, Waeytens A, Claeys C, et al. Staphylococcus aureus enterotoxin B regulates prostaglandin E2 synthesis, growth, and migration in nasal tissue fibroblasts. J Infect Dis 2008;197(7):1036–43.

80. Corriveau MN, Zhang N, Holtappels G, et al. Detection of Staphylococcus aureus in nasal tissue with peptide nucleic acid-fluorescence in situ hybridization. Am J Rhinol Allergy 2009;23(5):461–5.

81. Parvez N, Jinadatha C, Fader R, et al. Universal MRSA nasal surveillance: characterization of outcomes at a tertiary care center and implications for infection control. South Med J 2010;103(11):1084–91.

82. Jervis-Bardy J, Foreman A, Field J, et al. Impaired mucosal healing and infection associated with Staphylococcus aureus after endoscopic sinus surgery. Am J Rhinol Allergy 2009;23(5):549–52.

83. Foreman A, Holtappels G, Psaltis AJ, et al. Adaptive immune responses in Staphylococcus aureus biofilm-associated chronic rhinosinusitis. Allergy 2011; 66(11):1449–56.

84. Lebeaux D, Ghigo JM, Beloin C. Biofilm-related infections: bridging the gap between clinical management and fundamental aspects of recalcitrance toward antibiotics. Microbiol Mol Biol Rev 2014;78(3):510–43.

85. Psaltis AJ, Weitzel EK, Ha KR, et al. The effect of bacterial biofilms on post–sinus surgical outcomes. Am J Rhinol 2008;22(1):1–6.

86. Sabini P, Josephson GD, Reisacher WR, et al. The role of endoscopic sinus surgery in patients with acquired immune deficiency syndrome. Am J Otolaryngol 1998;19(6):351–6.

87. Godoy JM, Godoy AN, Ribalta G, et al. Bacterial pattern in chronic sinusitis and cystic fibrosis. Otolaryngol Head Neck Surg 2011;145(4):673–6.

88. Hansen SK, Rau MH, Johansen HK, et al. Evolution and diversification of pseudomonas aeruginosa in the paranasal sinuses of cystic fibrosis children have implications for chronic lung infection. ISME J 2012;6(1):31–45.

89. Carenfelt C, Lundberg C. The role of local gas composition in pathogenesis of maxillary sinus empyema. Acta Otolaryngol 1978;85(1–2):116–21.

90. Jousimies-Somer HR, Savolainen S, Ylikoski JS. Macroscopic purulence, leukocyte counts, and bacterial morphotypes in relation to culture findings for sinus secretions in acute maxillary sinusitis. J Clin Microbiol 1988;26(10):1926–33.

91. Siqueira JF, Rôças IN. Community as the unit of pathogenicity: an emerging concept as to the microbial pathogenesis of apical periodontitis. Oral Surg Oral Med Oral Pathol Oral Radiol Endod 2009;107(6):870–8.

92. Coyne MJ, Zitomersky NL, McGuire AM, et al. Evidence of extensive DNA transfer between bacteroidales species within the human gut. MBio 2014;5(3): e01305–14.

93. McKay TL, Ko J, Bilalis Y, et al. Mobile genetic elements of Fusobacterium nucleatum. Plasmid 1995;33(1):15–25.

94. Davies J, Davies D. Origins and evolution of antibiotic resistance. Microbiol Mol Biol Rev 2010;74(3):417–33.

95. Iwase T, Uehara Y, Shinji H, et al. Staphylococcus epidermidis Esp inhibits Staphylococcus aureus biofilm formation and nasal colonization. Nature 2010; 465(7296):346–9.

96. Leatham MP, Banerjee S, Autieri SM, et al. Precolonized human commensal Escherichia coli strains serve as a barrier to E. coli O157:H7 growth in the streptomycin-treated mouse intestine. Infect Immun 2009;77(7):2876–86.

97. Fabich AJ, Jones SA, Chowdhury FZ, et al. Comparison of carbon nutrition for pathogenic and commensal Escherichia coli strains in the mouse intestine. Infect Immun 2008;76(3):1143–52.

98. Hauser LJ, Ir D, Kingdom TT, et al. Investigation of bacterial repopulation after sinus surgery and perioperative antibiotics. Int Forum Allergy Rhinol 2016; 6(1):34–40.

99. Munyaka PM, Khafipour E, Ghia JE. External influence of early childhood establishment of gut microbiota and subsequent health implications. Front Pediatr 2014;2:109.

100. Goodrich JK, Waters JL, Poole AC, et al. Human genetics shape the gut microbiome. Cell 2014;159(4):789–99.

101. Knudson AG. Mutation and cancer: statistical study of retinoblastoma. Proc Natl Acad Sci U S A 1971;68(4):820–3.

102. Mukerji SS, Pynnonen MA, Kim HM, et al. Probiotics as adjunctive treatment for chronic rhinosinusitis: a randomized controlled trial. Otolaryngol Head Neck Surg 2009;140(2):202–8.

103. Cleland EJ, Drilling A, Bassiouni A, et al. Probiotic manipulation of the chronic rhinosinusitis microbiome. Int Forum Allergy Rhinol 2014;4(4):309–14.

104. Rudmik L, Soler ZM. Medical therapies for adult chronic sinusitis: a systematic review. JAMA 2015;314(9):926–39.

105. Rosenfeld RM, Piccirillo JF, Chandrasekhar SS, et al. Clinical practice guideline (update): adult sinusitis. Otolaryngol Head Neck Surg 2015;152(Suppl 2): S1–39.

106. Dellamonica P, Choutet P, Lejeune JM, et al. Efficacy and tolerance of cefotiam hexetil in the super-infected chronic sinusitis. A randomized, double-blind study in comparison with cefixime. Ann Otolaryngol Chir Cervicofac 1994;111(4): 217–22 [in French].

107. Legent F, Bordure P, Beauvillain C, et al. A double-blind comparison of ciprofloxacin and amoxycillin/clavulanic acid in the treatment of chronic sinusitis. Chemotherapy 1994;40(Suppl 1):8–15.

108. Huck W, Reed BD, Nielsen RW, et al. Cefaclor vs amoxicillin in the treatment of acute, recurrent, and chronic sinusitis. Arch Fam Med 1993;2(5):497–503.

109. Martinez-Devesa P, Patiar S. Oral steroids for nasal polyps. Cochrane Database Syst Rev 2011;(7):CD005232.

110. van Zele T, Gevaert P, Holtappels G, et al. Oral steroids and doxycycline: two different approaches to treat nasal polyps. J Allergy Clin Immunol 2010; 125(5):1069–76.e4.

111. Wallwork B, Coman W, Mackay-Sim A, et al. A double-blind, randomized, placebo-controlled trial of macrolide in the treatment of chronic rhinosinusitis. Laryngoscope 2006;116(2):189–93.

112. Videler WJ, Badia L, Harvey RJ, et al. Lack of efficacy of long-term, low-dose azithromycin in chronic rhinosinusitis: a randomized controlled trial. Allergy 2011;66(11):1457–68.

113. Soler ZM, Oyer SL, Kern RC, et al. Antimicrobials and chronic rhinosinusitis with or without polyposis in adults: an evidenced-based review with recommendations. Int Forum Allergy Rhinol 2013;3(1):31–47.

Biofilm and Osteitis in Refractory Chronic Rhinosinusitis

Yi Chen Zhao, MBBS, PhD, FRACS,
Peter-John Wormald, MD, FRACS, FRCS, MBChB*

KEYWORDS

- Biofilm • Osteitis • Refractory rhinosinusitis • Endoscopic surgery

KEY POINTS

- Biofilm is a sessile colony of bacteria with unique phenotypic expressions that interacts with the immune system, producing inflammation and contributing to the disease's refractory nature.
- Osteitis is predominately an inflammation of bone that is associated with refractory chronic rhinosinusitis (CRS).
- Both osteitis and biofilm are poor prognostic markers and are part of the inflammatory load.
- Surgery is currently the cornerstone of treatment for CRS; reducing inflammatory load with maximal ventilation of the affected paranasal sinuses facilitates postoperative medical treatment.
- Adjunctive treatments are currently being investigated with topical antibiotics being shown to be effective against biofilm.

BIOFILM IN REFRACTORY CHRONIC RHINOSINUSITIS
Definition of Biofilm

Chronic rhinosinusitis (CRS) is a multifactorial inflammatory condition of the upper respiratory tract that results from a complex interplay between the host immune response and multiple extrinsic environmental and disease-causing factors.[1] Bacteria and fungi have long been implicated as pathogens in the development of CRS, although the specific mechanism remains unclear. These microbes can exist either as a planktonic "free-floating" state or as a biofilm.

Financial conflict of interest: P.-J. Wormald receives royalties from Medtronic, Integra and Scopis and is a consultant for Neilmed.

Department of Surgery - Otolaryngology Head & Neck Surgery, The University of Adelaide, Adelaide, Queen Elizabeth Hospital 28 Woodville Rd, Woodville South, South Australia 5011, Australia

* Corresponding author. Department of Otolaryngology Head & Neck Surgery, Queen Elizabeth Hospital, Woodville South, South Australia 5011, Australia.

E-mail address: peterj.wormald@adelaide.edu.au

Otolaryngol Clin N Am 50 (2017) 49–60
http://dx.doi.org/10.1016/j.otc.2016.08.005
0030-6665/17/© 2016 Elsevier Inc. All rights reserved.

oto.theclinics.com

Biofilm is defined as a microbial-derived sessile community characterized by cells irreversibly attached to a surface or to each other, embedded within a matrix and exhibiting an altered phenotype with respect to growth and gene transcription.[2] Within a biofilm, the microbes are surrounded by an extracellular matrix of polysaccharides, nucleic acids, and proteins. The bacteria and the extracellular polymeric substance form microcolonies with water channels conveying fluid and nutrients.[3] This matrix confers characteristics of biofilm that allows it to adhere to surfaces, evade the immune response, increase resistance to antimicrobials, and provide a reservoir for recalcitrant infections.[2] The ability of the biofilm to evade the host immune response and confer antibiotic resistance are some of the key pathologic features of a biofilm. Not only does the extracellular matrix provide a physical barrier to antibiotics, some of the bacteria in biofilm exists in a hypometabolic, slow-growing state making them more resistant to antibiotic treatment.[4] The bacteria within a biofilm communicate via quorum sensing with small signal molecules that allow for rapid coordination of behavior to the environment.[5,6] The close proximity of the bacteria within the biofilm also allows frequent gene transfer that, combined with recurrent antibiotic exposure, leads to the development of antibiotic resistance.[6]

Biofilm in CRS was first discovered in 2004 using scanning electron microscopy[7] with subsequent studies showing confocal scanning microscopy to be the best method of detection.[8] Since then, numerous studies have demonstrated the presence of biofilm in CRS patients, with the reported prevalence ranging from 44% to 92%.[9]

Detection of Biofilm

In terms of detection of biofilm, current techniques include the use of scanning electron microscopy, transmission electron microscopy, confocal laser scanning microscopy using BacLight staining, fluorescence in situ hybridization, and molecular techniques. Confocal scanning laser microscopy has been shown to have the greatest sensitivity and specificity for biofilm detection (**Fig. 1**).[8]

Characterization of biofilm

Identification of the microorganism that forms the biofilm has been demonstrated by using fluorescence in situ hybridization probes (**Figs. 2 and 3**). *Staphylococcus aureus*[10] biofilms are the most commonly identified bacterial biofilm. *Pseudomonas aeruginosa, Haemophilus influenza,*[9] and *Streptococcus pnuemoniae* may also be

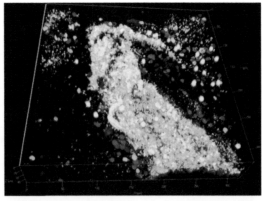

Fig. 1. Example of BacLight detection of biofilm. Red dots indicate sinonasal epithelium and green dots indicate bacterial colonies and biofilm matrix. Notice the concentration of the microcolonies with the extracellular matrix.

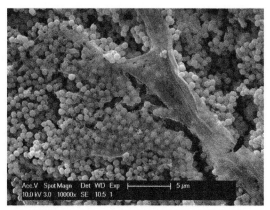

Fig. 2. Biofilm detected using scanning electron microscopy demonstrating small round bacteria surrounded by extracellular matrix.

represented in CRS biofilm formation.[11] These studies have identified a high proportion of polymicrobial biofilm, including the presence of fungal biofilm in up to 50% of cases.[9,10] Inoculation with *S aureus* or a cilia toxin–producing mucosal injury may be a prerequisite for formation of fungal biofilm.[9,10]

Limitation of current techniques

Although the fluorescence in situ hybridization technique is very accurate, only a limited number of probes can be applied; therefore, researchers need to presumptively decide which organisms to target with the probes. Newer molecular-based polymerase chain reaction techniques can identify DNA of all microorganisms present that make up the complex microbiome of the sinonasal cavity.[11] These findings reinforce the interplay between not just the host and the microbes, but also the interplay between the microorganisms as well.[10] Moreover, a practical test for biofilm detection in the clinical setting is not available currently.

Pathophysiology of Biofilm and Its Role in Refractory Chronic Rhinosinusitis

Does biofilm equal disease?

The pathophysiology of biofilm in CRS has not been elucidated fully. Some studies have indicated that biofilms are not uniformly present in patients with CRS,[12–14]

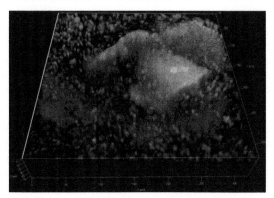

Fig. 3. Detection of biofilm using fluorescence in situ hybridization technique. Red dots indicate sinonasal epithelial cells. Green dots indicate bacterial colonies and biofilm.

whereas other studies have found biofilm in healthy controls.[9,13] Limitations in detection and sampling methods may partly explain this discrepancy. For instance, scanning electron microscopy may not reliably differentiate between biofilm and mucous, resulting in false-positive biofilm detection.[11] These findings emphasize that biofilm is just 1 factor in the multifactorial pathogenesis of CRS.

The effect of biofilm on disease seems to be at least partly related to the nature of the comprising organisms. In particular, S aureus biofilm represents a poor prognostic indicator. Multiple studies have demonstrated that S aureus biofilm-positive disease have worse postoperative outcomes in both objective and subjective scores compared with biofilm-negative disease.[14–17] S aureus biofilm patients have higher burden of disease with higher symptom scores and Lund-Mackay computed tomography (CT) scores. They are also more likely to have persistent disease postoperatively with worse subjective scores and objective assessments. In contrast, patients with an H influenza biofilm behave more like biofilm-negative patients and have a higher success rate with conventional treatment.[14,18,19]

How does biofilm contribute to refractory chronic rhinosinusitis?

Biofilm contributes to the refractory nature of some patients with CRS by its highly resistant nature to both antibiotic treatment and the host immune response. Defects within the innate immune response have been found in patients with biofilm-positive CRS. These are characterized by the downregulation of lactoferrin, which prevents bacterial aggregation[20] and MUC7, an antimicrobial glycoprotein. In addition, there is an upregulation of sialic acid, which exposes more adherent sites for bacteria.[21] The presence of the biofilm leads to significant destruction of the cilia in the epithelial layer of the mucosa, resulting in disruption in the mucociliary blanket.[22] Mucous stasis within the sinus cavity then results, which predisposes to further biofilm formation. The presence of biofilm also elicits a local inflammatory response with elevation of T lymphocytes and macrophage numbers.[23] The life cycle of the biofilm provides a local reservoir of bacteria with shedding of bacteria into planktonic form and leading to recurrent infections. In the case of S aureus biofilms, there is continued release of superantigenic molecules. There are also associations between biofilm and local markers of recalcitrant disease, such as intracellular bacterial infections[24] and osteitis.[25] In addition to the changes in the local environment, biofilm alters the host's adaptive immune function, with skewing toward a T-helper cell 2 profile and elevated levels of interleukin-5, interleukin-6, and eosinophilic cationic proteins.[26]

Treatment of Biofilm

The effective treatment of biofilm in refractory CRS is challenging. At present, there is no consensus of the optimal treatment modality, although local and topical treatment of sinus cavities has an intuitive appeal. Unfortunately, although some treatments have shown promise, none have been able to provide reliable long-term control. In addition, some potential biofilm treatments having been found to be ciliary toxic.[27]

Surgery

Endoscopic sinus surgery may have a role in biofilm-related refractory CRS. Surgically opening the involved sinuses serves the dual purpose of establishing maximal sinus ventilation and providing a conduit for the postoperative application of topical therapies. Limited study has suggested that surgery may reduce significantly the density of the biofilm.[28] Mechanical disruption of biofilm by irrigation during surgery may also be applied. The efficacy of topical therapy may depend on the successful reduction of the inflammatory load contributed by the biofilm.[29] The principles of functional surgery should be observed to avoid unnecessary mucosal stripping, because doing so would lead to dysfunctional postoperative mucociliary clearance.

Topical steroids
Topical treatment with corticosteroids is one of the cornerstones of treatment of CRS, although its role in biofilm-related disease has not been fully established. The benefit may be greatest in the postoperative setting. In vitro studies have found that it reduces S aureus biofilm.[30] Higher than standard doses of topical steroids may be required, such as budesonide 750 to 2000 mg/2 mL, fluticasone 400 mg/200 mL, or mometasone 300 to 400 mg/200 mL.

Topical antibiotics
The postoperative use of topical antibiotics has shown some promise in treating biofilm disease. A study by Ha and colleagues[31] showed that standard antibiotics needed very high doses in a toxic range to achieve biofilm removal. In contrast, nonabsorbed topical antibiotics such as mupirocin were effective in standard concentrations.[31,32] An in vitro study of topical antibiotics has suggested that mupirocin of 125 mg/mL can reduce biofilm mass by more than 90%.[31] Subsequently, a randomized control trial demonstrated twice-daily mupirocin rinses were effective in short-term eradication of S aureus compared with normal saline rinses.[32] Unfortunately, the relapse with recurrent infection occurred in up to 74% of patients treated with mupirocin over a 12-month follow-up period.[32]

Surfactants
Topical surfactants such as citric acid zwitterionic surfactant (Medtronic ENT, Jacksonville, FL), Johnson's Baby Shampoo (Johnson & Johnson, New Brunswick, NJ), and SinuSurf (NeilMed Pharmaceuticals, Santa Rosa, CA) have shown promise. Johnson's Baby Shampoo diluted to 1% solution was found to improve symptoms of mucus thickness and postnasal drip,[33] but had side effects of nasal irritation[34] and increased mucociliary clearance time.[35] SinuSurf (NeilMed Pharmaceuticals) was found to be initially helpful but was subsequently withdrawn owing to the side effect of anosmia.[36] Citric acid zwitterionic surfactant was found to be ciliary toxic and is not recommended for use.[27]

Other experimental treatments
Although there is not yet a definitive antibiofilm agent, there are a number of avenues are under investigation. In a sheep model, irrigation with Maunka honey (active ingredient methylglyoxal) was found to be safe to mucosa and efficacious against S aureus biofilm when used at a concentration of 0.9 to 1.8 mg/mL.[37] However, it was toxic to the cilia at concentrations greater than this level. Similarly, another in vitro study demonstrated the usefulness of colloidal silver for reduction of biofilm compared with control with maximal effect noted at a concentration of 100 to 150 μL.[38]

Nonconventional antimicrobial treatment has also been investigated. N,N-dichloro-2,2-dimethyltaurine, is a broad-spectrum antimicrobial agent, has been investigated in a sheep model and demonstrated significant biofilm reduction compared with saline.[39]

Bacteriophages are viruses that directly target and destroy bacteria. Early results with the use of S aureus-specific bacteriophages have been shown to be effective against clinical isolates of S aureus with reduction of biofilm mass.[40]

Photodynamic therapy with treatment of in vitro bacterial colonies with methylene blue trihydrate and subsequent exposure to 664 nm of light demonstrated 99% reduction after a single treatment[41] with no histologic evidence of side effect.[42] Low-frequency ultrasound treatment at 40 kHz, 0.5 W/cm^2 sound pressure on in vitro nasal polyp has found significant reduction in biofilm and inflammatory cells.[43]

OSTEITIS IN REFRACTORY CHRONIC RHINOSINUSITIS
Definitions of Osteitis

Osteitis is inflammation of bone without marrow space. It is characterized by neo-osteogenesis with new woven bone formation and thickening of the mucosa.[44] Although infectious mechanisms have been implicated in osteitis, it is predominately a disease of inflammation and bone remodeling There is, however, contention regarding the exact role of osteitis in CRS and its role in refractory disease.[45]

Prevalence of Osteitis

Although osteitis has been described since 1992, the exact prevalence is variable with studies citing an incidence of 36% to 53% depending on the radiologic or histologic criteria used in the study.[46,47] In patients with refractory CRS who have undergone multiple surgeries, the incidence of osteitis has been reported to be as high as 64%.[48]

Pathophysiology of Osteitis

Early experimental studies demonstrated localized periosteal reaction and bone changes as early as 4 days after inoculation of bacteria.[49] These studies demonstrated that infections can infiltrate through the mucosa, inducing an inflammatory reaction. This not only occurs in the underlying bone, but also at distal sites through widening of the bony vascular network and Harversian canal system.[50,51] The cycle of mucosal and bony infection and inflammation can theoretically act as a persisting nidus of disease.[52] However, more recent human studies have presented conflicting findings with some studies showing an absence of bacteria within the bone itself[44,53] and other studies showing bacterial microcolonies existing in the bone without an osteitis reaction.[54]

Biofilm association

Biofilm is certainly associated with osteitis, with the volume of biofilm present correlating with the degree of osteitis.[25] Biofilm potentially also acts as a reservoir for bacteria that cause bony inflammation through a release of eosinophilic inflammatory mediators implicated in the formation of osteitis.[55] The inflammation that occurs in osteitis leads to continuous remodeling of bone with histologic findings of new woven bone formation, periosteal thickening, bone resorption, and finally fibrosis in the most severe case of CRS.[56]

Disease Severity and Osteitis

There is a clear correlation between disease severity and osteitis. From a radiologic perspective, the degree of osteitis correlates with the Lund-Mackay score.[46] From a clinical perspective, patients with osteitis exhibited a greater severity of inflammatory CRS findings on endoscopy.[57] These patients are also more resistant to medical treatment[58] as well as surgical treatment with more severe osteitis in patients undergoing revision surgery than primary.[44] One of the perplexing factors regarding osteitis is that stripping of the mucosa or periosteum in multiple surgeries can also lead to underlying bone changes with worsening of CT grades of osteitis. This raises the question of whether the osteitis is causing recalcitrant disease necessitating further surgery, or alternatively that surgery may play a role in osteitis.[44,47] Ultimately, osteitis may represent an irreversible common endpoint of recalcitrant CRS disease with inflammatory involvement of both the mucosa and underlying bone.[45]

Diagnosis of Osteitis

Computed tomography scan

Although histology is considered the most accurate way of diagnosing osteitis, radiologic studies are the more commonly used investigations. CT scan was first used by Biedlingmaier[58] to diagnose osteitis and correlated well with histologic findings especially in more severe cases (**Fig. 4**).

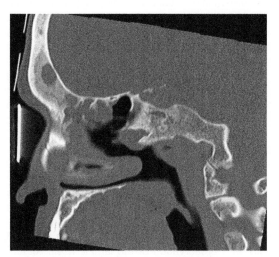

Fig. 4. Significant osteitis within the frontal sinus after surgery.

Scoring system

Unfortunately, the most commonly used CT staging system for CRS, the Lund-Mackay score, does not account for bony changes. Several scoring systems have been developed to further characterize osteitis. Lee and colleagues[46] measured the thickness of bony partitions to determine severity and, more recently, Georgalas and colleagues[48] proposed a Global Osteitis Scoring Scale that created an aggregate score depending on bony thickness and percentage of wall involvement in each of the sinuses. This score was found to correlate highly with the Lund-Mackay score, duration of symptoms and previous surgery.

Single-photon emission computed tomography

An alternative to CT scan is single-photon emission CT, which incorporates the radioactive isotope ^{99}technetium-methylene diphosphonate. Single-photon emission CT has been shown to have a 94% sensitivity toward detection of histologic osteitis.[59] Increased radioisotope uptake is also noted in patients with refractory CRS postoperatively.[58,60] However, the use of radioactive isotopes and the costs associated with the test limit the use of single-photon emission CT in clinical practice.

Histology

Although animal studies demonstrate inflammatory involvement of the bone matrix in osteitis, human studies have not shown significant inflammation or infection. In fact, there have not be any studies that demonstrate the presence of bacteria within the bone of patients with osteitis.[61] In early histologic study by Kennedy and colleagues,[62] significantly greater bone activity in patients with osteitis was demonstrated using radiolabeled tetracycline. Other histologic studies since have demonstrated similar findings of varying degree of woven bone formation, periosteal thickening, and fibrosis.[46,56,63,64]

Implication for Treatment of Osteitis

Surgery

It is unclear whether repeated surgery leads to osteitis, or the presence of osteitis leads to refractory disease requiring repeated surgery. Nevertheless, surgery remains the cornerstone of treatment of osteitis. Like biofilm, osteitis is part of disease load and may represent irreversible changes within severely diseased mucosa. It is therefore important to maximally remove osteitic bone when present. It is also important, during standard endoscopic sinus surgery, to preserve healthy mucosa and avoid stripping of the periosteum to avoid inducing surgically related bone changes; therefore, preservation of healthy mucosa is also paramount in sinus surgery. The presence of osteitis should also favor more aggressive and radical approaches to complete removal of bone to avoid recurrence.[52] In recalcitrant CRS, the bony ethmoid partitions are more frequently involved in osteitis compared with the lamina papyracea. Sinuses that become chronically obstructed such as the frontal, sphenoid, and maxillary sinuses, will on occasions develop osteitic changes.[46]

In patients with a high disease load (Lund Makay score of >16), it is important to remove as much of the disease as possible with clearance of polyps from all the sinuses but with preservation of the periostium. This facilitates regrowth of normal healthy mucosa postoperatively. It is also important to widely open all the sinus ostia to facilitate access to topical medical treatment postoperatively. When there are osteitic changes in the ethmoid septations on the lamina papyracea, these should be removed carefully with preservation of the lamina itself. Although it may not be safe to aggressively remove osteitic bone over the lateral wall of the sphenoid sinus, the anterior face and sphenoid septation can be drilled away. Osteitic changes in the lateral wall of the maxillary are usually not removed; however, a high disease load (polyps, fungus eosinophilic mucous) must be completely cleared from the sinus and the sinus ostium should be maximized.

The presence of osteitis is a poor prognostic indicator for outcomes after surgery.[57] In patients with osteitis, there is a greater incidence of disease recurrence[65] as well as an increased chance of postsurgical stenosis in patients undergoing a Draf III procedure.[66]

Antibiotics

Antibiotic treatment has been considered for osteitis because bacterial infection was thought to be a major cause.[67] However, despite initial experimental studies, microorganisms have not been consistently demonstrated within clinical osteitic bone. Macrolide antibiotics have been used but as an anti-inflammatory agent. By inhibiting interleukin-1β, macrolides may prevent the differentiation between the nasal fibroblasts to osteoblasts and may prevent progression of osteitis.[68] However, there is little overall evidence to support the use of antibiotics in osteitis. Although there is a study demonstrating a dose-dependent response in both mucosa and underlying bone in the use of topical tobramycin in a rabbit model of sinusitis,[69] there has been little research into the use of topical antibiotics in the treatment of osteitis specifically.

SUMMARY

Biofilm and osteitis are important factors that contribute toward CRS recalcitrance and resistance to traditional medical and surgical treatments. Biofilm contributes to CRS via its innate characteristics of antibiotic resistance, adherence to surfaces, and acting as a nidus for ongoing or recurrent infection. It also has interaction with the innate immune system leading to local inflammation as well as the adaptive immune system by promoting eosinophilic inflammation. Biofilm from *S aureus* is particularly damaging compared with other types of biofilm and is often found with concomitant fungal growth. The polymicrobial nature of biofilms is only beginning to be understood as further research is carried out into the microbiome of the sinonasal cavity.

The contribution of osteitis is less clear. It is hypothesized that osteitis results from overlying mucosal inflammation and acts as a nidus for ongoing inflammation. Although it has a strong association with refractory disease and need for revision surgery, it is unclear whether surgery exacerbates the formation of osteitis, or if its formation is a reflection of the extent of inflammatory disease load.

Despite research into biofilm and osteitis, mechanical removal of biofilm and accessible foci of osteitis through surgery followed by ongoing medical therapy remain the cornerstone of management. It is important to recognize that biofilm and osteitis are poor prognostic factors, which may require aggressive and sometimes radical surgery to control. Ultimately, they are part of the inflammatory load that if insufficiently reduced may lead to refractory disease.[29] Adjunctive treatments such as topical antibiotics have demonstrated a role in control of biofilm though not in osteitis. There is also a concept that early aggressive treatment in CRS may prevent irreversible mucosal change, although this has not been proven in clinical trials.[70] Further research is currently being carried out to identify other agents that can supplement surgery in the control of the refractory CRS.

REFERENCES

1. Jain R, Douglas R. When and how should we treat biofilms in chronic sinusitis? Curr Opin Otolaryngol Head Neck Surg 2014;22:16–21.
2. Donlan RM, Costerton JW. Biofilms: survival mechanisms of clinically relevant microorganisms. Clin Microbiol Rev 2002;15:167–93.
3. Stoodley P, Lewandowski Z. Liquid flow in biofilm systems. Appl Environ Microbiol 1994;60:2711–6.
4. Foreman A, Jervis-Bardy J, Wormald PJ. Do biofilms contribute to the initiation and recalcitrance of chronic rhinosinusitis? Laryngoscope 2011;121:1085–91.
5. Galloway WR, Hodgkinson JT, Bowden SD, et al. Quorum sensing in Gram-negative bacteria: small-molecule modulation of AHL and AI-2 quorum sensing pathways. Chem Rev 2010;111:28–67.
6. Harvey R, Lund V. Biofilms and chronic rhinosinusitis: systematic review of evidence, current concepts and directions for research. Rhinology 2007;45:3.
7. Cryer J, Schipor I, Perloff JR, et al. Evidence of bacterial biofilms in human chronic sinusitis. ORL J Otorhinolaryngol Relat Spec 2004;66:155–8.
8. Foreman A, Singhal D, Psaltis AJ, et al. Targeted imaging modality selection for bacterial biofilms in chronic rhinosinusitis. Laryngoscope 2010;120:427–31.
9. Healy DY, Leid JG, Sanderson AR, et al. Biofilms with fungi in chronic rhinosinusitis. Otolaryngol Head Neck Surg 2008;138:641–7.
10. Foreman A, Psaltis AJ, Tan LW, et al. Characterization of bacterial and fungal biofilms in chronic rhinosinusitis. Am J Rhinol Allergy 2009;23:556–61.
11. Foreman A, Boase S, Psaltis A, et al. Role of Bacterial And Fungal Biofilms In Chronic Rhinosinusitis. Curr Allergy Asthma Rep 2012;12:127–35.
12. Ramadan HH. Chronic rhinosinusitis and bacterial biofilms. Curr Opin Otolaryngol Head Neck Surg 2006;14:183–6.

13. Sanderson AR, Leid JG, Hunsaker D. Bacterial biofilms on the sinus mucosa of human subjects with chronic rhinosinusitis. Laryngoscope 2006;116:1121–6.
14. Singhal D, Psaltis AJ, Foreman A, et al. The impact of biofilms on outcomes after endoscopic sinus surgery. Am J Rhinol Allergy 2010;24:169–74.
15. Hochstim CJ, Masood R, Rice DH. Biofilm and persistent inflammation in endoscopic sinus surgery. Otolaryngol Head Neck Surg 2010;143:697–8.
16. Psaltis AJ, Weitzel EK, Ha KR, et al. The effect of bacterial biofilms on post-sinus surgical outcomes. Am J Rhinol 2008;22:1–6.
17. Zhang Z, Kofonow JM, Finkelman BS, et al. Clinical factors associated with bacterial biofilm formation in chronic rhinosinusitis. Otolaryngol Head Neck Surg 2011;144:457–62.
18. Foreman A, Wormald PJ. Different biofilms, different disease? A clinical outcomes study. Laryngoscope 2010;120:1701–6.
19. Singhal D, Foreman A, Bardy J-J, et al. Staphylococcus aureus biofilms. Laryngoscope 2011;121:1578–83.
20. Psaltis AJ, Wormald PJ, Ha KR, et al. Reduced levels of lactoferrin in biofilm-associated chronic rhinosinusitis. Laryngoscope 2008;118:895–901.
21. Tan L, Psaltis A, Baker LM, et al. Aberrant mucin glycoprotein patterns of chronic rhinosinusitis patients with bacterial biofilms. Am J Rhinol Allergy 2010;24:319–24.
22. You H, Zhuge P, Li D, et al. Factors affecting bacterial biofilm expression in chronic rhinosinusitis and the influences on prognosis. Am J Otolaryngol 2011;32:583–90.
23. Wood AJ, Fraser J, Swift S, et al. Are biofilms associated with an inflammatory response in chronic rhinosinusitis? Int Forum Allergy Rhinol 2011;1:335–9.
24. Tan NCW, Foreman A, Jardeleza C, et al. Intracellular Staphylococcus aureus: the Trojan horse of recalcitrant chronic rhinosinusitis? Int Forum Allergy Rhinol 2013;3:261–6.
25. Dong D, Yulin Z, Xiao W, et al. Correlation between bacterial biofilms and osteitis in patients with chronic rhinosinusitis. Laryngoscope 2014;124:1071–7.
26. Foreman A, Holtappels G, Psaltis AJ, et al. Adaptive immune responses in Staphylococcus aureus biofilm–associated chronic rhinosinusitis. Allergy 2011;66:1449–56.
27. Valentine R, Jervis-Bardy J, Psaltis A, et al. Efficacy of using a hydrodebrider and of citric acid/zwitterionic surfactant on a Staphylococcus aureus bacterial biofilm in the sheep model of rhinosinusitis. Am J Rhinol Allergy 2011;25:323–6.
28. Hai PVT, Lidstone C, Wallwork B. The effect of endoscopic sinus surgery on bacterial biofilms in chronic rhinosinusitis. Otolaryngol Head Neck Surg 2010;142:S27–32.
29. Bassiouni A, Naidoo Y, Wormald P-J. When FESS fails: the inflammatory load hypothesis in refractory chronic rhinosinusitis. Laryngoscope 2012;122:460–6.
30. Goggin R, Jardeleza C, Wormald PJ, et al. Corticosteroids directly reduce Staphylococcus aureus biofilm growth: an in vitro study. Laryngoscope 2014;124:602–7.
31. Ha KR, Psaltis AJ, Butcher AR, et al. Vitro activity of mupirocin on clinical isolates of staphylococcus aureus and its potential implications in chronic rhinosinusitis. Laryngoscope 2008;118:535–40.
32. Jervis-Bardy J, Boase S, Psaltis A, et al. A randomized trial of mupirocin sinonasal rinses versus saline in surgically recalcitrant staphylococcal chronic rhinosinusitis. Laryngoscope 2012;122:2148–53.

33. Chiu AG, Palmer JN, Woodworth BA, et al. Baby shampoo nasal irrigations for the symptomatic post–functional endoscopic sinus surgery patient. Am J Rhinol 2008;22:34–7.

34. Farag AA, Deal AM, McKinney KA, et al. Single-blind randomized controlled trial of surfactant vs hypertonic saline irrigation following endoscopic endonasal surgery. In: International forum of allergy & rhinology. Wiley Online Library; 2013. p. 276–80.

35. Isaacs S, Fakhri S, Luong A, et al. The effect of dilute baby shampoo on nasal mucociliary clearance in healthy subjects. Am J Rhinol Allergy 2011;25:e27–9.

36. Rosen PL, Palmer JN, O'Malley BW Jr, et al. Surfactants in the management of rhinopathologies. Am J Rhinol Allergy 2013;27:177.

37. Paramasivan S, Drilling AJ, Jardeleza C, et al. Methylglyoxal-augmented manuka honey as a topical anti–Staphylococcus aureus biofilm agent: safety and efficacy in an in vivo model. In: International forum of allergy & rhinology. Wiley Online Library; 2014. p. 187–95.

38. Goggin R, Jardeleza C, Wormald PJ, et al. Colloidal silver: a novel treatment for Staphylococcus aureus biofilms?. In: International forum of allergy & rhinology. Wiley Online Library; 2014. p. 171–5.

39. Singhal PD, Jekle PA, Debabov PD, et al. Efficacy of NVC-422 against Staphylococcus aureus biofilms in a sheep biofilm model of sinusitis. Int Forum Allergy Rhinol 2012;2:309–15.

40. Drilling A, Morales S, Jardeleza C, et al. Bacteriophage reduces biofilm of Staphylococcus aureus ex vivo isolates from chronic rhinosinusitis patients. Am J Rhinol Allergy 2014;28:3–11.

41. Biel MA, Sievert C, Usacheva M, et al. Antimicrobial photodynamic therapy treatment of chronic recurrent sinusitis biofilms. Int Forum Allergy Rhinol 2011;1:329–34.

42. Biel MA, Jones JW, Pedigo L, et al. The effect of antimicrobial photodynamic therapy on human ciliated respiratory mucosa. Laryngoscope 2012;122:2628–31.

43. Karosi T, Sziklai I, Csomor P. Low-frequency ultrasound for biofilm disruption in chronic rhinosinusitis with nasal polyposis: In vitro pilot study. Laryngoscope 2013;123:17–23.

44. Bhandarkar ND, Sautter NB, Kennedy DW, et al. Osteitis in chronic rhinosinusitis: a review of the literature. Int Forum Allergy Rhinol 2013;3:355–63.

45. Leung N, Mawby TA, Turner H, et al. Osteitis and chronic rhinosinusitis: a review of the current literature. Eur Arch Otorhinolaryngol 2016;273:2917–23.

46. Lee JT, Kennedy DW, Palmer JN, et al. The incidence of concurrent osteitis in patients with chronic rhinosinusitis: a clinicopathological study. Am J Rhinol 2006; 20:278–82.

47. Snidvongs K, McLachlan R, Sacks R, et al. Correlation of the Kennedy Osteitis Score to clinico-histologic features of chronic rhinosinusitis. Int Forum Allergy Rhinol 2013;3:369–75.

48. Georgalas C, Videler W, Freling N, et al. Global Osteitis Scoring Scale and chronic rhinosinusitis: a marker of revision surgery. Clin Otolaryngol 2010;35: 455–61.

49. Norlander T, Forsgren K, Pontus Stierna JK, et al. Cellular regeneration and recovery of the maxillary sinus mucosa: an experimental study in rabbits. Acta Otolaryngol 1992;112:33–7.

50. Bolger WE, Leonard D, Dick EJ, et al. Gram negative sinusitis: a bacteriologic and histologic study in rabbits. Am J Rhinol 1997;11:15–25.

51. Khalid AN, Hunt J, Perloff JR, et al. The role of bone in chronic rhinosinusitis. Laryngoscope 2002;112:1951–7.
52. Sethi N. The significance of osteitis in rhinosinusitis. Eur Arch Otorhinolaryngol 2015;272:821–6.
53. Lee JM, Chiu AG. Role of maximal endoscopic sinus surgery techniques in chronic rhinosinusitis. Otolaryngol Clin North Am 2010;43:579–89.
54. Wood AJ, Fraser J, Amirapu S, et al. Bacterial microcolonies exist within the sphenoid bone in chronic rhinosinusitis and healthy controls. In: International forum of allergy & rhinology. Wiley Online Library; 2012. p. 116–21.
55. Snidvongs K, McLachlan R, Chin D, et al. Osteitic bone: a surrogate marker of eosinophilia in chronic rhinosinusitis. Rhinology 2012;50:299–305.
56. Giacchi RJ, Lebowitz RA, Yee HT, et al. Histopathologic evaluation of the ethmoid bone in chronic sinusitis. Am J Rhinol 2001;15:193–7.
57. Bhandarkar ND, Mace JC, Smith TL. The impact of osteitis on disease severity measures and quality of life outcomes in chronic rhinosinusitis. Int Forum Allergy Rhinol 2011;1:372–8.
58. Biedlingmaier JF, Whelan P, Zoarski G, et al. Histopathology and CT analysis of partially resected middle turbinates. Laryngoscope 1996;106:102–4.
59. Catalano PJ, Dolan R, Romanow J, et al. Correlation of bone SPECT scintigraphy with histopathology of the ethmoid bulla: preliminary investigation. Ann Otol Rhinol Laryngol 2007;116:647–52.
60. Jang Y, Koo T, Chung S, et al. Bone involvement in chronic rhinosinusitis assessed by 99mTc-MDP bone SPECT. Clin Otolaryngol Allied Sci 2002;27:156–61.
61. Snidvongs K, Earls P, Dalgorf D, et al. Osteitis is a misnomer: a histopathology study in primary chronic rhinosinusitis. Int Forum Allergy Rhinol 2014;4:390–6.
62. Kennedy DW, Senior BA, Gannon FH, et al. Histology and histomorphometry of ethmoid bone in chronic rhinosinusitis. Laryngoscope 1998;108:502–7.
63. Cho SH, Min HJ, Han HX, et al. CT analysis and histopathology of bone remodeling in patients with chronic rhinosinusitis. Otolaryngol Head Neck Surg 2006;135:404–8.
64. Georgalas C. Osteitis and paranasal sinus inflammation: what we know and what we do not. Curr Opin Otolaryngol Head Neck Surg 2013;21:45–9.
65. Telmesani LM, Al-Shawarby M. Osteitis in chronic rhinosinusitis with nasal polyps: a comparative study between primary and recurrent cases. Eur Arch Otorhinolaryngol 2010;267:721–4.
66. Ye T, Hwang PH, Huang Z, et al. Frontal ostium neo-osteogenesis and patency after Draf III procedure: a computer-assisted study. Int Forum Allergy Rhinol 2014;4:739–44.
67. Kacker A, Huang C, Anand V. Incidence of chronic hyperostotic rhinosinusitis in patients undergoing primary sinus surgery compared to revision surgery. Rhinology 2002;40:80–2.
68. Park C-S, Park Y-S, Park Y-J, et al. The inhibitory effects of macrolide antibiotics on bone remodeling in chronic rhinosinusitis. Otolaryngol Head Neck Surg 2007;137:274–9.
69. Antunes MB, Feldman MD, Cohen NA, et al. Dose-dependent effects of topical tobramycin in an animal model of Pseudomonas sinusitis. Am J Rhinol 2007;21:423–7.
70. Bassiouni A, Naidoo Y, Wormald PJ. Does mucosal remodeling in chronic rhinosinusitis result in irreversible mucosal disease? Laryngoscope 2012;122:225–9.

Refractory Chronic Rhinosinusitis with Nasal Polyposis

Benjamin P. Hull, MD, MHA, Rakesh K. Chandra, MD*

KEYWORDS

- Polyps • Asthma • Allergy • Superantigen • Innate immunity • Cystic fibrosis
- Allergic fungal sinusitis

KEY POINTS

- Chronic rhinosinusitis with nasal polyposis (CRSwNP) is an aggressive, refractory disease process with multiple causes.
- Patients should be screened for allergic conditions and asthma and tested appropriately.
- Cystic fibrosis should be considered in children, patients with a family history, or patients who manifest the constellation of symptoms.
- Effective treatment requires surgery with an individualized medical regimen and long-term surveillance.

Chronic rhinosinusitis (CRS) describes the family of disease processes that result in inflammation of the paranasal sinuses.[1] The causes of these processes vary, but they all share an identical common endpoint—inflammation.[2] CRS affects nearly 31 million Americans annually[3] and is responsible for approximately 20 million annual office visits[3] and 200,000 sinus surgeries a year.[4] Treatment for CRS is also responsible for approximately 6 billion dollars in annual direct and indirect health care costs.[3] The disease process has a significant functional and emotional impact on those who suffer from it.[3] Patients with CRS have demonstrated quality-of-life scores lower than patients with congestive heart failure, angina, chronic obstructive pulmonary disease, and low back pain.[5] CRS can be divided into 2 categories: chronic rhinosinusitis with nasal polyposis (CRSwNP) and chronic rhinosinusitis without nasal polyposis (CRSsNP). This article discusses various forms of CRSwNP that are refractory to medical and surgical therapy.

CHRONIC RHINOSINUSITIS WITH NASAL POLYPOSIS

CRSwNP represents a unique set of disease processes. It is less common than CRSsNP, as demonstrated by a prevalence ranging from 0.5% to 4.3% in national

Department of Otolaryngology-Head & Neck Surgery, Vanderbilt University, 1215 21st Ave S, 7209 MCE-S, Nashville, TN 37232-8605, USA
* Corresponding author.
E-mail address: Rakesh.chandra@vanderbilt.edu

Otolaryngol Clin N Am 50 (2017) 61–81
http://dx.doi.org/10.1016/j.otc.2016.08.006
0030-6665/17/© 2016 Elsevier Inc. All rights reserved.

Abbreviations	
ABPA	Allergic bronchopulmonary aspergillosis
AFS	Allergic fungal sinusitis
CF	Cystic fibrosis
CFTR	Conductance regulator protein
CRS	Chronic rhinosinusitis
CRSsNP	Chronic rhinosinusitis without nasal polyposis
CRSwNP	Chronic rhinosinusitis with nasal polyposis
CT	Computed tomography
CTIG	CT image guidance
IgE	Immunoglobulin E
IL-22RI	IL-22 receptor-1
IL-5	Interleukin-5
MRSA	Methicillin-resistant *Staphylococcus aureus*
NO	Nitric oxide
SEA	Staphylococcal enterotoxin-A
SEB	Staphylococcal enterotoxin-B
TLR	Toll-like receptor

population surveys.[6] However, it commonly results in the need for revision surgery, as demonstrated by the observation that 38% to 69% of cases requiring revision endoscopic sinus surgery are due to CRSwNP.[3,7–9] Patients with CRSwNP commonly describe olfactory impairment[10,11] and are also likely to endorse nasal obstruction.[12] CRSwNP appears to be a more refractory and aggressive form of CRS (**Fig. 1**). The presence of nasal polyposis is statistically associated with the presence of asthma, inhalant allergy, and aspirin sensitivity.[3] Patients with CRSwNP have been observed to have worse subjective symptoms (as evidenced by higher Sino-Nasal Outcome Test-20 scores), objective symptoms (demonstrated by Lund-McKay computed tomography [CT] scores), and more frequently require revision surgery than patients with CRSsNP.[3] Patients with CRSwNP have also been observed to have greater disease severity on preoperative nasal endoscopy[8,13,14] and to demonstrate more improvement after surgery than nonpolyp patients based on endoscopic scores. However, the final postoperative endoscopic scores were still higher for patients with CRSwNP.[3] These observations corroborate the observation that CRSwNP is associated with a greater burden of disease.[3,8]

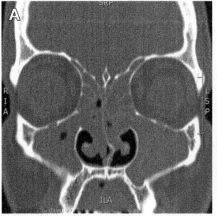 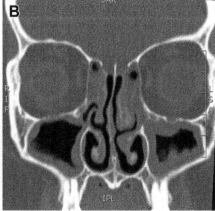

Fig. 1. (*A*) CRSwNP. (*B*) CRSsNP.

The development of CRSwNP is multifactorial. It is a complex disease with suspected contributions from multiple genetic and environmental factors.[15] A family history of nasal polyposis has been reported in 14% of patients with CRSwNP.[16] Certain forms of CRSwNP, like allergic fungal sinusitis (AFS), have been shown to be more common in specific parts of the United States,[17] although the intrinsic mechanism behind AFS remains to be clarified.

Nasal polyp tissue itself has been examined to elucidate histopathologic and immunohistochemical clues to the cause of CRS. Polyp tissue has demonstrated a significantly greater spontaneous release of inflammatory cytokines than control mucosa,[18] suggesting the polyps actively promote inflammation, rather than simply resulting from it. In Western countries, more than 70% of polyp tissue have shown tissue eosinophilia,[19] suggesting association with allergy and Th-2 processes. Neutrophilic inflammation has been more commonly observed in polyps from patients with cystic fibrosis (CF) and in patients in Asian countries.[1,11,20] Eosinophilic polyps demonstrate less glandularity, more edema, and minimal collagen deposition except at the basement membrane, as opposed to their noneosinophilic counterparts, which display glandular hypertrophy, more fibrosis, denser collagen deposition, and a mononuclear cellular infiltrate.[21] Grossly eosinophilic polyps are friable and readily disintegrate, whereas noneosinophilic polyps have been described as rubbery.[21] Noneosinophilic polyps have also been shown to have an increase in transcripts for vascular endothelial growth factor, suggesting that hypoxia due to obstruction of sinus ostia may be a driving force.[21] These histologic and immunohistochemical observations have augmented the understanding of the processes driving CRSwNP.

CRSwNP can be refractory to medical and surgical therapy for many different reasons. Recalcitrant forms have been associated with eosinophilia, asthma, and allergy and have also been associated with deficiencies in mucociliary dysfunction, as in CF.[3] Some have proposed that variations in innate immunity may predict and modify more aggressive disease.[3] Superantigens have also been implicated in recalcitrant CRSwNP.[3] This article discusses each of these in more detail. Aspirin-exacerbated respiratory disorder, a well-known aggressive form of CRSwNP, is discussed elsewhere.

ASTHMA, ALLERGY, AND EOSINOPHILIA

Asthma and allergy are 2 common conditions that are associated with CRSwNP. Both disease processes are directed by helper T cells[2] and are characterized by an abundance of eosinophils. Eosinophils are the primary effector cell in the pathophysiology of both upper airway sinusitis and allergy, and lower airway asthma.[22] Although asthma and allergy are associated with each other, for reasons not entirely clear, they do not always coexist. Higher levels of eosinophilia, immunoglobulin E (IgE), and interleukin-5 (IL-5; an eosinophil survival and differentiation factor[8]) have been observed in CRSwNP compared with CRSsNP,[23] and greater levels of eosinophilia have been observed in patients with more aggressive CRSwNP.[24,25] In fact, total IgE level is considered by some as a marker for upper and lower airway inflammatory disease and has been implicated in CRS.[26–28]

Eosinophilia has been observed peripherally and in tissue specimens from patients with CRSwNP. The amount of eosinophilia in nasal polyp tissue was found to relate to eosinophilia in peripheral blood, but not to elevated serum IgE.[29] Patients with elevated peripheral eosinophil counts have also been observed to be more likely to experience postoperative sinus infections, experience recurrence of polyps, and need revision sinus surgery.[30] In addition, increased peripheral eosinophilia has been shown to correlate with more severe radiographic sinus disease.[31] Tissue eosinophilia has also been associated with more advanced CRS by radiographic, endoscopic, and smell identification metrics.[7] Patients with elevated mucosal eosinophilia also demonstrated fewer improvements in quality of life after endoscopic sinus surgery than noneosinophilic patients.[32] Tissue eosinophilia also appears to correlate with histologic findings; basement membrane thickness was found to correlate with epithelial and subepithelial infiltration of eosinophils in nasal polyp tissue.[33] These findings all support the conclusion that eosinophilia is intimately involved in CRSwNP.

Allergy is an exaggerated immune-mediated response with objective and reproducible symptoms or signs initiated by exposure to a defined stimulus at a dose tolerated by normal subjects.[34] Allergy is common in CRS and is observed in 25% to 70% of cases.[35,36] One study found that 39% of patients who required revision sinus surgery demonstrated inhalant allergy.[3] Tan and colleagues[37] reported that although allergy was common to CRSwNP and CRWsNP, patients with polyps had more positive skin tests, and patients with medically refractory sinusitis were more likely to have multiple positive skin tests and asthma.[37] Although allergy has not been shown to predict polyposis,[3] it does worsen the impact of nasal polyposis on quality of life.[38] The identification and appropriate management of allergy are important to effective treatment of CRSwNP.

CRS is common in asthmatics, as evidenced by the observation that up to 80% of asthmatics have some form of radiologic evidence of sinusitis.[39] More severe asthma is often associated with more severe radiographic disease,[8] although radiologic severity is weakly associated with patient-reported symptom scores.[40] Staikuniene and colleagues[8] observed that 40% of patients with CRS had asthma, and Batra and colleagues[3] observed that 48% of patients who required revision sinus surgery had asthma. Asthma is also associated with CRSwNP[9,22]; it was observed in approximately 15% of CRS patients with polyps and only 3.5% of patients with CRSsNP.[3] The prevalence of asthma in patients with CRSwNP may in fact be somewhat higher; Klossek and colleagues[41] observed wheezing and respiratory discomfort in 31% and 42% of CRSwNP patients, respectively, but the formal diagnosis of asthma was reported in only 26% of those patients. Furthermore, Batra and colleagues[3] reported that asthma was the only comorbidity that predicted the presence of polyposis in CRS, reinforcing the strength of this association. This interrelationship is not surprising, because asthma and nasal polyps both manifest an inflammatory response with characteristic predominance of eosinophils, goblet cell hyperplasia, and Th-2 cell immune response.[42] Aggressive medical and surgical management of CRS has been shown to reduce the frequency of asthma attacks, usage of inhalers, and steroid requirement, thereby decreasing the severity of a patient's asthma.[43–46] Effective management of CRSwNP requires looking for the coexistence of asthma and treating it appropriately when present. A multimodality approach is often required.

ALLERGIC FUNGAL SINUSITIS

AFS is a distinct disease process with an aggressive form of CRSwNP. Its discovery began in 1976 when Safirstein[47] described a patient suffering from allergic bronchopulmonary aspergillosis (ABPA) with nasal obstruction, hard and blood-tinged nasal casts, nasal polyposis, and cultures positive for *Aspergillus fumigatus*.[47] In 1981, Millar and colleagues[48] recognized a histologic resemblance between specimens of patients with chronic fungal sinusitis and expectorated plugs from patients with ABPA. Katzenstein and colleagues[49,50] noted fungal hyphae in ABPA and this variant of CRS and coined the term allergic Aspergillus sinusitis. In 1994, Bent and Kuhn were credited with defining the disease with 5 criteria (**Box 1**).[51]

AFS has been reported to account for up to 8% of CRS requiring surgery,[51] although this is significantly affected by geography.[52] It is much more prevalent in the humid river basins and coastal regions of the southeastern United States.[17] The mean age at presentation ranges from 20 to 35 years old,[52] and men and women appear to be equally affected.[52] Most patients present with nasal obstruction (often unilateral), olfactory dysfunction, and expulsion of nasal casts, and some patients present with extrasinus complications.[51,52] Aspirin sensitivity is rarely observed in AFS,[51] and there are mixed reports suggesting a relationship with asthma.[2,51] The pathophysiology of the disease remains largely unknown.[51] It has been suggested that patients with ostiomeatal complex disease without the propensity to develop AFS in whom fungus becomes trapped develop a mycetoma, whereas those who are atopic are more likely to develop AFS.[51] Much remains to be discovered about the exact pathophysiologic mechanism driving AFS.

Patients with AFS demonstrate evidence of type 1 hypersensitivity.[51] Allergy to fungus is present, although it is not necessarily to the same species detected in the eosinophilic mucin.[52] Interestingly, a significant portion of CRS patients have fungal allergy but do not have the syndrome of AFS,[52] suggesting additional factors must be driving this process. Bent and Kuhn[51] observed that AFS patients have either a strong history of allergy (inhalant or fungal), increased total IgE, and positive skin-prick testing or radioallergosorbent testing,[51] and nonfungal allergy is common.[52] Peripheral eosinophilia has also been observed,[51] as has increased expression of fungal and nonfungal IgE in sinus tissues of patients with AFS.[17] Nasal polyposis is universal to AFS[51,52] and is characterized by tissue eosinophilia.[21] Furthermore, AFS tissue specimens show the presence of fungus without tissue invasion. Some reports suggest that Bipolaris is more common than other species,[53,54] although Aspergillus, Alternaria, Cladosporidium, Curvularia, Drechslera, and Helminthosporidium have also been identified.[52]

Imaging studies for AFS are characteristic, as are the eosinophilic mucin associated with them. CT scans demonstrate serpiginous areas of increased attenuation (**Fig. 2**), which is thought to be due to ferromagnetic elements produced by fungi and inspissated secretions.[51,55,56] Most CT scans demonstrate some degree of bone erosion, and extension of sinus disease into adjacent sites is also not uncommon.[51,52] One series reported that 98% of patients had expansion of sinuses, and 93% had erosion of a sinus wall.[56] Eosinophilic mucin of AFS is a thick, tenacious, highly viscous substance that has been described as the consistency of peanut butter or axle grease.[8] It contains Charcot-Leyden crystals, made up of the breakdown products of necrotic eosinophils.[51] Although eosinophilic mucin is not specific to AFS, it does represent a hallmark characteristic of the disease.

Box 1
Bent and Kuhn criteria
Type 1 hypersensitivity
Nasal polyposis
Characteristic CT findings
Eosinophilic mucin
Fungal stain

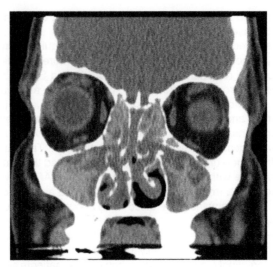

Fig. 2. AFS; notice the double densities.

The goal of treatment of AFS is to provide relief from the extensive polyposis of the disease and to prevent recurrences.[55] Surgical removal of all the disease is necessary, and special attention is required to remove all of the fungal mucin driving the local tissue response.[8] Large surgical outflow tracts should be created to improve drainage and ventilation of the sinuses and to facilitate improved delivery of topical therapies.[55] Cultures are routinely obtained as well as both tissue and mucin abnormality to definitively confirm the diagnosis. Oral and topical corticosteroids have proven effective at retarding recurrences,[55] although recurrence of polyps and eosinophilic mucin is high and patients should be counseled accordingly.[52] Oral corticosteroids should be administered in the immediate postoperative period, and the patient should be transitioned to topical corticosteroids to control the inflammation long term.[55] Immunotherapy has been shown to demonstrate variable efficacy,[57] although it is recommended when possible.[8,55] A recent review of topical and systemic antifungal therapies for AFS showed no benefit,[58] and side effects (particularly in systemic antifungals) can be significant.[55]

CYSTIC FIBROSIS

CF is the most common life-shortening autosomal-recessive disease process,[59–61] with a prevalence of 1:3500 live births and a carrier frequency of 1:25 people.[61,62] The pathogenesis of CF is due to the mutation of the gene on chromosome 7 that results in a defect in the CF transmembrane conductance regulator protein (CFTR) associated with this chloride-ion channel.[60,61,63–66] This defect results in viscous secretions with decreased water content,[65,66] and therefore, impairs the function of the mucociliary apparatus. A broad spectrum of phenotypes has been associated with different CFTR gene mutations.[67] In the United States, approximately half of CF is due to mutational homozygosity at codon 508, termed the ΔF508 mutation.[68,69] This mutation has been correlated with clinical disease severity and nasal polyposis on endoscopy.[70]

The diagnosis of CF relies on the sweat chloride test and genotyping.[71] Diagnosis requires clinical symptoms in at least one affected organ system as well as evidence of CFTR dysfunction (via sweat chloride or genotype analysis).[60] CRS, with or without nasal polyps, is universal to patients with CF by either clinical or radiographic evaluation.[59,61,65,72] Patients typically present with olfactory dysfunction.[66] Nasal obstruction is commonly described if polyps are present, and headaches are more common when mucoceles are present.[72] Often these symptoms arise in childhood.[72] Up to two-thirds of CF patients will develop nasal polyps,[65,73,74] many of which present in childhood. Polyps in CF tend to be more neutrophilic and less eosinophilic,[1,61] which reflects the excessive inspissated mucous and stasis of secretions produced in this disorder that drives the sinonasal inflammation.[63,65] This phenomenon results in colonization of the sinuses with noncommensal bacteria and biofilm formation.[61] For example, *Pseudomonas aeruginosa* is a commonly cultured bacterium from CF patients' sinuses.[75,76] Furthermore, the inflammatory sinonasal process associated with CF results in a cycle of infection, remodeling, glandular hyperplasia, and recurrent infection.[21] In addition, radiographic evaluation commonly demonstrates underdeveloped sinuses (**Fig. 3**).[2,77] Interestingly, Steinke and colleagues[61] described increased levels of extracellular DNA in CF tissue specimens. DNA has been shown to make secretions more viscous,[61] and CF patients who underwent revision sinus surgery demonstrated improved quality of life in association with the administration of dornase alpha, a synthetic protein that degrades DNA present in secretions.[78] Although strides have been made in treating CRS due to CF, it still often remains a challenge for both the physician and the patient.

Some evidence has been suggestive that the CF carrier state is related to the development of CRS in the general population.[79–81] In 2000, Wang and colleagues[79] discovered that adult CRS patients were more likely to harbor a mutation associated with CF than a control group. In 2002, Raman and colleagues[80] found the same to be true in children with CRS. In 2005, Wang and colleagues[81] demonstrated that known CF carriers had a higher prevalence of CRS than the general population. Although this does not explain all forms of CRS, it may explain some forms given the high prevalence of CF carrier status. Furthermore, the phenotypic variability of CF may correspond with a tendency for carriers of the same genes to develop CRS. Further investigation is warranted.

Although controversial, treatment of the sinuses in CF patients may benefit pulmonary function. In 1990, it was noticed that aggressive sinonasal management decreased the frequency of pulmonary exacerbations.[82] It has been suggested that

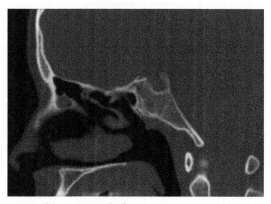

Fig. 3. CT scan of 14-year-old CF patient before surgery; notice the underdeveloped sinuses. (*Courtesy of* Frank Virgin, MD, Nashville, TN.)

the paranasal sinuses may act as a reservoir for pathogens that are responsible for acute exacerbations of sinusitis as well as seeding the lungs.[65] The findings of Holzmann and colleagues[76] demonstrated a significant correlation in lung transplant patients between the sinus aspirates and bronchoalveolar lavage specimens, lending support to this proposed mechanism. Furthermore, they found that successful management of the sinuses led to fewer pneumonias and episodes of tracheobronchitis.[76] Surgical treatment of the sinuses has also been shown to significantly improve nasal obstruction, rhinorrhea, olfactory dysfunction, cough, and congestion,[83,84] and to improve quality of life.[85] Virgin and colleagues[73] demonstrated that CF patients who underwent surgical therapy with modified endoscopic medial maxillectomies had improved symptoms scores, endoscopic scores, and fewer hospital admissions due to pulmonary exacerbations, although the forced expiratory volume in 1 second did not change. Although surgery does not offer a cure, it does facilitate better medical management of the sinuses. Still, many CF patients will require revision surgery with some estimates ranging from 37% to 58%.[74,86] Medical management for CF includes frequent sinonasal irrigations to help facilitate the mucociliary apparatus.[87] Topical steroids have been shown to improve endoscopic findings, but have not altered symptoms.[65] However, they are still often recommended. Topical dornase alfa has been shown to improve symptoms and endoscopic findings.[65] One of the largest breakthroughs in CF treatment is the use of ivacaftor and lumacaftor, a potentiator and corrector of the CFTR channels, respectively.[88] They are only approved for 10 mutations carried by approximately 7% of the CF population, but preliminary results are promising. To date, no large studies exist focusing specifically on their effect on CRS associated with CF.

A more in-depth discussion of CF can be found elsewhere in this issue.

INNATE IMMUNITY AND CYTOKINES

The innate immune system is evolutionarily old.[89] In the sinonasal cavity, it is made up of epithelial cells, pattern recognition receptors, and other cytokines that work in concert as a nonspecific defense mechanism. It does not function independently of the adaptive immune system, but the innate immune system serves as the body's initial defense. Lane and colleagues[90] suggested that "the ultimate common pathway of immune activation that characterizes CRS is an abnormal response to a trigger at the mucosal surface." Impairment of the innate immune system renders the mucosal surface vulnerable to insult, that stimulates the adaptive changes observed in CRS.[90,91] Sinonasal epithelial cells serve several functions in host defense. They form a mechanical barrier and facilitate mucociliary clearance,[90] which has been suggested to be the primary mechanism of sinonasal innate immunity.[91] Epithelial cells also express pattern recognition receptors to allow for identification of pathogens in the form of toll-like receptors (TLR),[92] transmembrane receptors that interact with pathogen ligands and are involved in signal transduction.[93] Recent studies investigating the relationship of certain TLRs to CRSwNP provided evidence linking innate immunity with CRS. Patients with surgically recalcitrant CRSwNP have been shown to have lower levels of TLR-9 activity, contributing to the hypothesis that the underactivity of the innate immune system in sinonasal mucosa may play a role in the perpetuation of Th2 inflammation and failure to restore the Th1-Th2 balance in CRSwNP.[89] It has also been shown that patients with CRSwNP who develop early recurrence of polyps after surgery had a lower level of TLR-2 (recognizes peptidoglycan) and TLR-9 (recognizes bacterial/viral DNA) than surgically responsive counterparts.[90] Furthermore, Ramanathan and colleagues[94] demonstrated that exposure of sinonasal epithelial cells from non-CRS patients to IL-4 or IL-13, 2 cytokines associated with Th2-inflammatory disease, resulted in decreased expression of TLR-9 genes, suggesting a link between Th2-inflammation and genes associated with innate immunity. It has been suggested that the downregulation of TLR-9 in recalcitrant CRSwNP may contribute to colonization of the sinuses with noncommensal organisms,[89] because there is evidence to suggest increased colonization with bacteria and fungi.[95] TLRs appear to be an important link between innate immunity and CRSwNP and represent an exciting newer area of research.

In addition to TLRs, cytokines and cell signaling molecules play a large role in mediating innate and adaptive immunity. Interleukins have been shown to mediate CRS—specifically, IL-3, IL-5, IL-6, IL-8, and IL-13 are involved in the activation of eosinophils in nasal polyps.[96–98] Staikuniene and colleagues[8] suggested that eotaxin-3, a known indicator of eosinophil chemotaxis and activation, may be a driver of CRSwNP via recruitment of eosinophils,[99] IL-25 and IL-33 have also been identified in CRSwNP.[99] IL-33 is a cytokine that is normally retained in the nucleus of basal epithelial cells.[100] When tissue damage occurs, various intracellular molecules are released that broadly elicit an innate immune response.[100] Tissue damage has been shown to be a nonspecific trigger of epithelial IL-33 in recalcitrant nasal polyps.[100,101] IL-16 is a cytokine that functions as a potent chemoattractant for eosinophils.[102] Elevated serum and tissue levels of IL-16 have been found to be associated with CRSwNP.[102] IL-22 is a T-helper cell-derived cytokine that has been speculated to play a role in innate immunity.[103] Polarization of T cells toward a Th2 phenotype has been shown to lower IL-22 production.[104] Stimulation of IL-22 receptor-1 (IL-22R1) has been shown to nonspecifically increase the innate immune response in skin and bowel inflammatory diseases,[104] and CRSwNP tissue demonstrated decreased expression of the IL-22R1 compared with CRSsNP.[104] Interestingly, in the same study, IL-22 levels of recalcitrant CRSwNP were elevated compared with those of controls and medically responsive CRSwNP, although without statistical significance.[104] This observation suggests another link between innate immunity and the Th2 phenotype commonly observed in CRSwNP. Further discussion of various cytokines can be found in this issue.

Nitric oxide (NO) is another chemical that aids in innate immunity. The paranasal sinuses have been shown to be a reservoir of NO.[105] Levels of exhaled NO are decreased in patients with CF, CRS (with and without polyposis), and acute rhinosinusitis, and levels have been shown to increase after successful treatment of CRS with surgery.[106] NO functions as a vasodilator, smooth muscle relaxer, and regulator of inflammation and innate immunity.[105] It has been shown to be involved in ciliary motion in that low NO is associated with ciliary dyskinesia.[105,107,108] NO has also been shown to be involved in antibacterial defense; it can diffuse inside of cells and change bacterial DNA, enzymes, and lipids on membranes.[107] In vitro studies have also shown that NO is bactericidal against *P aeruginosa*.[109] NO remains a potential site of intervention to improve sinonasal health in patients with CRS.

STAPHYLOCOCCAL SUPERANTIGENS

The development of CRSwNP has long been suggested to be due to allergy and infection. Some have suggested that there may be a link between the 2,[110] and that the microbes themselves may be amplifying the immune response in unique ways,[111] lending support to the concept of superantigen participation in CRSwNP. Superantigens are molecules that trigger an inordinately large T-cell response and have been implicated in CRSwNP. They have been suggested to participate in the pathophysiology of other chronic disease processes that are characterized by inflammation[112]:

rheumatoid arthritis, diabetes mellitus, rheumatic fever, Kawasaki disease, and toxic shock syndrome.[113,114] They are 10,000 times more potent than conventional antigens.[111] Superantigens do not require processing by antigen-presenting cells, instead binding directly to the MHC complex.[112–114] Simultaneously,[111,112] they bind to the T-cell receptor outside the typical antigen-binding site to form a "clamp" between the T cell and the antigen-presenting cell.[112,114] This action results in a massive release of Th-1 and Th-2 cytokines.[110] Activation of up to 30% of all host T cells can occur in response to superantigens[113,115] because many superantigens are capable of binding to several T-cell receptor variable beta gene motifs.[111]

S aureus is a ubiquitous bacterium. Reports have suggested that approximately 29% of the population in the United States is colonized with S aureus, and 1.5% is colonized with methicillin-resistant Staphylococcus aureus (MRSA), although they are asymptomatic.[116,117] Approximately 25% of people have been found to be nasal carriers of S aureus,[19] and up to 60% of patients with CRSwNP have been found to be colonized with S aureus.[118] MRSA has been reported in 2% to 21% of sinonasal culture isolates.[119] It is one of the most common bacteria to colonize the paranasal sinuses in both asymptomatic postoperative and operative patients with CRS.[120,121] The process of autogenous infection is supported by the observation of 80% concordance between S aureus isolated from the infection site and the anterior nasal cavity.[122–126] Some have suggested that carriers are genetically asymptomatic, whereas those who develop signs and symptoms of sinusitis are genetically susceptible.[119]

S aureus superantigens have been implicated in the development of asthma and allergy[127] and have been suggested to participate in the development of CRSwNP.[128] S aureus is known to have 6 groups of enterotoxins (SAEs): Staphylococcal enterotoxin-A (SEA), Staphylococcal enterotoxin-B (SEB), Staphylococcal enterotoxin-C, Staphylococcal enterotoxin-D, Staphylococcal enterotoxin-E, and Toxic Shock Syndrome Toxin-1.[129,130] SEB has been shown to polarize mucosal inflammation to a Th-2 pattern.[18,131] This observation has led to the concept that in a genetically susceptible host, superantigen production may drive inflammatory patterns implicated in CRSwNP.[111] Several studies lend support to this possibility. High levels of SEA and SEB have been observed in the nasal secretions of patients with CRS and asthma.[132] Corriveau and colleagues[133] reported a higher rate of intramucosal colonization of S aureus in patients with CRSwNP compared with controls and patients with CRSsNP.[131] A meta-analysis with 340 cases demonstrated a higher culture-positive rate in patients with CRSwNP compared with controls.[129] Immunologic mediators have been used to demonstrate the presence of superantigens in CRSwNP. Staphylococcal IgE antibodies have been detected in 78% of cases of CRSwNP,[110] and Bachert and colleagues[134] found that 50% of sinonasal tissue from patients with CRSwNP demonstrated IgE antibodies directed at SEA and SEB. A meta-analysis in 2014 showed that S aureus superantigens and their specific IgE were detected in higher concentrations in patients with CRSwNP.[129] Some research has focused on specifics in immunology. For example, in vitro studies in mice have shown that S aureus superantigens have been shown to augment isotype switching and synthesis.[1,52,135] The immunoglobulin variable beta chain region appears to be involved in enterotoxin stimulation of the immunoglobulin response. Bernstein and colleagues[115] showed that the clonal expansion of the variable beta chain correlated with the observed enterotoxin. Another study demonstrated that T-cell receptor variable beta chain expansion was noted in 58% of patients with CRSwNP.[136] Both findings suggest that T-cell receptors with specific variable beta chains are expanded and activated, whereas those without the T-cell receptor variable beta chain are excluded.[112]

Superantigens have also been observed to directly affect sinonasal mucosa. Min and colleagues[137] demonstrated that in rabbit sinonasal mucosa SEA induces subepithelial edema and inflammatory cell infiltrate and decreases ciliary beat frequency. Another study showed that polyp tissue from patients exhibiting an immune response to SAEs had higher levels of cysteinyl leukotrienes, lipoxin A-4, and leukotriene B-4 compared with enterotoxin IgE-negative nasal polyps.[138] Stimulation of human nasal epithelial cells with SEB has been associated with an increased presence of proinflammatory mediators and prolonged eosinophil survival.[139] The effect of SAEs on sinonasal mucosa in CRS (and nasal polyps) establishes a link between the immune response observed in CRS and the microbiology observed in CRS.

Although most studies investigating S aureus superantigens appear to corroborate their contribution to the development of CRSwNP, some studies do not. Damm and colleagues[140] showed that the nasal Staphylococcal culture rate in patients with CRSwNP were no higher than the control group, and the carrier condition was not a risk factor of disease extent and severity. Furthermore, a relationship between S aureus superantigen genes and the severity of nasal polyposis was not identified.[141,142]

Most of the evidence suggests that superantigens are involved in CRSwNP, but much still needs to be learned about their treatment. It is crucial for the clinician to obtain a culture and sensitivity because there are differences in community-acquired bacteria compared with hospital-acquired counterparts.[119] Many different regimens have been proposed for the treatment of S aureus (including MRSA). McCoul and colleagues[119] comparatively reviewed systemic antibiotics, topical mupirocin, nebulized solutions, and chlorhexidine baths. No regimen was found to be statistically superior. Steroids have long been a mainstay of management of CRSwNP. Some have suggested that superantigens may participate in steroid insensitivity.[19] Wang and colleagues[143] further expounded on this concept. Tissue samples obtained from patients with CRSwNP and CRSsNP were exposed to Staphylococcus exotoxins and tested for a glucocorticoid receptor. Among polyp patients, 72% of recurrent polyp patients and 55% of primary polyp patients tested positive for the receptor, whereas only 6% of patients with CRSsNP tested positive, and no controls tested positive. These results suggest that more refractory CRSwNP may be related to the presence of a glucocorticoid receptor that is induced by Staphylococcal exotoxins, resulting in steroid insensitivity.

Much still remains to be learned about S aureus superantigen. Although its presence has certainly been associated with CRSwNP, the appropriate management regimens remain to be elucidated.

TREATMENT

It is imperative that the treating otolaryngologist attempts to elucidate the pathophysiology that is driving this process and tailor the treatment accordingly. In many cases, patients will require a multidisciplinary approach with other clinicians (eg, allergists/immunologists and pulmonologists). The most effective treatment for the difficult CRSwNP patient is most often endoscopic sinus surgery followed by individualized long-term medical management that should be dictated by the patient's disease process.[3]

The overall goal of endoscopic sinus surgery is to remove polyp tissue with care to avoid generating scar tissue along the uninvolved mucosa while creating widely patent outflow tracts that facilitate the delivery of topical therapy. To this end, the surgeon must familiarize himself or herself with the patient's CT scan and anatomy because CRSwNP can distort sinonasal anatomy, elevating the risk of surgery.[144,145] Polyp removal is often associated with higher blood loss than nonpolyp sinus surgery. Hemostasis facilitates improved visualization and aids in safer dissection. Many techniques are used to improve hemostasis. Hathorn and colleagues[146] demonstrated that placing the patient in reverse Trendelenburg can decrease operative blood loss by several hundred milliliters and improves visualization. Although preoperative systemic steroids have been shown to decrease intraoperative blood loss, as shown by Wright and Agrawal,[147] the amount is clinically insignificant. The use of preoperative steroid use should be left to the discretion of the treating otolaryngologist, as anecdotal reports suggest they aid in facilitating an easier dissection. Higgins and colleagues[148] showed that topical vasoconstriction with oxymetazoline or epinephrine does decrease blood loss and can improve visualization during sinus surgery. The injection of local anesthesia mixed with epinephrine may do the same, with some studies showing no benefit.[149,150] Careful consideration to both practices should be given.

Revision sinus surgery is common in CRSwNP and differs from primary sinus surgery. Surgical landmarks are often absent or distorted. Accurate identification of landmarks allows the surgeon to systematically perform safe endoscopic sinus surgery, and the lack of clearly recognizable landmarks can make surgery more challenging and increase risk to the patient. A preoperative CT scan can assist the surgeon in developing a roadmap for the case. The surgeon may also intermittently refer to the scan intraoperatively. CT image guidance (CTIG) technology can facilitate intraoperative review of images and can correlate endoscopic findings with radiographic structures, although the surgeon should rely on knowledge of anatomy when there is discordance among the 2. One of the indications for CTIG is revision sinus surgery.[151] Revision surgery also warrants consideration of variations in surgical technique. For example, often the middle turbinate is resected due to extensive polyposis. Soler and colleagues[152] demonstrated that resection of bilateral middle turbinates is associated with slight improvement in endoscopy scores and olfaction, but the decision to resect the middle turbinate should be left to the discretion of the operating surgeon. Finally, revision surgery can be challenging and should be performed only by experienced high-volume sinus surgeons.

The mainstay of medical management of CRSwNP is treatment with steroids. Patients with a suspected eosinophilic process should be treated with oral steroids when possible, because oral steroids have been shown to reduce polyp size in the short term and provide symptomatic relief.[153] Oral steroids have also been shown to decrease the expression of inflammatory cytokines and increase the expression of some innate immune genes.[154] Furthermore, oral steroids have been shown to induce apoptosis of eosinophils.[155,156] Topical nasal steroids are also imperative for long-term management. A *Cochrane Review* has shown that topical steroids improve symptoms, decrease polyp size, prevent recurrences after surgery, and are associated with only minor adverse events.[157] A common off-label nasal steroid that is often used for polypoid cases is topical budesonide, which can be added to a sinonasal rinse, nebulized, or applied in the Mygind's position. Although this is not a US Food and Drug Administration–approved application of the medication, topical budesonide has been shown to improve patient sinus scores and reduce hyposmia in chronic eosinophilic sinusitis.[158] Steroids have also been shown to increase the levels of proteins involved in innate immunity. For example, Salman and colleagues[159] demonstrated that oral steroid use was associated with upregulation of various surfactant proteins; surfactant proteins modulate T-cell responses to inhaled allergens and pathogens and promote bacterial clearance. Given the diffuse prevalence of inflammation in patients with CRSwNP, the use of steroids is imperative to prevent recurrence of disease.

Other medical therapies are available. Culture-directed antibiotic therapy has been advocated for years, and in some cases, intravenous medications may be required. Tabaee and colleagues[116] described how some refractory strains of MRSA required intravenous antibiotic therapy to eradicate. Doxycycline has been shown to significantly reduce levels of myeloperoxidase, eosinophilic cationic protein, and matrix metalloproteinase-9 in nasal secretions, all of which are associated with Th-2 inflammation.[160,161] Macrolides have been shown to be anti-inflammatory and more beneficial in patients with low IgE more than those with high IgE.[2] These patients are typically those with CRSsNP,[162] so their use should not be first line for CRSwNP. However, not all nasal polyps are associated with elevated IgE and their use should be considered in those cases. Patients with allergic sinonasal disease with nasal polyposis should undergo allergy testing and be considered for immunotherapy. Immunotherapy has been shown to suppress the Th-2-mediated responses[163] and can be a powerful adjunct to the management of refractory CRSwNP. Of course, saline irrigations should be used in the immediate postoperative period to facilitate removal of debris, blood, and crusts, although its use was not associated with a distinct alteration in the proportional abundance of commensal bacteria in CRSwNP.[164]

SUMMARY

CRSwNP remains a diverse family of diseases. The current understanding clearly demonstrates that there is variability in the pathophysiology, and an understanding of the different types of disease processes is important in creating an individualized treatment regimen. Effective treatment involves careful surgical eradication of disease and appropriate postoperative medical management, which almost always includes oral and topical steroids. Recidivism is not uncommon, and patients with CRSwNP need long-term follow-up to treat recurrences in the early stages. Patients should be counseled accordingly.

REFERENCES

1. van Drunen CM, Reinartz S, Wigman J, et al. Inflammation in chronic rhinosinusitis and nasal polyposis. Immunol Allergy Clin North Am 2009;29:621–9.

2. Han JK. Subclassification of chronic rhinosinusitis. Laryngoscope 2013; 123(Suppl 2):S15–27.

3. Batra PS, Tong L, Citardi MJ. Analysis of comorbidities and objective parameters in refractory chronic rhinosinusitis. Laryngoscope 2013;123(Suppl 7): S1–11.

4. Hemmerdinger SA, Jacobs JB, Lebowitz RA. Accuracy and cost analysis of image-guided sinus surgery. Otolaryngol Clin North Am 2005;38:453–60.

5. Senior BA, Glaze C, Benninger MS. Use of the Rhinosinusitis Disability Index (RSDI) in rhinologic disease. Am J Rhinol 2001;15:15–20.

6. Fokkens W, Lund V, Mullol J, et al. European position paper on rhinosinusitis and nasal polyps 2007. Rhinol Suppl 2007;(20):1–136.

7. Soler ZM, Sauer DA, Mace J, et al. Relationship between clinical measures and histopathologic findings in chronic rhinosinusitis. Otolaryngol Head Neck Surg 2009;141:454–61.

8. Staikūniene J, Vaitkus S, Japertiene LM, et al. Association of chronic rhinosinusitis with nasal polyps and asthma: clinical and radiological features, allergy and inflammation markers. Medicina (Kaunas) 2008;44:257–65.

9. Pearlman AN, Chandra RK, Chang D, et al. Relationships between severity of chronic rhinosinusitis and nasal polyposis, asthma, and atopy. Am J Rhinol Allergy 2009;23:145–8.

10. Raherison C, Montaudon M, Stoll D, et al. How should nasal symptoms be investigated in asthma? A comparison of radiologic and endoscopic findings. Allergy 2004;59:821–6.

11. Van Zele T, Claeys S, Gevaert P, et al. Differentiation of chronic sinus diseases by measurement of inflammatory mediators. Allergy 2006;61:1280–9.

12. Agius AM. Long-term follow-up of patients with facial pain in chronic rhinosinusitis–correlation with nasal endoscopy and CT. Rhinology 2010;48:65–70.

13. Smith TL, Mendolia-Loffredo S, Loehrl TA, et al. Predictive factors and outcomes in endoscopic sinus surgery for chronic rhinosinusitis. Laryngoscope 2005;115:2199–205.

14. Kountakis SE, Arango P, Bradley D, et al. Molecular and cellular staging for the severity of chronic rhinosinusitis. Laryngoscope 2004;114:1895–905.

15. Platt MP, Soler Z, Metson R, et al. Pathways analysis of molecular markers in chronic sinusitis with polyps. Otolaryngol Head Neck Surg 2011;144:802–8.

16. Greisner WA, Settipane GA. Hereditary factor for nasal polyps. Allergy Asthma Proc 1996;17:283–6.

17. Ahn CN, Wise SK, Lathers DM, et al. Local production of antigen-specific IgE in different anatomic subsites of allergic fungal rhinosinusitis patients. Otolaryngol Head Neck Surg 2009;141:97–103.

18. Patou J, Gevaert P, Van Zele T, et al. Staphylococcus aureus enterotoxin B, protein A, and lipoteichoic acid stimulations in nasal polyps. J Allergy Clin Immunol 2008;121:110–5.

19. Zhang N, Gevaert P, van Zele T, et al. An update on the impact of Staphylococcus aureus enterotoxins in chronic sinusitis with nasal polyposis. Rhinology 2005;43:162–8.

20. Zhang N, Van Zele T, Perez-Novo C, et al. Different types of T-effector cells orchestrate mucosal inflammation in chronic sinus disease. J Allergy Clin Immunol 2008;122:961–8.

21. Payne SC, Early SB, Huyett P, et al. Evidence for distinct histologic profile of nasal polyps with and without eosinophilia. Laryngoscope 2011;121:2262–7.

22. Lin DC, Chandra RK, Tan BK, et al. Association between severity of asthma and degree of chronic rhinosinusitis. Am J Rhinol Allergy 2011;25:205–8.

23. Dietz de Loos DA, Hopkins C, Fokkens WJ. Symptoms in chronic rhinosinusitis with and without nasal polyps. Laryngoscope 2013;123:57–63.

24. Braunstahl GJ, Fokkens W. Nasal involvement in allergic asthma. Allergy 2003;58:1235–43.

25. Bousquet J, Chanez P, Lacoste JY, et al. Eosinophilic inflammation in asthma. N Engl J Med 1990;323:1033–9.

26. Newman LJ, Platts-Mills TA, Phillips CD, et al. Chronic sinusitis. Relationship of computed tomographic findings to allergy, asthma, and eosinophilia. JAMA 1994;271:363–7.

27. Baroody FM, Suh SH, Naclerio RM. Total IgE serum levels correlate with sinus mucosal thickness on computerized tomography scans. J Allergy Clin Immunol 1997;100:563–8.

28. Lal D, Baroody FM, Weitzel EK, et al. Total IgE levels do not change 1 year after endoscopic sinus surgery in patients with chronic rhinosinusitis. Int Arch Allergy Immunol 2006;139:146–8.
29. Kim JW, Hong SL, Kim YK, et al. Histological and immunological features of non-eosinophilic nasal polyps. Otolaryngol Head Neck Surg 2007;137:925–30.
30. Zadeh MH, Banthia V, Anand VK, et al. Significance of eosinophilia in chronic rhinosinusitis. Am J Rhinol 2002;16:313–7.
31. Poznanovic SA, Kingdom TT. Total IgE levels and peripheral eosinophilia: correlation with mucosal disease based on computed tomographic imaging of the paranasal sinus. Arch Otolaryngol Head Neck Surg 2007;133:701–4.
32. Soler ZM, Sauer D, Mace J, et al. Impact of mucosal eosinophilia and nasal polyposis on quality-of-life outcomes after sinus surgery. Otolaryngol Head Neck Surg 2010;142:64–71.
33. Saitoh T, Kusunoki T, Yao T, et al. Relationship between epithelial damage or basement membrane thickness and eosinophilic infiltration in nasal polyps with chronic rhinosinusitis. Rhinology 2009;47:275–9.
34. Johansson SG, Hourihane JO, Bousquet J, et al. A revised nomenclature for allergy. An EAACI position statement from the EAACI nomenclature task force. Allergy 2001;56:813–24.
35. Settipane GA. Nasal polyps: epidemiology, pathology, immunology, and treatment. Am J Rhinol 1987;1:119–26.
36. Mygind N, Dahl R, Bachert C. Nasal polyposis, eosinophil dominated inflammation, and allergy. Thorax 2000;55(Suppl 2):S79–83.
37. Tan BK, Zirkle W, Chandra RK, et al. Atopic profile of patients failing medical therapy for chronic rhinosinusitis. Int Forum Allergy Rhinol 2011;1:88–94.
38. Alobid I, Benítez P, Valero A, et al. The impact of atopy, sinus opacification, and nasal patency on quality of life in patients with severe nasal polyposis. Otolaryngol Head Neck Surg 2006;134:609–12.
39. Slavin RG. Asthma and sinusitis. J Allergy Clin Immunol 1992;90:534–7.
40. Zheng Y, Zhao Y, Lv D, et al. Correlation between computed tomography staging and quality of life instruments in patients with chronic rhinosinusitis. Am J Rhinol Allergy 2010;24:e41–5.
41. Klossek JM, Neukirch F, Pribil C, et al. Prevalence of nasal polyposis in France: a cross-sectional, case-control study. Allergy 2005;60:233–7.
42. Pezato R, Balsalobre L, Lima M, et al. Convergence of two major pathophysiologic mechanisms in nasal polyposis: immune response to Staphylococcus aureus and airway remodeling. J Otolaryngol Head Neck Surg 2013;42:27.
43. Okano M, Fujiwara T, Kariya S, et al. Cellular responses to Staphylococcus aureus alpha-toxin in chronic rhinosinusitis with nasal polyps. Allergol Int 2014;63:563–73.
44. Dhong HJ, Jung YS, Chung SK, et al. Effect of endoscopic sinus surgery on asthmatic patients with chronic rhinosinusitis. Otolaryngol Head Neck Surg 2001;124:99–104.
45. Dunlop G, Scadding GK, Lund VJ. The effect of endoscopic sinus surgery on asthma: management of patients with chronic rhinosinusitis, nasal polyposis, and asthma. Am J Rhinol 1999;13:261–5.
46. Awad OG, Fasano MB, Lee JH, et al. Asthma outcomes after endoscopic sinus surgery in aspirin-tolerant versus aspirin-induced asthmatic patients. Am J Rhinol 2008;22:197–203.
47. Safirstein BH. Allergic bronchopulmonary aspergillosis with obstruction of the upper respiratory tract. Chest 1976;70:788–90.

48. Millar J, Johnston A, Lamb D. Allergic aspergillosis of the maxillary sinuses. Thorax 1981;36:710.
49. Katzenstein AL, Sale SR, Greenberger PA. Allergic Aspergillus sinusitis: a newly recognized form of sinusitis. J Allergy Clin Immunol 1983;72:89–93.
50. Katzenstein AL, Sale SR, Greenberger PA. Pathologic findings in allergic aspergillus sinusitis. A newly recognized form of sinusitis. Am J Surg Pathol 1983;7: 439–43.
51. Bent JP, Kuhn FA. Diagnosis of allergic fungal sinusitis. Otolaryngol Head Neck Surg 1994;111:580–8.
52. Pant H, Schembri MA, Wormald PJ, et al. IgE-mediated fungal allergy in allergic fungal sinusitis. Laryngoscope 2009;119:1046–52.
53. Allphin AL, Strauss M, Abdul-Karim FW. Allergic fungal sinusitis: problems in diagnosis and treatment. Laryngoscope 1991;101:815–20.
54. Manning SC, Schaefer SD, Close LG, et al. Culture-positive allergic fungal sinusitis. Arch Otolaryngol Head Neck Surg 1991;117:174–8.
55. Marple BF. Allergic fungal rhinosinusitis: current theories and management strategies. Laryngoscope 2001;111:1006–19.
56. Mukherji SK, Figueroa RE, Ginsberg LE, et al. Allergic fungal sinusitis: CT findings. Radiology 1998;207:417–22.
57. Mabry RL, Manning SC, Mabry CS. Immunotherapy in the treatment of allergic fungal sinusitis. Otolaryngol Head Neck Surg 1997;116:31–5.
58. Ryan MW, Clark CM. Allergic fungal rhinosinusitis and the unified airway: the role of antifungal therapy in AFRS. Curr Allergy Asthma Rep 2015;15:75.
59. Gysin C, Alothman GA, Papsin BC. Sinonasal disease in cystic fibrosis: clinical characteristics, diagnosis, and management. Pediatr Pulmonol 2000;30:481–9.
60. Boyle MP. Nonclassic cystic fibrosis and CFTR-related diseases. Curr Opin Pulm Med 2003;9:498–503.
61. Steinke JW, Payne SC, Chen PG, et al. Etiology of nasal polyps in cystic fibrosis: not a unimodal disease. Ann Otol Rhinol Laryngol 2012;121:579–86.
62. Davis PB, Drumm M, Konstan MW. Cystic fibrosis. Am J Respir Crit Care Med 1996;154:1229–56.
63. Voter KZ, Ren CL. Diagnosis of cystic fibrosis. Clin Rev Allergy Immunol 2008; 35:100–6.
64. Davis PB. Cystic fibrosis since 1938. Am J Respir Crit Care Med 2006;173: 475–82.
65. Liang J, Higgins TS, Ishman SL, et al. Surgical management of chronic rhinosinusitis in cystic fibrosis: a systematic review. Int Forum Allergy Rhinol 2013;3: 814–22.
66. Ramsey B, Richardson MA. Impact of sinusitis in cystic fibrosis. J Allergy Clin Immunol 1992;90:547–52.
67. Rowntree RK, Harris A. The phenotypic consequences of CFTR mutations. Ann Hum Genet 2003;67:471–85.
68. Noone PG, Knowles MR. 'CFTR-opathies': disease phenotypes associated with cystic fibrosis transmembrane regulator gene mutations. Respir Res 2001;2: 328–32.
69. Farrell PM, Rosenstein BJ, White TB, et al. Guidelines for diagnosis of cystic fibrosis in newborns through older adults: Cystic Fibrosis Foundation consensus report. J Pediatr 2008;153:S4–14.
70. Jorissen MB, De Boeck K, Cuppens H. Genotype-phenotype correlations for the paranasal sinuses in cystic fibrosis. Am J Respir Crit Care Med 1999;159: 1412–6.

71. Stewart B, Zabner J, Shuber AP, et al. Normal sweat chloride values do not exclude the diagnosis of cystic fibrosis. Am J Respir Crit Care Med 1995;151: 899–903.
72. Gentile VG, Isaacson G. Patterns of sinusitis in cystic fibrosis. Laryngoscope 1996;106:1005–9.
73. Virgin FW, Rowe SM, Wade MB, et al. Extensive surgical and comprehensive postoperative medical management for cystic fibrosis chronic rhinosinusitis. Am J Rhinol Allergy 2012;26:70–5.
74. Yung MW, Gould J, Upton GJ. Nasal polyposis in children with cystic fibrosis: a long-term follow-up study. Ann Otol Rhinol Laryngol 2002;111:1081–6.
75. Murray TS, Egan M, Kazmierczak BI. Pseudomonas aeruginosa chronic colonization in cystic fibrosis patients. Curr Opin Pediatr 2007;19:83–8.
76. Holzmann D, Speich R, Kaufmann T, et al. Effects of sinus surgery in patients with cystic fibrosis after lung transplantation: a 10-year experience. Transplantation 2004;77:134–6.
77. Rutland J, Cole PJ. Nasal mucociliary clearance and ciliary beat frequency in cystic fibrosis compared with sinusitis and bronchiectasis. Thorax 1981;36: 654–8.
78. Mainz JG, Schiller I, Ritschel C, et al. Sinonasal inhalation of dornase alfa in CF: a double-blind placebo-controlled cross-over pilot trial. Auris Nasus Larynx 2011;38:220–7.
79. Wang X, Moylan B, Leopold DA, et al. Mutation in the gene responsible for cystic fibrosis and predisposition to chronic rhinosinusitis in the general population. JAMA 2000;284:1814–9.
80. Raman V, Clary R, Siegrist KL, et al. Increased prevalence of mutations in the cystic fibrosis transmembrane conductance regulator in children with chronic rhinosinusitis. Pediatrics 2002;109:E13.
81. Wang X, Kim J, McWilliams R, et al. Increased prevalence of chronic rhinosinusitis in carriers of a cystic fibrosis mutation. Arch Otolaryngol Head Neck Surg 2005;131:237–40.
82. Umetsu DT, Moss RB, King VV, et al. Sinus disease in patients with severe cystic fibrosis: relation to pulmonary exacerbation. Lancet 1990;335:1077–8.
83. Mainz JG, Koitschev A. Management of chronic rhinosinusitis in CF. J Cyst Fibros 2009;8(Suppl 1):S10–4.
84. Halvorson DJ, Dupree JR, Porubsky ES. Management of chronic sinusitis in the adult cystic fibrosis patient. Ann Otol Rhinol Laryngol 1998;107:946–52.
85. Jones JW, Parsons DS, Cuyler JP. The results of functional endoscopic sinus (FES) surgery on the symptoms of patients with cystic fibrosis. Int J Pediatr Otorhinolaryngol 1993;28:25–32.
86. Rowe-Jones JM, Mackay IS. Endoscopic sinus surgery in the treatment of cystic fibrosis with nasal polyposis. Laryngoscope 1996;106:1540–4.
87. Davidson TM, Murphy C, Mitchell M, et al. Management of chronic sinusitis in cystic fibrosis. Laryngoscope 1995;105:354–8.
88. Kuk K, Taylor-Cousar JL. Lumacaftor and ivacaftor in the management of patients with cystic fibrosis: current evidence and future prospects. Ther Adv Respir Dis 2015;9:313–26.
89. Ramanathan M, Lee WK, Dubin MG, et al. Sinonasal epithelial cell expression of toll-like receptor 9 is decreased in chronic rhinosinusitis with polyps. Am J Rhinol 2007;21:110–6.

90. Lane AP, Truong-Tran QA, Schleimer RP. Altered expression of genes associated with innate immunity and inflammation in recalcitrant rhinosinusitis with polyps. Am J Rhinol 2006;20:138–44.

91. Lane AP. The role of innate immunity in the pathogenesis of chronic rhinosinusitis. Curr Allergy Asthma Rep 2009;9:205–12.

92. Vandermeer J, Sha Q, Lane AP, et al. Innate immunity of the sinonasal cavity: expression of messenger RNA for complement cascade components and toll-like receptors. Arch Otolaryngol Head Neck Surg 2004;130:1374–80.

93. Takeda K, Kaisho T, Akira S. Toll-like receptors. Annu Rev Immunol 2003;21: 335–76.

94. Ramanathan M, Lee WK, Spannhake EW, et al. Th2 cytokines associated with chronic rhinosinusitis with polyps down-regulate the antimicrobial immune function of human sinonasal epithelial cells. Am J Rhinol 2008;22:115–21.

95. Ferguson BJ, Seethala R, Wood WA. Eosinophilic bacterial chronic rhinosinusitis. Laryngoscope 2007;117:2036–40.

96. Aurora R, Chatterjee D, Hentzleman J, et al. Contrasting the microbiomes from healthy volunteers and patients with chronic rhinosinusitis. JAMA Otolaryngol Head Neck Surg 2013;139:1328–38.

97. Laberge S, Pinsonneault S, Varga EM, et al. Increased expression of IL-16 immunoreactivity in bronchial mucosa after segmental allergen challenge in patients with asthma. J Allergy Clin Immunol 2000;106:293–301.

98. Pullerits T, Lindén A, Malmhäll C, et al. Effect of seasonal allergen exposure on mucosal IL-16 and CD4+ cells in patients with allergic rhinitis. Allergy 2001;56: 871–7.

99. Lam M, Hull L, McLachlan R, et al. Clinical severity and epithelial endotypes in chronic rhinosinusitis. Int Forum Allergy Rhinol 2013;3:121–8.

100. Paris G, Pozharskaya T, Asempa T, et al. Damage-associated molecular patterns stimulate interleukin-33 expression in nasal polyp epithelial cells. Int Forum Allergy Rhinol 2014;4:15–21.

101. Reh DD, Wang Y, Ramanathan M, et al. Treatment-recalcitrant chronic rhinosinusitis with polyps is associated with altered epithelial cell expression of interleukin-33. Am J Rhinol Allergy 2010;24:105–9.

102. Lackner A, Raggam RB, Stammberger H, et al. The role of interleukin-16 in eosinophilic chronic rhinosinusitis. Eur Arch Otorhinolaryngol 2007;264:887–93.

103. Gurney AL. IL-22, a Th1 cytokine that targets the pancreas and select other peripheral tissues. Int Immunopharmacol 2004;4:669–77.

104. Ramanathan M, Spannhake EW, Lane AP. Chronic rhinosinusitis with nasal polyps is associated with decreased expression of mucosal interleukin 22 receptor. Laryngoscope 2007;117:1839–43.

105. Madeo J, Frieri M. Bacterial biofilms and chronic rhinosinusitis. Allergy Asthma Proc 2013;34:335–41.

106. Deroee AF, Naraghi M, Sontou AF, et al. Nitric oxide metabolites as biomarkers for follow-up after chronic rhinosinusitis surgery. Am J Rhinol Allergy 2009;23: 159–61.

107. Lee RJ, Cohen NA. Role of the bitter taste receptor T2R38 in upper respiratory infection and chronic rhinosinusitis. Curr Opin Allergy Clin Immunol 2015;15: 14–20.

108. Rolla G, Heffler E, Bommarito L, et al. Exhaled nitric oxide as a marker of diseases. Recenti Prog Med 2005;96:634–40 [in Italian].

109. Barraud N, Hassett DJ, Hwang SH, et al. Involvement of nitric oxide in biofilm dispersal of Pseudomonas aeruginosa. J Bacteriol 2006;188:7344–53.

110. Tripathi A, Conley DB, Grammer LC, et al. Immunoglobulin E to staphylococcal and streptococcal toxins in patients with chronic sinusitis/nasal polyposis. Laryngoscope 2004;114:1822–6.
111. Schubert MS. A superantigen hypothesis for the pathogenesis of chronic hypertrophic rhinosinusitis, allergic fungal sinusitis, and related disorders. Ann Allergy Asthma Immunol 2001;87:181–8.
112. Pezato R, Świerczyńska-Krępa M, Niżankowska-Mogilnicka E, et al. Role of imbalance of eicosanoid pathways and staphylococcal superantigens in chronic rhinosinusitis. Allergy 2012;67:1347–56.
113. Bernstein JM, Kansal R. Superantigen hypothesis for the early development of chronic hyperplastic sinusitis with massive nasal polyposis. Curr Opin Otolaryngol Head Neck Surg 2005;13:39–44.
114. Proft T, Fraser JD. Bacterial superantigens. Clin Exp Immunol 2003;133:299–306.
115. Bernstein JM, Ballow M, Schlievert PM, et al. A superantigen hypothesis for the pathogenesis of chronic hyperplastic sinusitis with massive nasal polyposis. Am J Rhinol 2003;17:321–6.
116. Tabaee A, Anand VK, Yoon C. Outpatient intravenous antibiotics for methicillin-resistant Staphylococcus aureus sinusitis. Am J Rhinol 2007;21:154–8.
117. Gorwitz RJ, Kruszon-Moran D, McAllister SK, et al. Changes in the prevalence of nasal colonization with Staphylococcus aureus in the United States, 2001-2004. J Infect Dis 2008;197:1226–34.
118. Van Zele T, Gevaert P, Watelet JB, et al. Staphylococcus aureus colonization and IgE antibody formation to enterotoxins is increased in nasal polyposis. J Allergy Clin Immunol 2004;114:981–3.
119. McCoul ED, Jourdy DN, Schaberg MR, et al. Methicillin-resistant Staphylococcus aureus sinusitis in nonhospitalized patients: a systematic review of prevalence and treatment outcomes. Laryngoscope 2012;122:2125–31.
120. Desrosiers M, Hussain A, Frenkiel S, et al. Intranasal corticosteroid use is associated with lower rates of bacterial recovery in chronic rhinosinusitis. Otolaryngol Head Neck Surg 2007;136:605–9.
121. Al-Shemari H, Abou-Hamad W, Libman M, et al. Bacteriology of the sinus cavities of asymptomatic individuals after endoscopic sinus surgery. J Otolaryngol 2007;36:43–8.
122. Coates T, Bax R, Coates A. Nasal decolonization of Staphylococcus aureus with mupirocin: strengths, weaknesses and future prospects. J Antimicrob Chemother 2009;64:9–15.
123. Pujol M, Peña C, Pallares R, et al. Nosocomial Staphylococcus aureus bacteremia among nasal carriers of methicillin-resistant and methicillin-susceptible strains. Am J Med 1996;100:509–16.
124. von Eiff C, Becker K, Machka K, et al. Nasal carriage as a source of Staphylococcus aureus bacteremia. Study Group. N Engl J Med 2001;344:11–6.
125. Kluytmans J, van Belkum A, Verbrugh H. Nasal carriage of Staphylococcus aureus: epidemiology, underlying mechanisms, and associated risks. Clin Microbiol Rev 1997;10:505–20.
126. Luzar MA, Coles GA, Faller B, et al. Staphylococcus aureus nasal carriage and infection in patients on continuous ambulatory peritoneal dialysis. N Engl J Med 1990;322:505–9.
127. Pastacaldi C, Lewis P, Howarth P. Staphylococci and staphylococcal superantigens in asthma and rhinitis: a systematic review and meta-analysis. Allergy 2011;66:549–55.

128. Kilty SJ, Desrosiers MY. Are biofilms the answer in the pathophysiology and treatment of chronic rhinosinusitis? Immunol Allergy Clin North Am 2009;29: 645–56.

129. Ou J, Wang J, Xu Y, et al. Staphylococcus aureus superantigens are associated with chronic rhinosinusitis with nasal polyps: a meta-analysis. Eur Arch Otorhinolaryngol 2014;271:2729–36.

130. Balaban N, Rasooly A. Staphylococcal enterotoxins. Int J Food Microbiol 2000; 61:1–10.

131. Sachse F, Becker K, von Eiff C, et al. Staphylococcus aureus invades the epithelium in nasal polyposis and induces IL-6 in nasal epithelial cells in vitro. Allergy 2010;65:1430–7.

132. Shiomori T, Yoshida S, Miyamoto H, et al. Relationship of nasal carriage of Staphylococcus aureus to pathogenesis of perennial allergic rhinitis. J Allergy Clin Immunol 2000;105:449–54.

133. Corriveau MN, Zhang N, Holtappels G, et al. Detection of Staphylococcus aureus in nasal tissue with peptide nucleic acid-fluorescence in situ hybridization. Am J Rhinol Allergy 2009;23:461–5.

134. Bachert C, Gevaert P, Holtappels G, et al. Total and specific IgE in nasal polyps is related to local eosinophilic inflammation. J Allergy Clin Immunol 2001;107: 607–14.

135. Bachert C, Zhang N, Patou J, et al. Role of staphylococcal superantigens in upper airway disease. Curr Opin Allergy Clin Immunol 2008;8:34–8.

136. Tripathi A, Kern R, Conley DB, et al. Staphylococcal exotoxins and nasal polyposis: analysis of systemic and local responses. Am J Rhinol 2005;19:327–33.

137. Min YG, Oh SJ, Won TB, et al. Effects of staphylococcal enterotoxin on ciliary activity and histology of the sinus mucosa. Acta Otolaryngol 2006;126:941–7.

138. Pérez-Novo CA, Claeys C, Van Zele T, et al. Eicosanoid metabolism and eosinophilic inflammation in nasal polyp patients with immune response to Staphylococcus aureus enterotoxins. Am J Rhinol 2006;20:456–60.

139. Huvenne W, Callebaut I, Reekmans K, et al. Staphylococcus aureus enterotoxin B augments granulocyte migration and survival via airway epithelial cell activation. Allergy 2010;65:1013–20.

140. Damm M, Quante G, Jurk T, et al. Nasal colonization with Staphylococcus aureus is not associated with the severity of symptoms or the extent of the disease in chronic rhinosinusitis. Otolaryngol Head Neck Surg 2004;131:200–6.

141. Van Zele T, Vaneechoutte M, Holtappels G, et al. Detection of enterotoxin DNA in Staphylococcus aureus strains obtained from the middle meatus in controls and nasal polyp patients. Am J Rhinol 2008;22:223–7.

142. Heymans F, Fischer A, Stow NW, et al. Screening for staphylococcal superantigen genes shows no correlation with the presence or the severity of chronic rhinosinusitis and nasal polyposis. PLoS One 2010;5:e9525.

143. Wang M, Shi P, Chen B, et al. Superantigen-induced glucocorticoid insensitivity in the recurrence of chronic rhinosinusitis with nasal polyps. Otolaryngol Head Neck Surg 2011;145:717–22.

144. Dessi P, Castro F, Triglia JM, et al. Major complications of sinus surgery: a review of 1192 procedures. J Laryngol Otol 1994;108:212–5.

145. Hopkins C, Browne JP, Slack R, et al. Complications of surgery for nasal polyposis and chronic rhinosinusitis: the results of a national audit in England and Wales. Laryngoscope 2006;116:1494–9.

146. Hathorn IF, Habib AR, Manji J, et al. Comparing the reverse Trendelenburg and horizontal position for endoscopic sinus surgery: a randomized controlled trial. Otolaryngol Head Neck Surg 2013;148:308–13.

147. Wright ED, Agrawal S. Impact of perioperative systemic steroids on surgical outcomes in patients with chronic rhinosinusitis with polyposis: evaluation with the novel Perioperative Sinus Endoscopy (POSE) scoring system. Laryngoscope 2007;117:1–28.

148. Higgins TS, Hwang PH, Kingdom TT, et al. Systematic review of topical vasoconstrictors in endoscopic sinus surgery. Laryngoscope 2011;121:422–32.

149. Javer AR, Gheriani H, Mechor B, et al. Effect of intraoperative injection of 0.25% bupivacaine with 1:200,000 epinephrine on intraoperative blood loss in FESS. Am J Rhinol Allergy 2009;23:437–41.

150. Wormald PJ, Athanasiadis T, Rees G, et al. An evaluation of effect of pterygopalatine fossa injection with local anesthetic and adrenalin in the control of nasal bleeding during endoscopic sinus surgery. Am J Rhinol 2005;19:288–92.

151. Han JK, Hwang PH, Smith TL. Contemporary use of image-guided systems. Curr Opin Otolaryngol Head Neck Surg 2003;11:33–6.

152. Soler ZM, Hwang PH, Mace J, et al. Outcomes after middle turbinate resection: revisiting a controversial topic. Laryngoscope 2010;120:832–7.

153. Martinez-Devesa P, Patiar S. Oral steroids for nasal polyps. Cochrane Database Syst Rev 2011;(7):CD005232.

154. Schleimer RP. Glucocorticoids suppress inflammation but spare innate immune responses in airway epithelium. Proc Am Thorac Soc 2004;1:222–30.

155. Druilhe A, Létuvé S, Pretolani M. Glucocorticoid-induced apoptosis in human eosinophils: mechanisms of action. Apoptosis 2003;8:481–95.

156. Ohta K, Yamashita N. Apoptosis of eosinophils and lymphocytes in allergic inflammation. J Allergy Clin Immunol 1999;104:14–21.

157. Kalish L, Snidvongs K, Sivasubramaniam R, et al. Topical steroids for nasal polyps. Cochrane Database Syst Rev 2012;(12):CD006549.

158. Steinke JW, Payne SC, Tessier ME, et al. Pilot study of budesonide inhalant suspension irrigations for chronic eosinophilic sinusitis. J Allergy Clin Immunol 2009;124:1352–4.e7.

159. Salman S, Akpinar ME, Yigit O, et al. Surfactant protein A and D in chronic rhinosinusitis with nasal polyposis and corticosteroid response. Am J Rhinol Allergy 2012;26:e76–80.

160. Van Zele T, Gevaert P, Holtappels G, et al. Oral steroids and doxycycline: two different approaches to treat nasal polyps. J Allergy Clin Immunol 2010;125:1069–76.e4.

161. Grammer LC. Doxycycline or oral corticosteroids for nasal polyps. J Allergy Clin Immunol Pract 2013;1:541–2.

162. Wallwork B, Coman W, Mackay-Sim A, et al. A double-blind, randomized, placebo-controlled trial of macrolide in the treatment of chronic rhinosinusitis. Laryngoscope 2006;116:189–93.

163. Tanaka A, Ohashi Y, Kakinoki Y, et al. Immunotherapy suppresses both Th1 and Th2 responses by allergen stimulation, but suppression of the Th2 response is a more important mechanism related to the clinical efficacy of immunotherapy for perennial allergic rhinitis. Scand J Immunol 1998;48:201–11.

164. Liu CM, Kohanski MA, Mendiola M, et al. Impact of saline irrigation and topical corticosteroids on the postsurgical sinonasal microbiota. Int Forum Allergy Rhinol 2015;5:185–90.

Aspirin-Exacerbated Respiratory Disease

Evan S. Walgama, MD, Peter H. Hwang, MD*

KEYWORDS

- Aspirin-exacerbated respiratory disease • Chronic rhinosinusitis • Nasal polyposis
- Sinus surgery

KEY POINTS

- AERD is a well-recognized subtype of difficult-to-control CRS. It has specific biomarkers and disease-specific treatment considerations.
- The clinical hallmark of AERD is an acquired sensitivity to ingestion of aspirin and other cyclooxygenase-1 (COX-1) inhibitors.
- Familiarity with aspirin desensitization is essential for sinus surgeons, although it is often performed by medical allergists.

INTRODUCTION

Aspirin-exacerbated respiratory disease (AERD) is an inflammatory condition characterized by the triad of asthma, rhinosinusitis, and sensitivity to aspirin. AERD is also referred to as Samter triad, and beyond these two designations, the literature has used several others including aspirin triad, aspirin-sensitive asthma, aspirin-induced asthma, and aspirin-intolerant asthma. For this article, AERD is the preferred nomenclature.

AERD is one of the best characterized subtypes of rhinosinusitis.[1] Disordered eicosanoid metabolism, the pathophysiologic mechanism underlying AERD, is unique to this disorder. The rhinosinusitis of AERD is typically severe and, among currently defined subtypes, one of the more difficult to control. Fortunately, there are specific treatment options available to patients with aspirin sensitivity, including aspirin desensitization, which may ameliorate the severity of upper and lower airway inflammatory disease.[2–7] In this sense AERD is a prototype for the application of precision medicine principles; it is a well-defined subtype of chronic rhinosinusitis (CRS) with individualized treatment strategies tailored to the underlying pathophysiologic mechanism.

Disclosure Statement: No disclosures (E.S. Walgama); Consultant: Olympus, Intersect, Arrinex, Sinuwave (P.H. Hwang).
Department of Otolaryngology/Head and Neck Surgery, Stanford School of Medicine, Stanford Sinus Center, 801 Welch Road, Palo Alto, CA 94304, USA
* Corresponding author.
E-mail address: hwangph@stanford.edu

Otolaryngol Clin N Am 50 (2017) 83–94
http://dx.doi.org/10.1016/j.otc.2016.08.007
0030-6665/17/© 2016 Elsevier Inc. All rights reserved.
oto.theclinics.com

With a proliferation of novel biologic agents to address specific components of the inflammatory cascade, AERD may serve as a model for how other types of difficult-to-control CRS are treated in the future.

CLINICAL PRESENTATION

AERD is an acquired disorder that typically presents in the third or fourth decade.[8,9] Patients usually do not report a previous history of atopy, rhinitis, or asthma, and may offer a history of tolerating aspirin or nonsteroidal anti-inflammatory drugs well into adulthood. This disorder affects approximately 0.5% of the population, and females twice as often as males.[10] Obesity and smoking are risk factors that are more associated with AERD than aspirin-tolerant asthma.[10]

The hallmark of AERD is an acquired sensitivity to ingestion of aspirin and other cyclooxygenase (COX)-1 inhibitors. Patients with AERD develop symptoms 30 to 120 minutes after ingestion of aspirin, resulting from proinflammatory effects of dysregulated cysteinyl leukotrienes on the upper and lower respiratory tracts (increased vascular permeability, bronchoconstriction, and eosinophil chemotaxis and activation). Patients typically experience acute onset of nasal congestion, conjunctivitis, throat tightness, and exacerbation of asthma. There can also be an associated anaphylactic-like reaction characterized by urticaria, gastrointestinal disturbance, or hypotension.[11] Because the drug reaction is not IgE-mediated, it is not considered true anaphylaxis. The severity of symptoms is variable, from minimal wheezing to severe respiratory compromise.

In the absence of an acute exposure to aspirin, patients who develop AERD still experience progressive upper and lower respiratory inflammatory symptoms because of abnormally elevated circulating levels of cysteinyl leukotrienes. The syndrome may unfold over a few years, with the first symptom to present usually being rhinitis.[8] The rhinitis is often reported to have originated as a "cold that never went away." It is associated with a clear discharge and may be resistant to standard therapies. Rhinitis progresses to CRS in 60% to 90% of cases.[8] CRS associated with AERD is characterized by hyperplastic mucosal remodeling with prominent eosinophilia, and ultimately, nasal polyposis.

An average of 2 years later, patients develop asthma.[8] Patients frequently have no prior history of childhood asthma or any prior problems with reactive airway disease. The asthma of AERD is typically moderate-severe to severe, by current classification standards. It is often difficult to control; compared with patients with aspirin-tolerant asthma, patients with AERD are more likely to have severe asthma, to require intensive care unit admission for asthma, to need oral steroids for asthma exacerbation, and to receive high-dose inhaled steroids for asthma control.[12] However, sometimes asthma is absent.[4]

Aspirin intolerance can develop at any point during this time course but frequently is the last part of the triad to develop. This happens on average 4 years after the onset of asthma.[8] Because most patients with CRS and comorbid asthma do not have aspirin sensitivity, taking a careful history regarding aspirin tolerance is important to discern patients with AERD from those without AERD. Still, in patients with asthmatic rhinosinusitis who have no history of adverse reaction to aspirin, 15% have a positive oral aspirin challenge.[8] Conversely, for patients with asthmatic rhinosinusitis who do report a history of adverse reaction to aspirin, 14% have a negative oral aspirin challenge.[13] Patients who report recurrent adverse reactions to aspirin, or who had a previous severe reaction to aspirin, have fewer negative oral aspirin challenges.

PATHOPHYSIOLOGY

AERD is an acquired disorder of arachidonic acid metabolism. The salient finding is a marked baseline overproduction of cysteinyl leukotriene metabolites, most notably LTE4, which is a potent proinflammatory lipid. Leukotrienes are produced by the metabolism of arachidonic acid via the 5-lipoxygenase (5-LO) pathway. Because LTE4 is constitutively overexpressed, irrespective of aspirin exposure, patient avoidance of aspirin does not modify the natural history of the asthmatic and sinonasal manifestations of the disease.[7]

Aspirin is a potent COX-1 inhibitor. COX-1 modulates an alternative route for the metabolism of arachidonic acid, resulting in the synthesis of prostaglandins, including prostaglandin E_2 (PGE2), an anti-inflammatory prostaglandin. PGE2 provides negative feedback to the 5-LO pathway, reducing the burden of LTE4.[14] For patients with AERD, the ingestion of aspirin or other COX-1 inhibitors blocks PGE2 production, which in turn bolsters the 5-LO pathway, causing a surge of proinflammatory leukotrienes.[15] During oral aspirin challenge, PGE2 levels are decreased, and LTE4 levels are increased.[16] The resulting surge of serum leukotrienes results in acute bronchoconstriction, vascular permeability, and eosinophil migration, manifesting clinically as acute rhinitis and asthma. Notably, the reaction that occurs after ingestion of aspirin is pseudoallergic, because it is not IgE-mediated. Furthermore, sensitivity to ingested aspirin is a marker of disease, not the cause of the disease.

In the clinical setting, LTE4 is measured by urine collection, and serves as a marker of overall production of proinflammatory leukotrienes. At baseline, without exposure to aspirin, patients with AERD have elevated LTE4 levels three to five times that of those with aspirin-tolerant asthma.[17] The magnitude of the surge in urinary LTE4 after aspirin challenge has been shown to correlate with the severity of the clinical reaction observed.[18] In patients with a positive oral aspirin challenge, testing of urinary LTE4 is not routinely necessary. But in patients with a negative oral aspirin challenge for whom there is still strong suspicion for AERD, an elevated urinary LTE4 may predict a therapeutic benefit for aspirin therapy.

Leukotrienes seem to play a dominant role in the pathophysiology of patients with AERD relative to aspirin-tolerant patients with asthma and CRS. After aspirin desensitization and continued aspirin therapy, sensitivity to inhaled LTE4 was noted to decrease 33-fold from the predesensitization state in patients with AERD, although there was no observed change in sensitivity in aspirin-tolerant patients.[19] In a double-blind placebo-controlled trial of patients with AERD, oral challenge with aspirin produced a six-fold increase in urinary LTE4 compared with placebo.[16] In patients with asthma who were tolerant to aspirin during oral aspirin challenge, this phenomenon was observed to a lesser degree. The observed differences in leukotriene sensitivity and production, at baseline and during aspirin challenge, support the primary relevance of leukotrienes in patients with AERD compared with those without AERD.

Platelets have also been implicated in the overproduction of leukotrienes observed in patients with AERD.[20,21] Transcellular synthesis of LTE4 occurs when leukocytes adhere to platelets to appropriate their cellular machinery for leukotriene production. These platelet-leukocyte aggregates are measurable in the research setting and have been correlated with the increase in urinary LTE4 seen in patients with AERD during oral aspirin challenge.[22] The inhibition of platelets by aspirin, and thus of the requisite machinery for leukotriene production, may be one mechanism by which aspirin therapy improves symptoms in patients with AERD.

There are differences in cytokine expression that distinguish AERD-related CRS from aspirin-tolerant CRS. Compared with aspirin-tolerant CRS with nasal polyposis, polyp tissue from patients with AERD contain higher levels of eosinophilic cationic protein, a marker of eosinophilia,[23] elevated expression of interleukin-5,[24] and interferon-γ.[25] In addition to 5-LO, leukotriene C4 synthetase is another enzyme that is upregulated in AERD, which drives not only LTE4 production, but also precursor leukotrienes types C4 and D4.[26]

ASTHMA IN ASPIRIN-EXACERBATED RESPIRATORY DISEASE

Approximately 7% of all people with asthma are aspirin intolerant.[27] In the subgroup of those with severe asthma, this proportion doubles to 14%.[27] Of people with asthma with nasal polyposis, 10% to 42% are aspirin intolerant.[13,27,28] Patients with AERD typically have moderate-severe to severe asthma and thus, by current guidelines recommendations, usually require regular use of inhaled corticosteroid in addition to long-term inhaled β-agonists.[29]

CHRONIC RHINOSINUSITIS IN ASPIRIN-EXACERBATED RESPIRATORY DISEASE

AERD is a severe subtype of CRS, characterized by chronic eosinophilic hyperplastic inflammation of the sinonasal mucosa. Nasal polyps are typically present. A total of 8% to 26% of all patients with CRS with polyps have AERD.[30] Thus, for all patients who have CRS with polyps, it is important to elicit if there is a history of asthma, particularly adult-onset, or a history of adverse reaction to aspirin. Patients with AERD have worse sinonasal disease by computed tomography (CT) evaluation and are more likely to require revision surgery than aspirin-tolerant patients with CRS.[28,31]

TREATMENT OPTIONS FOR ASPIRIN-EXACERBATED RESPIRATORY DISEASE–RELATED CHRONIC RHINOSINUSITIS

Like all other patients with CRS, patients with AERD with symptomatic nasal polyposis should undergo a trial of medical therapy before pursuing surgical therapy. This usually includes saline irrigations, topical steroids, oral antibiotics, and judicious use of oral steroids.[32] Specifically for AERD, zileuton (see later) may be used preoperatively to reduce polyp burden, but this is not routine practice. It should be noted that as a subtype of CRS with nasal polyposis, AERD-related CRS is treated with standard therapies that are generally used for all subtypes of CRS with nasal polyposis. This discussion highlights specific strategies for management of AERD-related CRS, namely aspirin desensitization, and also reviews strategies for managing CRS with nasal polyposis generally, which are widely applied in clinical practice.

Antileukotriene Therapy

Two classes of drugs are available: leukotriene receptor competitive antagonists, which block the CysLT1 receptor; and 5-LO inhibitors, which block the rate-limiting step of arachidonic metabolism in the leukotriene pathway. To date, despite a plausible pathophysiologic rationale, there is no evidence that leukotriene receptor antagonists are beneficial for the treatment of CRS in the setting of AERD.[33] However, leukotriene receptor antagonists may benefit some patients with AERD in control of asthma and/or allergic rhinitis (independent of aspirin tolerance).

Drugs in the CysLT1 receptor antagonist class include montelukast, zafirlukast, and pranlukast. These drugs are indicated for asthma and are sometimes used in the treatment of allergic rhinitis. Some researchers have postulated that leukotriene receptor antagonists might have a role in preventing polyp regrowth after endoscopic sinus surgery, but studies of patients with nasal polyps, which included aspirin-tolerant CRS, have not shown leukotriene receptor antagonists to be effective as monotherapy when compared with topical mometasone.[34] In addition, there is no durable benefit for using montelukast as an additional therapy for symptom control in CRS with polyposis in patients already using topical nasal steroids.[35] These studies evaluated montelukast in the treatment of all CRS with nasal polyposis, not specifically AERD-associated CRS. A separate leukotriene receptor, CysLT2, has been shown to be upregulated in nasal polyp tissue, but the current leukotriene receptor antagonists do not affect these receptors.[36]

The only drug available in the 5-LO inhibitor class is zileuton, which is indicated for asthma. Ex vivo studies of nasal polyp tissue have shown increased inhibition of mast cell activation with the combination of zileuton plus montelukast compared with montelukast alone.[37] Currently no clinical studies directly evaluate use of this medication in patients with CRS.[38] A study of patients with asthma and AERD showed improved sense of smell and nasal peak inspiratory flow in the zileuton group compared with placebo to be a significant secondary outcome.[38] Use of this medication carries a small risk of hepatotoxicity and requires monitoring of liver function throughout its course.

For both classes of leukotriene-modifying medications, a rare but concerning potential side effect is psychiatric disturbance including suicidal ideation, particularly in adolescents, for which the Food and Drug Administration has issued warnings.

Antibiotic Therapy

Antibiotic therapy for AERD-associated rhinosinusitis is not an intuitive proposition given that the understood cause of AERD is inflammatory, not infectious. However, there is evidence that in all subtypes of CRS with nasal polyposis, the addition of 3 weeks of doxycycline to prednisone results in more durable reduction of disease by objective and subjective measures in patients with nasal polyps compared with prednisone alone.[39] The proposed mechanism of action of doxycycline is reduction of staphylococcal enterotoxin, to which nasal polyposis is associated with an IgE-mediated hypersensitivity. In patients with AERD, levels of antistaphylococcal enterotoxin IgE are elevated compared with aspirin-tolerant CRS with nasal polyposis, and may be responsible for the observed elevation of total IgE seen in patients with AERD without atopy.[40]

Omalizumab

Omalizumab, an anti-IgE monoclonal antibody, has been reported to be beneficial in the treatment of patients with AERD, even though the primary pathophysiologic disturbance of leukotriene overproduction and the adverse reaction to aspirin ingestion are not thought to be IgE-mediated.[41] Omalizumab is currently indicated for use in severe asthma. Aside from case reports, to date there are no large studies that have specifically addressed CRS and asthma in the setting of AERD. In patients with severe asthma who also have nasal polyposis, use of this medication is associated with improved control of CRS symptoms.[42] This effect seems to be independent of atopy status. In a prospective, uncontrolled study evaluating CRS and asthma symptoms in patients with severe asthma, patients receiving omalizumab had improved CRS symptom scores, decreased objective disease as measured on CT, improved asthma symptom scores, and reduced polyp burden.[43]

Oral Corticosteroids

No studies have specifically addressed oral steroid use in patients with AERD, but they are commonly used in clinical practice for AERD and for other subtypes of CRS with nasal polyposis. Oral corticosteroids are an effective short-term treatment of nasal polyps. The maximum effect is reached by approximately 2 to 3 weeks of therapy.[39] Although at times necessary, the short-term side effects of corticosteroid use include insomnia, anxiety, hyperglycemia, dyspepsia, and exacerbation of closed-angle glaucoma, if present. Long-term side effects include diabetes, osteoporosis, Cushing syndrome, adrenal insufficiency, and avascular necrosis of the femur. The prescribing of oral steroids for patients with CRS requires careful consideration, because of the potentially devastating adverse effects associated with their use.[44] Furthermore, use of oral steroid bursts even once yearly results in significant increase in the rate of diabetes and osteoporosis in patients with allergic rhinitis compared with those who do not receive systemic steroids.[45] Therefore, repeated use of steroids is not judicious as first-line therapy for most patients suffering from CRS.

Surgical Management

Endoscopic sinus surgery for patients with AERD with nasal polyps adheres to similar principles as with other types of CRS with nasal polyps. Surgery for AERD-associated rhinosinusitis is not minimally invasive in the sense that the goal is not merely to ventilate the sinuses at the ostiomeatal complex, considering that AERD and other forms of eosinophilic CRS are not caused by ostiomeatal obstruction of the sinuses.[46] Surgery should aim to remove polyps, remove any eosinophilic mucin that might stimulate ongoing inflammation, and yet preserve the mucosal lining of the surgical cavities. It should also facilitate access for postoperative irrigations. Thus, meticulous postoperative debridement is necessary to maintain widely patent sinuses.

Patients with AERD are more likely to have recurrence of nasal polyposis following surgery than patients with other forms of nasal polyposis. In one study, patients with AERD had an average of 10 times the number of sinus surgeries compared with aspirin-tolerant patients.[28] However, postoperative quality-of-life outcomes may actually be comparable between patients with and without AERD. Although patients with AERD have a higher preoperative disease burden by CT imaging, and worse postoperative endoscopy scores, there is no measurable difference in postoperative quality of life compared with patients with aspirin-tolerant CRS.[28,31] Surgical benefits seem to be preserved when performed in conjunction with aspirin desensitization (see next section). Patients with AERD with asthma and CRS who undergo sinus surgery have improved asthma control following surgery compared with the previous year.[47] Compared with the previous year before surgery, in the first postoperative year patients have fewer emergency room visits and improved asthma symptom scores.

Because patients with AERD have adverse reactions to COX-1 inhibitors, the management of postoperative pain must accommodate for drug intolerances. Aspirin cannot be used for pain control, and as for other strong COX-1 inhibitors, there is a 41% rate of cross-reactivity to ibuprofen, 4% cross-reactivity to naproxen, and 1% cross-reactivity to ketorolac.[48] Acetaminophen, commonly used in combination with narcotic medications, is actually a weak COX-1 inhibitor. At oral doses greater than 1000 mg of acetaminophen, one-third of patients with AERD experience an adverse reaction. Doses less than 500 mg are generally well tolerated.[49] COX-2 inhibitors, such as celecoxib, are generally tolerated but are not typically used in the postoperative period.[50]

Aspirin desensitization is usually performed 1 month after surgery, so as to avoid the risk of postoperative epistaxis from platelet inhibition and yet also to preempt early polyp regrowth. Aspirin therapy is not known to shrink the existing polyp burden, but it does seem to prevent polyp regrowth. Thus it is not recommended to pursue aspirin desensitization unless a thorough surgical removal of polyps has occurred first.

When patients who are already desensitized to aspirin require revision sinus surgery, the surgeon may elect to proceed with surgery with the patient on a reduced daily dose of 81 mg of aspirin, which maintains the desensitized state. The patient can then be re-escalated to therapeutic doses at home postoperatively without clinical supervision. Otherwise, if aspirin has been completely discontinued for more than 72 hours, the patient will likely need to repeat the complete process of desensitization from the beginning.

ASPIRIN CHALLENGE AND DESENSITIZATION

Aspirin challenge may be indicated if there is a history of adverse reaction to aspirin; if a patient has difficult-to-control asthmatic CRS (even without a previous history of aspirin sensitivity); or if desensitization is required for daily aspirin therapy, such as in the setting of coronary artery disease. A positive provocation test is required to establish the diagnosis of AERD. Establishing the diagnosis of AERD allows for the initiation of disease-specific therapy, usually the continuation of daily aspirin therapy to maintain a desensitized state.

Aspirin challenge is usually performed by medical allergy and immunology specialists. This may take the form of either bronchial, nasal, or oral testing, and sometimes a combination of these may be used. Each of these modalities has similar sensitivity and specificity.[51] Bronchial challenge is rarely performed because of increased risk for adverse pulmonary reactions.

Aspirin challenge testing in the United States typically involves titrating a dose of oral aspirin or nasal lysine spray, an aspirin derivative, until a reaction occurs as measured by symptom change and a reduction of nasal peak inspiratory flow or forced expiratory flow in 1 second (FEV_1). The most common criteria for an observed positive test are naso-ocular symptoms plus greater than 15% decline in FEV_1 (**Box 1**). Although most aspirin challenges are done on an outpatient basis, safe testing requires intravenous access, immediate availability of emergency resuscitative equipment, and a baseline FEV_1 greater than 70% of predicted or greater than 1.5 L.[52] Patients should stay on their regular asthma medications, and a leukotriene receptor antagonist, such as montelukast, should be initiated before testing if the patient is not already taking one, to reduce the severity of the expected reaction of a positive challenge.[53] When a positive reaction occurs, symptoms can be treated with appropriate medications, such as oxymetazoline nasal spray for nasal congestion, albuterol for wheezing, or ondansetron for nausea.

In case of a negative test, two possibilities exist: either the patient does not have AERD or they have what has been called "silent AERD," which refers to a

---

Box 1
Clinical parameters for positive oral aspirin challenge

1. Naso-ocular symptoms alone

2. Naso-ocular symptoms and a 15% or greater decline in FEV_1 (classic reaction)

3. Lower respiratory reaction only (FEV_1 declines by >20%)

4. Laryngospasm with or without any of the first three reactions

5. Systemic reactions: hives, flushing, gastric pain, hypotension

Adapted from Stevenson DD. Aspirin sensitivity and desensitization for asthma and sinusitis. Curr Allergy Asthma Rep 2009;9(2):157.

false-negative aspirin challenge.[54] In patients who test negative but have a strong history suggesting aspirin intolerance, the allergist may choose to pursue repeat testing after the patient has been taken off of leukotriene receptor antagonists. Another option is a short trial of aspirin therapy after the negative test to assess whether aspirin therapy results in improved symptoms of CRS and better asthma control, indicative of so-called silent AERD.

Numerous protocols for aspirin desensitization have been published that typically are performed by medical allergists over the course of 1 to 3 days.[52,55,56] Although formerly performed in critical care settings, aspirin desensitization is routinely performed in an outpatient clinic setting with appropriate monitoring and safety precautions. Initial doses begin with 20 mg to 40 mg of aspirin or, in some newer protocols, with intranasal lysine-aspirin or ketorolac spray. The dose of aspirin or aspirin derivative is gradually increased every 1 to 3 hours. After a positive test is confirmed, the goal is to repeat this dose and increase the dose until 325 mg of aspirin is tolerated without a reaction. At 325 mg, desensitization is complete. Patients who do not react to 325 mg will not react to 650 mg, and this final dose can be given at home.

Although 81 mg/day is a sufficient oral dose to maintain aspirin tolerance, patients with AERD seeking therapeutic benefits from aspirin desensitization require doses between 325 mg and 650 mg twice daily. In a randomized prospective crossover trial comparing these two doses,[57] approximately half the patients who started in the 650-mg group were able to decrease to 325 mg and without a reduction in clinical efficacy, and approximately half the patients who began in the 325-mg group received more symptom control after crossing over to 650 mg dose. There was no significant difference in the incidence of side effects at either dose. Thus, the authors of this study recommended starting at a dose of 650 mg twice daily, with an attempt to taper the dose by 325 mg daily after 1 month (975 mg/day), and again at 2 months (650 mg/day) while observing for continued symptom control.

OUTCOMES OF ASPIRIN DESENSITIZATION

The most prolific descriptions of outcomes of aspirin therapy in AERD come from investigators at the Scripps Clinic in La Jolla, California. In 1984 the group reported a double-blind, placebo-controlled crossover trial in which 25 patients, all with AERD, were enrolled.[6] After desensitization and 3 months of therapy with either aspirin or placebo, all patients underwent repeat randomization to desensitization with either aspirin or placebo, followed by 3 months of therapy with the same. In this difficult-to-perform study, there was a significant improvement in nasal symptoms and decreased nasal steroid use during aspirin therapy, although this study was not able to show a difference in asthma control.

A 1990 observational cohort study followed 66 patients who were orally desensitized to aspirin and 40 patients who avoided aspirin.[7] Compared with the control group who avoided aspirin, patients who were treated with aspirin had improved sense of smell, asthma control, fewer sinus surgeries, and decreased steroid use, at an average follow-up time of 3.8 years. At 2 years, 30 patients in the aspirin group had discontinued therapy. The most common reason was for gastrointestinal intolerance. The patients who discontinued aspirin still had significantly reduced hospitalizations and emergency room visits compared with the group who avoided aspirin.

A 1996 study by the same group followed 65 patients treated with aspirin desensitization therapy.[5] It compared those who had been treated between 1 and 3 years with those treated between 3 and 6 years, and showed that there was no decline in efficacy over time as long as patients remained on daily aspirin.

A 2003 study by the same group followed 173 patients by telephone survey and compared outcomes during the first year of aspirin desensitization with the prior year before desensitization.[2] On average patients had fewer hospitalizations and fewer sinus surgeries after desensitization. Fourteen percent had discontinued aspirin therapy during the first year because of side effects, the most common of which involved the gastrointestinal tract. Of the 16 patients who discontinued aspirin for lack of efficacy, 14 of 16 were reported to have severe atopy. The authors hypothesized that uncontrolled atopy may be a reason for clinical failure after aspirin desensitization.

In a long-term study of sinonasal outcomes in patients with AERD who underwent surgery followed by aspirin desensitization, most patients (93%) were successfully desensitized, and compared with the preoperative state, this group demonstrated sustained improvement at 33 months as measured by endoscopy and quality-of-life assessment as measured by the Sinonasal Outcome Test-22 measure.[58]

Although these studies highlight useful clinical information about patients with AERD undergoing aspirin therapy and suggest its efficacy, most have been criticized for lack of control groups of patients without AERD.[33] Specifically, it is hypothesized that the anti-inflammatory effects of aspirin may be responsible for the improvement in clinical symptoms, not maintenance of a desensitized state.[59] Recently, a double-blind, placebo-controlled trial was performed comparing patients with AERD with those with aspirin-tolerant asthma.[16] Both groups were subjected to an aspirin desensitization protocol followed by 6 months of aspirin therapy. Only the AERD group experienced improvement in quality of life for asthma and CRS and also in objective measurements of peak inspiratory nasal flow, spirometry, and decreased urinary LTE4. This supports the hypothesis that maintenance of a desensitized state is a unique therapeutic option for patients with AERD.

SUMMARY

AERD is a well-recognized subtype of difficult-to-control CRS. It has specific biomarkers and disease-specific treatment considerations; in this way it serves as a prototype for the future of multispecialty treatment of CRS. Familiarity with aspirin desensitization is essential for sinus surgeons who would use the full armamentarium of medical and surgical therapies for their difficult patients.

REFERENCES

1. Han JK. Subclassification of chronic rhinosinusitis. Laryngoscope 2013; 123(Suppl 2):S15–27.
2. Berges-Gimeno MP, Simon RA, Stevenson DD. Long-term treatment with aspirin desensitization in asthmatic patients with aspirin-exacerbated respiratory disease. J Allergy Clin Immunol 2003;111(1):180–6.
3. Fokkens WJ, Lund VJ, Mullol J, et al. European position paper on rhinosinusitis and nasal polyps 2012. Rhinol Suppl 2012;(23):1–298, 3 p preceding table of contents.
4. Lumry WR, Curd JG, Zeiger RS, et al. Aspirin-sensitive rhinosinusitis: the clinical syndrome and effects of aspirin administration. J Allergy Clin Immunol 1983; 71(6):580–7.
5. Stevenson DD, Hankammer MA, Mathison DA, et al. Aspirin desensitization treatment of aspirin-sensitive patients with rhinosinusitis-asthma: long-term outcomes. J Allergy Clin Immunol 1996;98(4):751–8.

6. Stevenson DD, Pleskow WW, Simon RA, et al. Aspirin-sensitive rhinosinusitis asthma: a double-blind crossover study of treatment with aspirin. J Allergy Clin Immunol 1984;73(4):500–7.

7. Sweet JM, Stevenson DD, Simon RA, et al. Long-term effects of aspirin desensitization–treatment for aspirin-sensitive rhinosinusitis-asthma. J Allergy Clin Immunol 1990;85(1 Pt 1):59–65.

8. Szczeklik A, Nizankowska E, Duplaga M. Natural history of aspirin-induced asthma. AIANE Investigators. European Network on Aspirin-Induced Asthma. Eur Respir J 2000;16(3):432–6.

9. Berges-Gimeno MP, Simon RA, Stevenson DD. The natural history and clinical characteristics of aspirin-exacerbated respiratory disease. Ann Allergy Asthma Immunol 2002;89(5):474–8.

10. Eriksson J, Ekerljung L, Bossios A, et al. Aspirin-intolerant asthma in the population: prevalence and important determinants. Clin Exp Allergy 2015;45(1):211–9.

11. Berkes EA. Anaphylactic and anaphylactoid reactions to aspirin and other NSAIDs. Clin Rev Allergy Immunol 2003;24(2):137–48.

12. Mascia K, Haselkorn T, Deniz YM, et al. Aspirin sensitivity and severity of asthma: evidence for irreversible airway obstruction in patients with severe or difficult-to-treat asthma. J Allergy Clin Immunol 2005;116(5):970–5.

13. Dursun AB, Woessner KA, Simon RA, et al. Predicting outcomes of oral aspirin challenges in patients with asthma, nasal polyps, and chronic sinusitis. Ann Allergy Asthma Immunol 2008;100(5):420–5.

14. Sestini P, Armetti L, Gambaro G, et al. Inhaled PGE2 prevents aspirin-induced bronchoconstriction and urinary LTE4 excretion in aspirin-sensitive asthma. Am J Respir Crit Care Med 1996;153(2):572–5.

15. Szczeklik A, Stevenson DD. Aspirin-induced asthma: advances in pathogenesis, diagnosis, and management. J Allergy Clin Immunol 2003;111(5):913–21 [quiz: 922].

16. Świerczyńska-Krepa M, Sanak M, Bochenek G, et al. Aspirin desensitization in patients with aspirin-induced and aspirin-tolerant asthma: a double-blind study. J Allergy Clin Immunol 2014;134(4):883–90.

17. Micheletto C, Visconti M, Tognella S, et al. Aspirin induced asthma (AIA) with nasal polyps has the highest basal LTE4 excretion: a study vs AIA without polyps, mild topic asthma, and normal controls. Eur Ann Allergy Clin Immunol 2006;38(1):20–3.

18. Daffern PJ, Muilenburg D, Hugli TE, et al. Association of urinary leukotriene E4 excretion during aspirin challenges with severity of respiratory responses. J Allergy Clin Immunol 1999;104(3 Pt 1):559–64.

19. Arm JP, O'Hickey SP, Spur BW, et al. Airway responsiveness to histamine and leukotriene E4 in subjects with aspirin-induced asthma. Am Rev Respir Dis 1989;140(1):148–53.

20. Mitsui C, Kajiwara K, Hayashi H, et al. Platelet activation markers overexpressed specifically in patients with aspirin-exacerbated respiratory disease. J Allergy Clin Immunol 2016;137(2):400–11.

21. Laidlaw TM, Boyce JA. Platelets in patients with aspirin-exacerbated respiratory disease. J Allergy Clin Immunol 2015;135(6):1407–14 [quiz: 415].

22. Laidlaw TM, Kidder MS, Bhattacharyya N, et al. Cysteinyl leukotriene overproduction in aspirin-exacerbated respiratory disease is driven by platelet-adherent leukocytes. Blood 2012;119(16):3790–8.

23. Stevens WW, Ocampo CJ, Berdnikovs S, et al. Cytokines in chronic rhinosinusitis. Role in eosinophilia and aspirin-exacerbated respiratory disease. Am J Respir Crit Care Med 2015;192(6):682–94.

24. Perez-Novo CA, Watelet JB, Claeys C, et al. Prostaglandin, leukotriene, and lipoxin balance in chronic rhinosinusitis with and without nasal polyposis. J Allergy Clin Immunol 2005;115(6):1189–96.

25. Steinke JW, Liu L, Huyett P, et al. Prominent role of IFN-gamma in patients with aspirin-exacerbated respiratory disease. J Allergy Clin Immunol 2013;132(4): 856–65.e1-3.

26. Steinke JW, Borish L. Factors driving the aspirin exacerbated respiratory disease phenotype. Am J Rhinol Allergy 2015;29(1):35–40.

27. Rajan JP, Wineinger NE, Stevenson DD, et al. Prevalence of aspirin-exacerbated respiratory disease among asthmatic patients: a meta-analysis of the literature. J Allergy Clin Immunol 2015;135(3):676–81.e1.

28. Kim JE, Kountakis SE. The prevalence of Samter's triad in patients undergoing functional endoscopic sinus surgery. Ear Nose Throat J 2007;86(7):396–9.

29. National Asthma E, Prevention P. Expert panel report 3 (EPR-3): guidelines for the diagnosis and management of asthma-summary report 2007. J Allergy Clin Immunol 2007;120(5 Suppl):S94–138.

30. Graefe H, Roebke C, Schafer D, et al. Aspirin sensitivity and chronic rhinosinusitis with polyps: a fatal combination. J Allergy 2012;2012:817910.

31. Awad OG, Lee JH, Fasano MB, et al. Sinonasal outcomes after endoscopic sinus surgery in asthmatic patients with nasal polyps: a difference between aspirin-tolerant and aspirin-induced asthma? Laryngoscope 2008;118(7):1282–6.

32. Rosenfeld RM, Piccirillo JF, Chandrasekhar SS, et al. Clinical practice guideline (update): adult sinusitis. Otolaryngol Head Neck Surg 2015;152(2 Suppl):S1–39.

33. Bachert C, Zhang L, Gevaert P. Current and future treatment options for adult chronic rhinosinusitis: focus on nasal polyposis. J Allergy Clin Immunol 2015; 136(6):1431–40.

34. Vuralkan E, Saka C, Akin I, et al. Comparison of montelukast and mometasone furoate in the prevention of recurrent nasal polyps. Ther Adv Respir Dis 2012; 6(1):5–10.

35. Stewart RA, Ram B, Hamilton G, et al. Montelukast as an adjunct to oral and inhaled steroid therapy in chronic nasal polyposis. Otolaryngol Head Neck Surg 2008;139(5):682–7.

36. Smith TL, Sautter NB. Is montelukast indicated for treatment of chronic rhinosinusitis with polyposis? Laryngoscope 2014;124(8):1735–6.

37. Di Capite J, Nelson C, Bates G, et al. Targeting Ca2+ release-activated Ca2+ channel channels and leukotriene receptors provides a novel combination strategy for treating nasal polyposis. J Allergy Clin Immunol 2009;124(5): 1014–21.e1-3.

38. Dahlen B, Nizankowska E, Szczeklik A, et al. Benefits from adding the 5-lipoxygenase inhibitor zileuton to conventional therapy in aspirin-intolerant asthmatics. Am J Respir Crit Care Med 1998;157(4 Pt 1):1187–94.

39. Van Zele T, Gevaert P, Holtappels G, et al. Oral steroids and doxycycline: two different approaches to treat nasal polyps. J Allergy Clin Immunol 2010;125(5): 1069–76.e4.

40. Yoo HS, Shin YS, Liu JN, et al. Clinical significance of immunoglobulin E responses to staphylococcal superantigens in patients with aspirin-exacerbated respiratory disease. Int Arch Allergy Immunol 2013;162(4):340–5.

41. Bergmann KC, Zuberbier T, Church MK. Omalizumab in the treatment of aspirin-exacerbated respiratory disease. J Allergy Clin Immunol Pract 2015;3(3):459–60.

42. Gevaert P, Calus L, Van Zele T, et al. Omalizumab is effective in allergic and nonallergic patients with nasal polyps and asthma. J Allergy Clin Immunol 2013;131(1):110–6.e1.

43. Tajiri T, Matsumoto H, Hiraumi H, et al. Efficacy of omalizumab in eosinophilic chronic rhinosinusitis patients with asthma. Ann Allergy Asthma Immunol 2013; 110(5):387–8.

44. Poetker DM. Oral corticosteroids in the management of chronic rhinosinusitis with and without nasal polyps: risks and benefits. Am J Rhinol Allergy 2015;29(5): 339–42.

45. Aasbjerg K, Torp-Pedersen C, Vaag A, et al. Treating allergic rhinitis with depot-steroid injections increase risk of osteoporosis and diabetes. Respir Med 2013; 107(12):1852–8.

46. Snidvongs K, Chin D, Sacks R, et al. Eosinophilic rhinosinusitis is not a disease of ostiomeatal occlusion. Laryngoscope 2013;123(5):1070–4.

47. Awad OG, Fasano MB, Lee JH, et al. Asthma outcomes after endoscopic sinus surgery in aspirin-tolerant versus aspirin-induced asthmatic patients. Am J Rhinol 2008;22(2):197–203.

48. Szczeklik A, Gryglewski RJ, Czerniawska-Mysik G. Clinical patterns of hypersensitivity to nonsteroidal anti-inflammatory drugs and their pathogenesis. J Allergy Clin Immunol 1977;60(5):276–84.

49. Settipane RA, Stevenson DD. Cross sensitivity with acetaminophen in aspirin-sensitive subjects with asthma. J Allergy Clin Immunol 1989;84(1):26–33.

50. Martin-Garcia C, Hinojosa M, Berges P, et al. Safety of a cyclooxygenase-2 inhibitor in patients with aspirin-sensitive asthma. Chest 2002;121(6):1812–7.

51. Nizankowska-Mogilnicka E, Bochenek G, Mastalerz L, et al. EAACI/GA2LEN guideline: aspirin provocation tests for diagnosis of aspirin hypersensitivity. Allergy 2007;62(10):1111–8.

52. Stevenson DD. Aspirin sensitivity and desensitization for asthma and sinusitis. Curr Allergy Asthma Rep 2009;9(2):155–63.

53. White A, Ludington E, Mehra P, et al. Effect of leukotriene modifier drugs on the safety of oral aspirin challenges. Ann Allergy Asthma Immunol 2006;97(5): 688–93.

54. White AA, Bosso JV, Stevenson DD. The clinical dilemma of "silent desensitization" in aspirin-exacerbated respiratory disease. Allergy Asthma Proc 2013; 34(4):378–82.

55. Chen JR, Buchmiller BL, Khan DA. An hourly dose-escalation desensitization protocol for aspirin-exacerbated respiratory disease. J Allergy Clin Immunol Pract 2015;3(6):926–31.e1.

56. Lee RU, White AA, Ding D, et al. Use of intranasal ketorolac and modified oral aspirin challenge for desensitization of aspirin-exacerbated respiratory disease. Ann Allergy Asthma Immunol 2010;105(2):130–5.

57. Lee JY, Simon RA, Stevenson DD. Selection of aspirin dosages for aspirin desensitization treatment in patients with aspirin-exacerbated respiratory disease. J Allergy Clin Immunol 2007;119(1):157–64.

58. Cho KS, Soudry E, Psaltis AJ, et al. Long-term sinonasal outcomes of aspirin desensitization in aspirin exacerbated respiratory disease. Otolaryngol Head Neck Surg 2014;151(4):575–81.

59. Shah S, Mehta V. Controversies and advances in non-steroidal anti-inflammatory drug (NSAID) analgesia in chronic pain management. Postgrad Med J 2012; 88(1036):73–8.

Systemic and Odontogenic Etiologies in Chronic Rhinosinusitis

Edward C. Kuan, MD, MBA, Jeffrey D. Suh, MD*

KEYWORDS

- Chronic rhinosinusitis • Cystic fibrosis
- Eosinophilic granulomatosis with polyangiitis • Granulomatosis with polyangiitis
- Sarcoidosis • Primary ciliary dyskinesia • Odontogenic sinusitis

KEY POINTS

- Cystic fibrosis and primary ciliary dyskinesia result in pansinusitis and inspissated, thick mucopurulent secretions. Surgical therapy requires extended procedures to achieve antrostomies or ventilation and to treat obstructive polyposis.
- Patients with sinonasal sarcoidosis tend to present with nasal crusting, anosmia, and epistaxis. The nasal mucosa of the septum and turbinates may demonstrate nodules.
- Vasculitides present with lower respiratory tract disease. Medical therapy is the mainstay of therapy, with surgery indicated for severe symptoms, recurrent infections, and anatomic obstruction.
- Odontogenic sinusitis should be suspected in any patient with unilateral maxillary sinusitis with a longstanding history of maxillary dental problems or a recent history of a maxillary dental procedure.
- Otolaryngologists should personally review imaging studies to look for any bony dehiscence or anomalous connections between the maxillary sinus and the oral cavity.

INTRODUCTION

Although the majority of cases are largely attributed to local factors (ie, anatomic, allergic, immunologic, infectious), chronic rhinosinusitis (CRS) may also be caused by systemic or odontogenic disease. It is thus important for otolaryngologists to be aware of systemic and odontogenic etiologies of CRS, and to approach the management of these patients from a multidisciplinary standpoint. A thorough history, with

Conflicts of Interest: None.
Financial Disclosures: None.
Department of Head and Neck Surgery, University of California, Los Angeles (UCLA) Medical Center, 10833 Le Conte Avenue, 62-132 CHS, Los Angeles, CA 90095, USA
* Corresponding author.
E-mail address: jeffsuh@mednet.ucla.edu

Otolaryngol Clin N Am 50 (2017) 95–111
http://dx.doi.org/10.1016/j.otc.2016.08.008
0030-6665/17/© 2016 Elsevier Inc. All rights reserved.

special attention to comorbidities and medical conditions, should be elicited from each patient. Because all of these conditions have manifestations in multiple organ systems, consultations with other specialists should be sought in each case. In this review, we discuss the most common systemic diseases with distinguishing sinonasal manifestations, including cystic fibrosis (CF), sarcoidosis, vasculitides, primary ciliary dyskinesia (PCD), and odontogenic sinusitis.

SYSTEMIC ETIOLOGIES OF CHRONIC RHINOSINUSITIS
Cystic Fibrosis

CF is a relatively common autosomal-recessive genetic disorder involving a derangement in the gene encoding the CF transmembrane conductance regulator (*CFTR*). The most common mutation is ΔF508, or deletion of the phenylalanine codon at position 508, of which 1 out of 25 to 30 Caucasians are carriers.[1] This mutation results in restricted efflux of anions, such as chloride and bicarbonate, thus leading to thick, obstructive, inspissated sinobronchopulmonary secretions, further promoting mucosal inflammation and superinfections.[2] The pancreas and reproductive systems are also affected, frequently leading to exocrine insufficiency and male infertility, respectively. More recent studies have classified CF patients as either high or low risk based on *CFTR* genotype, with an apparent impact on prognosis.[3–7] Specifically, high-risk CF patients have an earlier age of diagnosis, worse pulmonary status (ie, lower forced expiratory volume at 1 second), increased colonization by *Pseudomonas aeruginosa*, increased sweat chloride, and worse overall survival.[8,9]

Patients tend to present with clinical manifestations of CF at a young age. A history of recurrent sinonasal and bronchopulmonary infections in a child should prompt consideration of a workup for CF. Similarly, the finding of nasal polyposis in a child is suggestive of unrecognized CF, occurring in one-third to one-half of patients.[10–12] On computed tomography (CT) imaging of the sinuses, CF patients tend to have hypoplasia of all sinuses (**Fig. 1**).[13,14] In a study by Ferril and colleagues,[9] comparison of high- and low-risk CF patients additionally found that high risk-patients are even more likely to have sinus hypoplasia. CF patients also tend to develop mucoceles.[15] Throughout their lives, CF patients require close care by pulmonologists, gastroenterologists, geneticists, otolaryngologists, respiratory therapists, and nutritionists to optimize their medical condition and preserve functional status.

Newborn screening for CF using serum immunoreactive trypsinogen and genetic testing for *CFTR* mutations is now nearly universal in the United States.[16,17] A diagnosis of CF can be made by (1) clinical signs and symptoms indicative of the diagnosis and (2) one of the following: (a) abnormal sweat chloride test on 2 separate occasions,

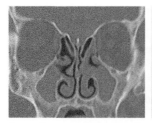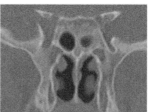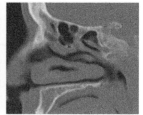

Fig. 1. Computed tomography image of the paranasal sinuses in a patient with cystic fibrosis showing maxillary (*left*), sphenoid (*center*), and frontal (*right*) sinus hypoplasia. Also note the significant bony thickening and osteitic changes surrounding the borders of each sinus, suggesting chronic inflammation.

(b) having 2 disease-causing mutations in *CFTR*, or (c) an abnormal nasal potential difference (less commonly used).[18] The most commonly used diagnostic tool is the sweat chloride test, which is deemed abnormal if 60 mmol/L or greater and borderline if between 40 (30 for age <6 months) and 59 mmol/L.[19] Although the test is generally reliable, it may nevertheless miss CF diagnoses up to 3 years of age.[20]

Management principles of CF-related CRS somewhat parallels that of non-CF CRS patients, although coordination with other disciplines is important. Medical therapy frequently involves nasal irrigations and dornase alfa (recombinant deoxyribonuclease) to clear thick secretions, topical and oral corticosteroids to ameliorate mucosal inflammation, and antibiotics for acute infections. Liang and colleagues[21] in a systematic review found that, of these therapies, dornase alfa and topical corticosteroids were associated with significant clinical improvement for CF-related CRS.

Surgical therapy for CF patients is individualized, and may be indicated for patients who have persistent symptoms after medical therapy, have obstructive nasal polyps and mucoceles, develop chronic or recurrent bronchopulmonary infections from rhinogenic flora, and prophylactically before lung transplantation. As opposed to reestablishing mucociliary clearance in non-CF patients, the role of surgery is to promote gravitational drainage of secretions. Often, this plan includes extended procedures such as a mega-antrostomy in place of a standard maxillary antrostomy. Several studies have highlighted significant improvements in quality-of-life after endoscopic sinus surgery (ESS).[22,23] This finding is corroborated by another systematic review by Liang and colleagues,[24] which found that ESS seems to improve symptoms and endoscopy scores, although the impact on lower airway disease is unknown. In the senior author's experience, ESS for CF patients seems to produce clinical improvement in pulmonary disease, and is thus recommended for medically suitable candidates. Most CF patients tolerate ESS in an outpatient setting. Soudry and colleagues[25] found in a cohort of 33 CF patients that postoperative pain, but not preoperative medical condition (eg, pulmonary function), was associated with inpatient admission after ESS for CF-related CRS, underscoring the importance of careful postoperative monitoring.

Another consideration is the impact of prophylactic ESS in CF patients before lung transplantation. Some experts have found that ESS not only seems to decrease *Pseudomonas* colonization and subsequent bronchopulmonary infections, but also decreases the risk of bronchiolitis obliterans and improves posttransplant survival.[26,27] In contrast, Leung and colleagues[28] found in a retrospective review of 87 CF lung transplant patients who underwent pretransplant ESS that bacterial recolonization occurred in 87% of cases within the course of several weeks postoperatively, with no change in survival as compared with those who did not undergo ESS. Prospective studies are required to define the clinical impact of ESS in patients with CF who undergo lung transplantation.

Both within the discipline of rhinology and beyond, novel therapeutic strategies for CF remain an active area of investigation. One proposed strategy to ameliorate the inflammatory consequences of CF-related CRS is through restoration of mucociliary clearance by administering "secretagogues," which promote transepithelial ionic transport. Recently, pharmacologic agents, especially those found naturally or within herbal medications, such as hesperidin,[29] chlorogenic acid,[30] Sinupret (Bionorica, Neumarkt, Germany),[31] quercetin,[32] and resveratrol, or *CFTR* modulators such as genistein, VRT-532, and UCCF-152,[33] have been demonstrated to have such properties based on both in vitro (human) and in vivo (murine and/or porcine) models. Using the same experimental models, tobacco smoke[34] and hypoxia[35] have been found to suppress transepithelial ion transport, worsening mucociliary clearance. Resveratrol in particular has been extensively studied and has been shown to restore mucociliary transport in a model of acquired CFTR deficiency (simulating CF).[36–38] Such therapies are extremely promising in expanding the arsenal of medical management for CF-related CRS.

Sarcoidosis

Sarcoidosis is a systemic granulomatous disease that primarily manifests in the respiratory tract, particularly the lungs in the form of bilateral, diffuse interstitial lung disease.[39] Other organs that may be involved include the skin, eye, heart, endocrine system, and gastrointestinal tract. Although it may affect all races, sarcoidosis is 3 to 4 times more common among blacks, and tends to be more severe in this population.[39] The pathophysiology is unclear, but involves genetic predisposition and modification by environmental factors, ultimately leading to immune dysfunction. Histopathologically, the hallmark of diagnosis is the presence of noncaseating granulomas. The standard workup should include chest radiography (bilateral hilar adenopathy) and laboratory testing (serum angiotensin converting enzyme), with biopsy considered for more accessible sites (eg, skin, nasal cavity), and the diagnosis is made through clinical, radiographic, and histopathologic data.

Sarcoidosis presenting in the sinonasal tract is rather rare, involving only approximately 1% of sarcoidosis cases.[40] CRS likely results through granulomatous destruction of nasal mucosa and surrounding structures (eg, cilia, olfactory fibers, vasculature), creating a drying effect and local tissue destruction (ulceration and perforation). Because the sinonasal signs and symptoms are rather nonspecific (nasal obstruction, crusting, epistaxis), rhinologic manifestations of sarcoidosis, especially at initial presentation, may be easily missed. In 1999, deShazo et al[41] proposed diagnostic criteria to aid in the diagnosis of sinonasal sarcoidosis: (1) radiologic evidence of sinusitis, (2) histopathologic confirmation of noncaseating granuloma in the sinus tissue supported by negative stains for fungus and acid-fast bacilli, (3) negative serologic test results for syphilis and antineutrophil cytoplasmic antibodies (ANCA), and (4) no clinical evidence of other disease processes associated with granulomatous nasal and sinus inflammation. The authors revisited this topic in 2010 and, in reviewing the most common rhinologic manifestations of 36 sarcoidosis patients, found that having 2 of the signs of nasal crusting, anosmia, and epistaxis in a patient with CRS was highly specific for sinonasal sarcoidosis.[42] Other reports have commented on the presence of a nodular appearance of the nasal mucosa overlying the septum and turbinates, which can be readily seen on endoscopy.[43,44]

The mainstay of treatment for sarcoidosis is medical, with symptomatic patients typically treated with systemic corticosteroids. Patients who have persistent disease refractory to corticosteroids may be tried on immunosuppressants (methotrexate, azathioprine, infliximab).[45] In a case control study, Aubart and colleagues[43] found that patients with sarcoidosis with sinonasal involvement tend to be more difficult to treat medically, requiring more frequent and longer durations of therapy. This observation was corroborated by Long and colleagues[46] in another retrospective study involving 6 patients with sinonasal sarcoidosis. Although no specific studies have examined this phenomenon, local medical treatments for the nasal cavity and sinuses may include nasal irrigations, corticosteroids (topical, intralesional, systemic), and antibiotic therapy (topical and systemic), although these therapies are secondary to primary systemic treatment.

The role of surgery for sarcoidosis-related CRS is limited, and should be reserved for patients with severe symptoms attributable to anatomic factors (eg, septal deviation, polyposis, ostiomeatal complex obstruction, scarring, mucocele) or recurrent infections (**Fig. 2**). The only study reviewing ESS for sarcoidosis patients included 6 patients, with symptomatic improvement and decreased steroid use in all cases.[47] In rare cases, patients with unrecognized sarcoidosis (asymptomatic or minimal symptoms) may have primary sinonasal complaints, and the diagnosis may be made after ESS. In the senior author's experience, sarcoidosis-related CRS patients tend to have a higher rate of synechiae formation, and thus the decision to consider surgery should be weighed against the potential need for vigilant postoperative care and the potential for an outcome that may be compromised by the patient's underlying inflammatory response. These patients should be referred to a pulmonologist for further workup and consideration of treatment, if indicated.

Eosinophilic Granulomatosis with Polyangiitis (Churg-Strauss Syndrome)

Previously known as Churg-Strauss syndrome or allergic granulomatosis and angiitis, eosinophilic granulomatosis with polyangiitis (EGPA) is an autoimmune vasculitic condition involving small- and medium-sized arteries.[48] Most commonly, EGPA affects the upper and lower respiratory tracts in the form of allergic rhinitis, CRS, and asthma, but can additionally involve the ear (otitis media, middle ear effusion), peripheral nervous system (neuropathy), heart (cardiomyopathy, pericarditis, arrhythmia), kidneys (acute renal insufficiency), and gastrointestinal tract (eosinophilic gastroenteritis).[49] In fact, sinonasal involvement is common ($\leq$70% of cases), and can manifest as nasal polyposis (60%–70%), crusting, rhinorrhea, anosmia, sneezing, mucopurulent discharge, epistaxis, and septal perforation.[50–53] The disease progresses in a distinct clinical pattern, although occasionally stages may overlap or not occur at all[54]:

1. Prodromal phase (allergic rhinitis, asthma)
2. Eosinophilic phase (serum eosinophilia, progressive pulmonary involvement)
3. Vasculitic phase (granulomatosis, constitutional symptoms)

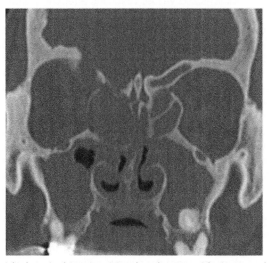

Fig. 2. A patient with chronic rhinosinusitis related to sarcoidosis. Note the thickened bone throughout the facial skeleton as a result of chronic inflammation. There are bilateral ethmoid mucoceles, with the right-sided mucocele causing compression and erosion of the medial orbital wall.

One of the hallmarks of EGPA is serum and tissue eosinophilia. Furthermore, approximately 50% of patients will test positive for ANCA (p-ANCA, or antimyeloperoxidase antibodies, in 70% of cases).[55,56] Although lung biopsy is the gold standard for tissue diagnosis, skin or nerve biopsy is less invasive and thus preferred. Based on the American College of Rheumatology guidelines, a diagnosis of EGPA is highly suggested (85% sensitivity, 99.7% specificity) with 4 or more of the following criteria: (1) asthma (history of and/or active wheezing), (2) greater than 10% eosinophils on differential leukocyte count, (3) peripheral neuropathy, (4) migratory or transient pulmonary opacities on radiologic imaging, (5) rhinosinusitis, and (6) a biopsy containing blood vessel showing eosinophilic accumulation in extravascular areas.[57] Consultation with a rheumatologist is recommended.

Similar to sarcoidosis, treatment is primarily medical, with systemic corticosteroids playing a key role. For patients with multiorgan involvement or severe disease, cyclophosphamide is added to corticosteroids.[58] Once remission is achieved, patients can be switched to maintenance therapy with less toxic immunosuppressants, such as methotrexate or azathioprine. Patients tend to respond well to treatment, with survival greater than 90% at 5 years based 1 study of 118 patients.[59] For sinonasal involvement, nasal irrigations, topical corticosteroids, and antibiotics may be indicated for symptomatic relief.

Because EGPA is a rare condition, no prospective or retrospective analyses of the impact of surgical therapy have been conducted. If the clinical history is suspicious and surgery is planned, surgically removed sinonasal contents should be sent for histopathologic analysis to seek a possible diagnosis.[60] An appropriate strategy for the management of patients with patients is aggressive, timely primary management of systemic disease, with ESS reserved for anatomic obstruction or recurrent infections.

Granulomatosis with Polyangiitis (Wegener's Granulomatosis)

Granulomatosis with polyangiitis (GPA), formerly known as Wegener's granulomatosis, is a small- and medium-sized vessel vasculitis affecting primarily the upper and lower respiratory tract and the renal system. The American College of Rheumatology criteria for GPA includes (1) nasal or oral inflammation (oral ulcers, nasal discharge), (2) abnormal chest radiograph showing nodules, infiltrates, or cavitations, (3) abnormal urinary sediment (microscopic hematuria with or without red cell casts), and (4) granulomatous inflammation on biopsy of a blood vessel or perivascular area.[61] Having 2 of these 4 criteria is 88% sensitive and 92% specific for a diagnosis of GPA.[61]

Laboratory testing should include serum PR3-ANCA (c [cytoplasmic]-ANCA), which is positive in nearly all cases of active, severe disease,[62] but less telling in cases of localized disease.[63] A recent study by Janisiewicz and colleagues[64] showed that higher c-ANCA titers are also associated with increased rheumatologic and otolaryngologic visits, suggesting more severe disease. Although the constellation of symptoms and laboratory results may point to the diagnosis, tissue biopsy, usually of the skin, kidney, or lungs, demonstrating granulomatous inflammation is preferable. Nasal mucosal biopsies are another potential option, though diagnostic yield is lower than biopsies from other sites.[65,66]

Sinonasal involvement in GPA is virtually universal (>90%), and typically manifests as nasal crusting, nasal obstruction, epistaxis, and septal perforation.[67,68] Progression of disease results in further granulomatous tissue inflammation, and cartilage destruction leading to saddle nose deformity (20%) is possible.[68,69] CT imaging of the paranasal sinuses may demonstrate mucosal thickening, septal destruction, osteitis, mucocele formation, neo-osteogenesis, and bone destruction (**Fig. 3**).[69–72]

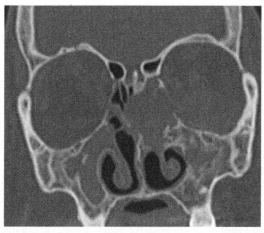

Fig. 3. A patient with chronic rhinosinusitis related to granulomatosis with polyangiitis (Wegener's granulomatosis). Note the extensive osteitic remodeling of the bilateral maxillary sinuses and the massive left ethmoid mucocele that has eroded through the inferior lamina papyracea, then further extends through the septum to the right nasal cavity.

Patients with GPA are initially treated with a combination of corticosteroids and methotrexate (mild disease, limited renal involvement) or cyclophosphamide (moderate to severe disease). Prognosis is generally related to the extent of renal involvement, with survival improving over the last several decades, likely owing to more effective medical therapies.[73] For sinonasal manifestations, local therapies such as nasal irrigations, topical corticosteroids, and antibiotics for infections are used. Once again, surgery may be considered for those patients with severe symptoms, especially those caused by anatomic or infectious factors.

Primary Ciliary Dyskinesia

PCD is a class of inherited disorders involving dysmotility (and sometimes, immotility) of cilia. Motile cilia are hairlike organelles protruding from the cell surface that play a role in transporting mucus and liquids over an epithelial surface through a "beating" motion. The most common mode of inheritance for PCD is autosomal recessive, although a multitude of genes may be affected.[74] Of these, the most common genetic mutation found in PCD patients is that coding for the motor protein dynein.[75] Kartagener syndrome is a subtype of PCD characterized by the triad of CRS, bronchiectasis, and situs inversus.

The direct rhinologic impact of poor ciliary motion is impaired mucociliary clearance, which predisposes patients to formation of thick, inspissated sinonasal secretions that are unable to be properly cleared from the sinuses. In addition, patients may also present with a history of recurrent bronchopulmonary and ear infections. In a retrospective review of 84 children diagnosed with PCD, the most common signs and symptoms were chronic suppurative cough (81%), CRS (71%), neonatal respiratory distress (57%), and recurrent otitis media (49%).[76] Once a diagnosis of PCD is made, consultation with genetics and pulmonology specialists should be sought to initiate appropriate counseling and provide long-term follow-up for monitoring pulmonary function, respectively. Because many patients with PCD are diagnosed in childhood, close collaboration with general and specialist pediatricians is equally critical in the care of PCD patients.

Traditionally, screening of PCD was conducted using the saccharin test, which assesses mucociliary clearance; however, the test is imprecise and thus no longer recommended as a diagnostic tool.[77] More recently, there has been evidence that nasal nitric oxide levels are decreased in PCD patients, and measurement of nitric oxide levels through sampling nasal air has thus supplanted the saccharin test for PCD screening.[78–80] To confirm the diagnosis, electron microscopy must be performed on nasal brush biopsies to evaluate ciliary structure.[81] Ciliary beat frequency and pattern can further be examined to assess motility.[82] CT imaging typically demonstrates pansinusitis, even after therapy (**Fig. 4**).

Owing to the rarity of the disease, there is no consensus statement for the management of sinonasal disease in patients with PCD, although treatment strategies are similar to that for CF-related sinonasal disease (ie, promotion of gravitational drainage). A systematic review by Mener and colleagues[83] found that management of sinonasal disease in children with PCD was highly variable and without adequate outcomes assessment. Medical therapies, including nasal irrigations, topical corticosteroid therapy, and systemic antibiotics for acute infections, are helpful in controlling mucosal inflammation and promoting mucociliary clearance. ESS is recommended for patients who fail to improve with medical therapy, or when patients develop recurrent pulmonary infections from a rhinologic source. Tympanostomy with pressure equalization tubes placement is indicated for recurrent middle ear infections.

ODONTOGENIC SINUSITIS

The floor of the maxillary sinus is in close proximity to the tooth roots of the maxillary molars (teeth #1–3 and #14–16) and, at its most anterior extent, may even be intimately associated with the premolars (teeth #4, #5, #12, and #13).[84] As such, periodontal disease or traumatic disruption of these tooth roots may erode the floor of the maxillary sinus, penetrate the periosteum and mucosa, and lead to maxillary sinusitis. The vast majority of cases (>75%) are unilateral,[85] although a unilateral source leading to sinusitis beyond the maxillary sinus or the contralateral sinus is possible.[86] The microbiology of such infections is quite distinct from that found in nonodontogenic sinusitis,

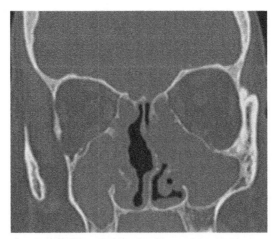

Fig. 4. A patient with primary ciliary dyskinesia after endoscopic sinus surgery. Despite having virtually all septations removed, there remains persistent severe mucosal inflammation producing pansinusitis.

and tends to be composed of a polymicrobial mix of anaerobes (eg, *Peptostreptococcus, Fusobacterium*).[87–89] In a metaanalysis of 770 odontogenic sinusitis cases, the molars are most commonly involved (91%), with overall rare involvement by the premolars (8%) and canines (1%).[90] In the same study, the most common cause was iatrogenic (eg, root canal, dental implants, sinus lift; **Fig. 5**) accounting for 56% of cases, followed by periodontic infections (40%) and odontogenic cysts (7%; **Fig. 6**).[90] Other dentoalveolar conditions such as osteonecrosis of the jaw (ie, bisphosphonate-related[91–94]) and malignancy, however rare, should also be considered in cases of isolated maxillary sinusitis (**Fig. 7**).[95]

Odontogenic sinusitis should be suspected in any patient with unilateral sinusitis with a recent history of dental procedures, especially those involving the upper teeth, or those patients with a longstanding history of dental problems. According to a retrospective review by Pokorny and Tataryn,[85] the most common presenting symptoms of odontogenic sinusitis are facial pain (88%), postnasal discharge (64%), nasal congestion (45%), toothache (39%), and foul drainage (15%). CT imaging of the paranasal sinuses typically reveals unilateral maxillary sinusitis, and careful inspection of the maxillary sinus floor for bone loss (ie, oroantral fistula), dehiscence, or foreign bodies should be performed. Matsumoto and colleagues[96] reviewed 190 CT scans of patients with unilateral sinus opacification and found that more than 70% were attributed to odontogenic infection. Another radiographic study by Bomeli and colleagues[97] found that the extent of maxillary sinus opacification was directly correlated with a concurrent dental source, with 79% of maxillary sinuses that are more than two-thirds opacified caused by an odontogenic infection.

Because odontogenic sinusitis provides a direct entry point for oral flora, it generally cannot be treated adequately with medical or sinonasal surgery alone.[98] Dental extraction, management of periodontal disease, or surgical repair of the oroantral fistula must be performed to resolve the infection.[99] If foreign materials or cystic lesions are implicated in worsening the infection, maxillary antrostomy may be performed to

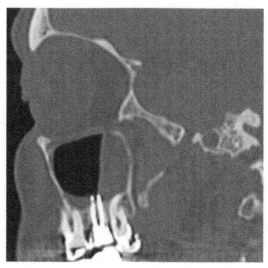

Fig. 5. Left odontogenic maxillary sinusitis in a patient who recently underwent a root canal procedure for tooth #15. Note that the root canal extends through the floor of the maxillary sinus and into the sinus itself.

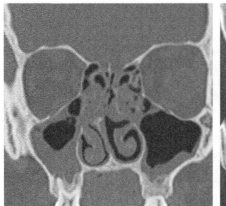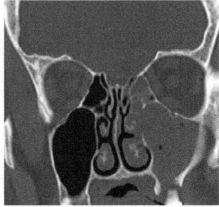

Fig. 6. Two separate patients with odontogenic sinusitis from a periodontal source. In the patient on the *left*, the labial root of tooth #3 has formed a periapical abscess and dehisced through the floor of the maxillary sinus. Also note that the left maxillary sinus and bilateral ethmoid sinuses are inflamed, although there was only one odontogenic source of infection. On the *right*, the patient has a left oroantral fistula from advanced periodontic disease.

gain access for retrieval and marsupialization, respectively.[100] For revision cases or those requiring wide or anterior access, an endoscopic medial maxillectomy (mega-antrostomy) may be performed.[101] Alternatively, a Caldwell-Luc approach may be undertaken, and has the advantage of direct access to the anterior wall of the maxillary sinus. Underdiagnosis and failure to recognize an odontogenic source of sinonasal infection are common, with many accounts in the literature of radiologists failing to mention odontogenic pathologies,[102,103] and, as such, odontogenic sinusitis is associated with a higher rate of revision surgery.[104,105]

Felisati and colleagues[106] presented a prospective series of 257 patients with odontogenic sinusitis, with recommendations for therapy based on the exact cause of the

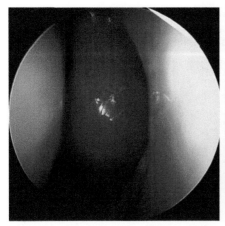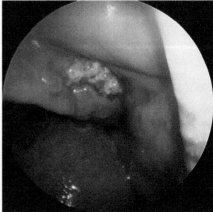

Fig. 7. A patient with left maxillary sinusitis from an odontogenic source. Endoscopy revealed frank mucopurulence in the middle meatus (*left*), and inspection of the oral cavity demonstrated osteonecrosis of the maxillary alveolar ridge (*right*).

odontogenic infection. They developed and followed an algorithm based on the cause, with an impressive 98.8% of patients deemed successfully treated. Their targeted treatment recommendations are as follows[106]:

- The maxillary sinus should be surgically addressed with ESS or a Caldwell-Luc approach in all cases.
- Patients with infection after implant or foreign material placement should have the material removed.
- Patients with oroantral communication should undergo surgical repair, such as with local flaps.

With appropriate treatment, disease resolution rates are high, with a low risk of recurrence. There seems to be no difference in the timing of whether odontogenic or sinonasal treatments are undertaken, as long as both disease processes are addressed. Many studies demonstrating improvement with therapy have significant follow-up times (>2 years).[106,107] Furthermore, because the microbiology is fundamentally different, odontogenic sinusitis requires a different antimicrobial treatment strategy. In the senior author's practice, broad coverage of polymicrobial, anaerobe-predominant organism populations are desired, with penicillins containing a beta-lactamase inhibitor (eg, amoxicillin/clavulanate) or clindamycin, and metronidazole combination therapy fulfilling both of those criteria.

SUMMARY

Recognition of systemic and odontogenic etiologies of CRS is of paramount importance in the care of patients presenting with sinonasal complaints. A comprehensive medical history, with attention to chronic, immunosuppressive conditions, is important. Many systemic etiologies may be diagnosed through certain specific clinical findings:

- CF should be suspected in any child with nasal polyposis, or in patients with recurrent or chronic sinopulmonary infections. These patients should be referred for genetic testing, or for workup of PCD.
- Patients with sarcoidosis may have a nodular appearance of the nasal mucosa and persistent nasal crusting. These patients should undergo chest imaging and laboratory testing for angiotensin-converting enzyme levels.
- Patients with GPA may present with both upper and lower airway disease and renal insufficiency, and the diagnosis is supported with a serum c-ANCA level.
- patients with EGPA tend to present with allergic rhinitis, asthma, and nasal polyposis; a p-ANCA level is helpful in suggesting the diagnosis.
- The otolaryngologist should always personally review imaging with special attention to the floor of the maxillary sinus in patients with unilateral sinusitis to identify a potential odontogenic source.

Treatment is geared toward the underlying condition, with local medical and surgical treatment of the sinonasal tract playing a more supplementary role. To optimize outcomes, otolaryngologists and rhinologists should communicate and coordinate with other disciplines involved in the care of these patients.

REFERENCES

1. Cutting GR, Kasch LM, Rosenstein BJ, et al. A cluster of cystic fibrosis mutations in the first nucleotide-binding fold of the cystic fibrosis conductance regulator protein. Nature 1990;346(6282):366–9.

2. Stoltz DA, Meyerholz DK, Welsh MJ. Origins of cystic fibrosis lung disease. N Engl J Med 2015;372(4):351–62.

3. Fanen P, Wohlhuter-Haddad A, Hinzpeter A. Genetics of cystic fibrosis: CFTR mutation classifications toward genotype-based CF therapies. Int J Biochem Cell Biol 2014;52:94–102.

4. Liechti-Gallati S, Bonsall I, Malik N, et al. Genotype/phenotype association in cystic fibrosis: analyses of the delta F508, R553X, and 3905insT mutations. Pediatr Res 1992;32(2):175–8.

5. McKone EF, Emerson SS, Edwards KL, et al. Effect of genotype on phenotype and mortality in cystic fibrosis: a retrospective cohort study. Lancet 2003; 361(9370):1671–6.

6. McKone EF, Goss CH, Aitken ML. CFTR genotype as a predictor of prognosis in cystic fibrosis. Chest 2006;130(5):1441–7.

7. Schibler A, Bolt I, Gallati S, et al. High morbidity and mortality in cystic fibrosis patients compound heterozygous for 3905insT and deltaF508. Eur Respir J 2001;17(6):1181–6.

8. Bonadia LC, de Lima Marson FA, Ribeiro JD, et al. CFTR genotype and clinical outcomes of adult patients carried as cystic fibrosis disease. Gene 2014;540(2): 183–90.

9. Ferril GR, Nick JA, Getz AE, et al. Comparison of radiographic and clinical characteristics of low-risk and high-risk cystic fibrosis genotypes. Int Forum Allergy Rhinol 2014;4(11):915–20.

10. De Gaudemar I, Contencin P, Van den Abbeele T, et al. Is nasal polyposis in cystic fibrosis a direct manifestation of genetic mutation or a complication of chronic infection? Rhinology 1996;34(4):194–7.

11. Weber SA, Ferrari GF. Incidence and evolution of nasal polyps in children and adolescents with cystic fibrosis. Braz J Otorhinolaryngol 2008;74(1):16–20.

12. Yung MW, Gould J, Upton GJ. Nasal polyposis in children with cystic fibrosis: a long-term follow-up study. Ann Otol Rhinol Laryngol 2002;111(12 Pt 1):1081–6.

13. Eggesbo HB, Sovik S, Dolvik S, et al. CT characterization of developmental variations of the paranasal sinuses in cystic fibrosis. Acta Radiol 2001;42(5): 482–93.

14. Woodworth BA, Ahn C, Flume PA, et al. The delta F508 mutation in cystic fibrosis and impact on sinus development. Am J Rhinol 2007;21(1):122–7.

15. Di Cicco M, Costantini D, Padoan R, et al. Paranasal mucoceles in children with cystic fibrosis. Int J Pediatr Otorhinolaryngol 2005;69(10):1407–13.

16. Cystic Fibrosis F, Borowitz D, Parad RB, et al. Cystic Fibrosis Foundation practice guidelines for the management of infants with cystic fibrosis transmembrane conductance regulator-related metabolic syndrome during the first two years of life and beyond. J Pediatr 2009;155(6 Suppl):S106–16.

17. Farrell PM, Rosenstein BJ, White TB, et al. Guidelines for diagnosis of cystic fibrosis in newborns through older adults: Cystic Fibrosis Foundation consensus report. J Pediatr 2008;153(2):S4–14.

18. Boyle MP. Nonclassic cystic fibrosis and CFTR-related diseases. Curr Opin Pulm Med 2003;9(6):498–503.

19. LeGrys VA, Yankaskas JR, Quittell LM, et al, Cystic Fibrosis Foundation. Diagnostic sweat testing: the Cystic Fibrosis Foundation guidelines. J Pediatr 2007;151(1):85–9.

20. Ooi CY, Castellani C, Keenan K, et al. Inconclusive diagnosis of cystic fibrosis after newborn screening. Pediatrics 2015;135(6):e1377–85.

21. Liang J, Higgins T, Ishman SL, et al. Medical management of chronic rhinosinusitis in cystic fibrosis: a systematic review. Laryngoscope 2014;124(6):1308–13.
22. Khalid AN, Mace J, Smith TL. Outcomes of sinus surgery in adults with cystic fibrosis. Otolaryngol Head Neck Surg 2009;141(3):358–63.
23. Virgin FW, Rowe SM, Wade MB, et al. Extensive surgical and comprehensive postoperative medical management for cystic fibrosis chronic rhinosinusitis. Am J Rhinol Allergy 2012;26(1):70–5.
24. Liang J, Higgins TS, Ishman SL, et al. Surgical management of chronic rhinosinusitis in cystic fibrosis: a systematic review. Int Forum Allergy Rhinol 2013; 3(10):814–22.
25. Soudry E, Mohabir PK, Miglani A, et al. Outpatient endoscopic sinus surgery in cystic fibrosis patients: predictive factors for admission. Int Forum Allergy Rhinol 2014;4(5):416–21.
26. Holzmann D, Speich R, Kaufmann T, et al. Effects of sinus surgery in patients with cystic fibrosis after lung transplantation: a 10-year experience. Transplantation 2004;77(1):134–6.
27. Vital D, Hofer M, Benden C, et al. Impact of sinus surgery on pseudomonal airway colonization, bronchiolitis obliterans syndrome and survival in cystic fibrosis lung transplant recipients. Respiration 2013;86(1):25–31.
28. Leung MK, Rachakonda L, Weill D, et al. Effects of sinus surgery on lung transplantation outcomes in cystic fibrosis. Am J Rhinol 2008;22(2):192–6.
29. Azbell C, Zhang S, Skinner D, et al. Hesperidin stimulates cystic fibrosis transmembrane conductance regulator-mediated chloride secretion and ciliary beat frequency in sinonasal epithelium. Otolaryngol Head Neck Surg 2010;143(3): 397–404.
30. Illing EA, Cho DY, Zhang S, et al. Chlorogenic acid activates CFTR-mediated Cl- Secretion in mice and humans: therapeutic implications for chronic rhinosinusitis. Otolaryngol Head Neck Surg 2015;153(2):291–7.
31. Zhang S, Skinner D, Hicks SB, et al. Sinupret activates CFTR and TMEM16A-dependent transepithelial chloride transport and improves indicators of mucociliary clearance. PLoS One 2014;9(8):e104090.
32. Zhang S, Smith N, Schuster D, et al. Quercetin increases cystic fibrosis transmembrane conductance regulator-mediated chloride transport and ciliary beat frequency: therapeutic implications for chronic rhinosinusitis. Am J Rhinol Allergy 2011;25(5):307–12.
33. Conger BT, Zhang S, Skinner D, et al. Comparison of cystic fibrosis transmembrane conductance regulator (CFTR) and ciliary beat frequency activation by the CFTR Modulators Genistein, VRT-532, and UCCF-152 in primary sinonasal epithelial cultures. JAMA Otolaryngol Head Neck Surg 2013;139(8):822–7.
34. Alexander NS, Blount A, Zhang S, et al. Cystic fibrosis transmembrane conductance regulator modulation by the tobacco smoke toxin acrolein. Laryngoscope 2012;122(6):1193–7.
35. Blount A, Zhang S, Chestnut M, et al. Transepithelial ion transport is suppressed in hypoxic sinonasal epithelium. Laryngoscope 2011;121(9):1929–34.
36. Woodworth BA. Resveratrol ameliorates abnormalities of fluid and electrolyte secretion in a hypoxia-Induced model of acquired CFTR deficiency. Laryngoscope 2015;125(Suppl 7):S1–13.
37. Zhang S, Blount AC, McNicholas CM, et al. Resveratrol enhances airway surface liquid depth in sinonasal epithelium by increasing cystic fibrosis transmembrane conductance regulator open probability. PLoS One 2013;8(11):e81589.

38. Alexander NS, Hatch N, Zhang S, et al. Resveratrol has salutary effects on mucociliary transport and inflammation in sinonasal epithelium. Laryngoscope 2011;121(6):1313–9.
39. Thomas KW, Hunninghake GW. Sarcoidosis. JAMA 2003;289(24):3300–3.
40. McCaffrey TV, McDonald TJ. Sarcoidosis of the nose and paranasal sinuses. Laryngoscope 1983;93(10):1281–4.
41. deShazo RD, O'Brien MM, Justice WK, et al. Diagnostic criteria for sarcoidosis of the sinuses. J Allergy Clin Immunol 1999;103(5 Pt 1):789–95.
42. Reed J, deShazo RD, Houle TT, et al. Clinical features of sarcoid rhinosinusitis. Am J Med 2010;123(9):856–62.
43. Aubart FC, Ouayoun M, Brauner M, et al. Sinonasal involvement in sarcoidosis: a case-control study of 20 patients. Medicine (Baltimore) 2006;85(6):365–71.
44. Braun JJ, Gentine A, Pauli G. Sinonasal sarcoidosis: review and report of fifteen cases. Laryngoscope 2004;114(11):1960–3.
45. Iannuzzi MC, Rybicki BA, Teirstein AS. Sarcoidosis. N Engl J Med 2007;357(21):2153–65.
46. Long CM, Smith TL, Loehrl TA, et al. Sinonasal disease in patients with sarcoidosis. Am J Rhinol 2001;15(3):211–5.
47. Kay DJ, Har-El G. The role of endoscopic sinus surgery in chronic sinonasal sarcoidosis. Am J Rhinol 2001;15(4):249–54.
48. Churg J, Strauss L. Allergic granulomatosis, allergic angiitis, and periarteritis nodosa. Am J Pathol 1951;27(2):277–301.
49. Conron M, Beynon HL. Churg-Strauss syndrome. Thorax 2000;55(10):870–7.
50. Srouji I, Lund V, Andrews P, et al. Rhinologic symptoms and quality-of-life in patients with Churg-Strauss syndrome vasculitis. Am J Rhinol 2008;22(4):406–9.
51. Olsen KD, Neel HB 3rd, Deremee RA, et al. Nasal manifestations of allergic granulomatosis and angiitis (Churg-Strauss syndrome). Otolaryngol Head Neck Surg (1979) 1980;88(1):85–9.
52. Bacciu A, Bacciu S, Mercante G, et al. Ear, nose and throat manifestations of Churg-Strauss syndrome. Acta Otolaryngol 2006;126(5):503–9.
53. Bacciu A, Buzio C, Giordano D, et al. Nasal polyposis in Churg-Strauss syndrome. Laryngoscope 2008;118(2):325–9.
54. Lanham JG, Elkon KB, Pusey CD, et al. Systemic vasculitis with asthma and eosinophilia: a clinical approach to the Churg-Strauss syndrome. Medicine (Baltimore) 1984;63(2):65–81.
55. Sinico RA, Di Toma L, Maggiore U, et al. Prevalence and clinical significance of antineutrophil cytoplasmic antibodies in Churg-Strauss syndrome. Arthritis Rheum 2005;52(9):2926–35.
56. Sable-Fourtassou R, Cohen P, Mahr A, et al. Antineutrophil cytoplasmic antibodies and the Churg-Strauss syndrome. Ann Intern Med 2005;143(9):632–8.
57. Masi AT, Hunder GG, Lie JT, et al. The American College of Rheumatology 1990 criteria for the classification of Churg-Strauss syndrome (allergic granulomatosis and angiitis). Arthritis Rheum 1990;33(8):1094–100.
58. Sinico RA, Bottero P. Churg-Strauss angiitis. Best Pract Res Clin Rheumatol 2009;23(3):355–66.
59. Samson M, Puechal X, Devilliers H, et al. Long-term outcomes of 118 patients with eosinophilic granulomatosis with polyangiitis (Churg-Strauss syndrome) enrolled in two prospective trials. J Autoimmun 2013;43:60–9.
60. van den Boer C, Brutel G, de Vries N. Is routine histopathological examination of FESS material useful? Eur Arch Otorhinolaryngol 2010;267(3):381–4.

61. Leavitt RY, Fauci AS, Bloch DA, et al. The American College of Rheumatology 1990 criteria for the classification of Wegener's granulomatosis. Arthritis Rheum 1990;33(8):1101–7.
62. Finkielman JD, Lee AS, Hummel AM, et al. ANCA are detectable in nearly all patients with active severe Wegener's granulomatosis. Am J Med 2007;120(7): 643.e9-14.
63. Borner U, Landis BN, Banz Y, et al. Diagnostic value of biopsies in identifying cytoplasmic antineutrophil cytoplasmic antibody-negative localized Wegener's granulomatosis presenting primarily with sinonasal disease. Am J Rhinol Allergy 2012;26(6):475–80.
64. Janisiewicz AM, Klau MH, Keschner DB, et al. Higher antineutrophil cytoplasmic antibody (C-ANCA) titers are associated with increased overall healthcare use in patients with sinonasal manifestations of granulomatosis with polyangiitis (GPA). Am J Rhinol Allergy 2015;29(3):202–6.
65. Del Buono EA, Flint A. Diagnostic usefulness of nasal biopsy in Wegener's granulomatosis. Hum Pathol 1991;22(2):107–10.
66. Devaney KO, Travis WD, Hoffman G, et al. Interpretation of head and neck biopsies in Wegener's granulomatosis. A pathologic study of 126 biopsies in 70 patients. Am J Surg Pathol 1990;14(6):555–64.
67. Srouji IA, Andrews P, Edwards C, et al. General and rhinosinusitis-related quality of life in patients with Wegener's granulomatosis. Laryngoscope 2006;116(9): 1621–5.
68. Cannady SB, Batra PS, Koening C, et al. Sinonasal Wegener granulomatosis: a single-institution experience with 120 cases. Laryngoscope 2009;119(4): 757–61.
69. Zycinska K, Wardyn KA, Piotrowska E, et al. Rhinologic and sinonasal changes in PR3 ANCA pulmonary vasculitis. Eur J Med Res 2010;15(Suppl 2):241–3.
70. Yang C, Talbot JM, Hwang PH. Bony abnormalities of the paranasal sinuses in patients with Wegener's granulomatosis. Am J Rhinol 2001;15(2):121–5.
71. Lohrmann C, Uhl M, Warnatz K, et al. Sinonasal computed tomography in patients with Wegener's granulomatosis. J Comput Assist Tomogr 2006;30(1): 122–5.
72. Grindler D, Cannady S, Batra PS. Computed tomography findings in sinonasal Wegener's granulomatosis. Am J Rhinol Allergy 2009;23(5):497–501.
73. Wallace ZS, Lu N, Unizony S, et al. Improved survival in granulomatosis with polyangiitis: a general population-based study. Semin Arthritis Rheum 2016;45(4): 483–9.
74. Horani A, Ferkol TW, Dutcher SK, et al. Genetics and biology of primary ciliary dyskinesia. Paediatr Respir Rev 2016;18:18–24.
75. Zariwala MA, Knowles MR, Omran H. Genetic defects in ciliary structure and function. Annu Rev Physiol 2007;69:423–50.
76. Hosie PH, Fitzgerald DA, Jaffe A, et al. Presentation of primary ciliary dyskinesia in children: 30 years' experience. J Paediatr Child Health 2015;51(7):722–6.
77. Barbato A, Frischer T, Kuehni CE, et al. Primary ciliary dyskinesia: a consensus statement on diagnostic and treatment approaches in children. Eur Respir J 2009;34(6):1264–76.
78. Knowles MR, Daniels LA, Davis SD, et al. Primary ciliary dyskinesia. Recent advances in diagnostics, genetics, and characterization of clinical disease. Am J Respir Crit Care Med 2013;188(8):913–22.
79. Walker WT, Jackson CL, Lackie PM, et al. Nitric oxide in primary ciliary dyskinesia. Eur Respir J 2012;40(4):1024–32.

80. Walker WT, Liew A, Harris A, et al. Upper and lower airway nitric oxide levels in primary ciliary dyskinesia, cystic fibrosis and asthma. Respir Med 2013;107(3): 380–6.

81. Stannard WA, Chilvers MA, Rutman AR, et al. Diagnostic testing of patients suspected of primary ciliary dyskinesia. Am J Respir Crit Care Med 2010;181(4): 307–14.

82. O'Callaghan C, Sikand K, Chilvers MA. Analysis of ependymal ciliary beat pattern and beat frequency using high speed imaging: comparison with the photomultiplier and photodiode methods. Cilia 2012;1(1):8.

83. Mener DJ, Lin SY, Ishman SL, et al. Treatment and outcomes of chronic rhinosinusitis in children with primary ciliary dyskinesia: where is the evidence? A qualitative systematic review. Int Forum Allergy Rhinol 2013;3(12):986–91.

84. Lawson W, Patel ZM, Lin FY. The development and pathologic processes that influence maxillary sinus pneumatization. Anat Rec (Hoboken) 2008;291(11): 1554–63.

85. Pokorny A, Tataryn R. Clinical and radiologic findings in a case series of maxillary sinusitis of dental origin. Int Forum Allergy Rhinol 2013;3(12):973–9.

86. Saibene AM, Pipolo GC, Lozza P, et al. Redefining boundaries in odontogenic sinusitis: a retrospective evaluation of extramaxillary involvement in 315 patients. Int Forum Allergy Rhinol 2014;4(12):1020–3.

87. Brook I. Microbiology of acute and chronic maxillary sinusitis associated with an odontogenic origin. Laryngoscope 2005;115(5):823–5.

88. Brook I. Microbiology of acute sinusitis of odontogenic origin presenting with periorbital cellulitis in children. Ann Otol Rhinol Laryngol 2007;116(5):386–8.

89. Saibene AM, Vassena C, Pipolo C, et al. Odontogenic and rhinogenic chronic sinusitis: a modern microbiological comparison. Int Forum Allergy Rhinol 2016;6(1):41–5.

90. Arias-Irimia O, Barona-Dorado C, Santos-Marino JA, et al. Meta-analysis of the etiology of odontogenic maxillary sinusitis. Med Oral Patol Oral Cir Bucal 2010; 15(1):e70–3.

91. Khan AM, Sindwani R. Bisphosphonate-related osteonecrosis of the skull base. Laryngoscope 2009;119(3):449–52.

92. Koulocheris P, Weyer N, Liebehenschel N, et al. Suppurative maxillary sinusitis in patients with bisphosphonate-associated osteonecrosis of the maxilla: report of 2 cases. J Oral Maxillofac Surg 2008;66(3):539–42.

93. Mast G, Otto S, Mucke T, et al. Incidence of maxillary sinusitis and oro-antral fistulae in bisphosphonate-related osteonecrosis of the jaw. J Craniomaxillofac Surg 2012;40(7):568–71.

94. Maurer P, Sandulescu T, Kriwalsky MS, et al. Bisphosphonate-related osteonecrosis of the maxilla and sinusitis maxillaris. Int J Oral Maxillofac Surg 2011;40(3): 285–91.

95. Troeltzsch M, Pache C, Kaeppler G, et al. Etiology and clinical characteristics of symptomatic unilateral maxillary sinusitis: a review of 174 cases. J Craniomaxillofac Surg 2015;43(8):1522–9.

96. Matsumoto Y, Ikeda T, Yokoi H, et al. Association between odontogenic infections and unilateral sinus opacification. Auris Nasus Larynx 2015;42(4):288–93.

97. Bomeli SR, Branstetter BF 4th, Ferguson BJ. Frequency of a dental source for acute maxillary sinusitis. Laryngoscope 2009;119(3):580–4.

98. Longhini AB, Branstetter BF, Ferguson BJ. Unrecognized odontogenic maxillary sinusitis: a cause of endoscopic sinus surgery failure. Am J Rhinol Allergy 2010; 24(4):296–300.

99. Wang KL, Nichols BG, Poetker DM, et al. Odontogenic sinusitis: a case series studying diagnosis and management. Int Forum Allergy Rhinol 2015;5(7): 597–601.
100. Costa F, Emanuelli E, Robiony M, et al. Endoscopic surgical treatment of chronic maxillary sinusitis of dental origin. J Oral Maxillofac Surg 2007;65(2):223–8.
101. Konstantinidis I, Constantinidis J. Medial maxillectomy in recalcitrant sinusitis: when, why and how? Curr Opin Otolaryngol Head Neck Surg 2014;22(1):68–74.
102. Longhini AB, Ferguson BJ. Clinical aspects of odontogenic maxillary sinusitis: a case series. Int Forum Allergy Rhinol 2011;1(5):409–15.
103. Longhini AB, Branstetter BF, Ferguson BJ. Otolaryngologists' perceptions of odontogenic maxillary sinusitis. Laryngoscope 2012;122(9):1910–4.
104. Lopatin AS, Sysolyatin SP, Sysolyatin PG, et al. Chronic maxillary sinusitis of dental origin: is external surgical approach mandatory? Laryngoscope 2002; 112(6):1056–9.
105. Albu S, Baciut M. Failures in endoscopic surgery of the maxillary sinus. Otolaryngol Head Neck Surg 2010;142(2):196–201.
106. Felisati G, Chiapasco M, Lozza P, et al. Sinonasal complications resulting from dental treatment: outcome-oriented proposal of classification and surgical protocol. Am J Rhinol Allergy 2013;27(4):e101–6.
107. Kim SJ, Park JS, Kim HT, et al. Clinical features and treatment outcomes of dental implant-related paranasal sinusitis: a 2-year prospective observational study. Clin Oral Implants Res 2015. [Epub ahead of print]. Available at: http://www.ncbi.nlm.nih.gov/pubmed/25675967.

Office Procedures in Refractory Chronic Rhinosinusitis

Andrew Thamboo, MD, MHSc, FRCSC, Zara M. Patel, MD*

KEYWORDS

- Office-based rhinology • Office procedures for rhinosinusitis
- Office procedures for sinusitis • Office sinus surgery • Office-based sinus surgery

KEY POINTS

- Choosing the appropriately tolerant patient to undergo office procedures will increase your chances for success.
- Procedures commonly done in the operating room can be performed in the office, if the appropriate anesthetic and patient monitoring is in place.
- Knowing the relative contraindications for specific in-office procedures will help to avoid complications.
- The office setting provides patients with refractory chronic rhinosinusitis an option to consider procedures done awake versus undergoing a general anesthetic.

INTRODUCTION

There is good evidence that patients with recalcitrant chronic rhinosinusitis (CRS) benefit from surgical therapy compared with medical therapy.[1] Delaying surgical intervention not only affects symptomatology, but productivity as well. The costs associated with lost productivity for CRS patients can be substantial.[2] Consequently, patients often seek immediate solutions whenever possible. For a number of reasons, including rapid return to work, avoidance of general anesthesia, decreased procedural costs, patient factors, or the simplicity of the procedure, patients or surgeons may prefer that procedures be performed in an office setting. There is no standard algorithm for determining whether a patient should be managed by an in-office procedure; therefore, a surgeon must provide an individualized approach to each patient based on their

Disclosure Statement: Dr A. Thamboo does not have any relevant commercial or financial conflicts of interests or funding sources. Dr. Z.M. Patel has served as a consultant for Medtronic and Patara Pharma and is on the Intersect ENT Speakers Bureau.
Department of Otolaryngology-Head and Neck Surgery, Stanford University School of Medicine, 801 Welch Road, Stanford, CA 94305-5739, USA
* Corresponding author.
E-mail address: zmpatel@stanford.edu

clinical presentation and objective findings. Depending on the presenting problem, surgeon skill set, and required equipment, many patients can successfully tolerate sinonasal surgery in the office setting under local anesthesia. A solid grasp of the complex sinonasal anatomy and its relationship to vital structures, in addition to an understanding of the pathophysiology of presenting symptoms, will allow the surgeon to choose the best surgical approach to address the problem. Most in-office procedures are first mastered in the operating room before the clinic setting, which results in a better patient experience. With time and experience, a competent and skilled surgeon is able to provide patients with outcomes in the clinic setting comparable with those of the operating room for specific procedures.

PROCEDURE ROOM SETUP

The ability to perform any of the procedures described herein requires proper procedural setup. The surgeon should be able to perform the procedure comfortably and all assistants involved should be aware of their role in the procedure. Most surgical procedures are performed with the patient sitting semirecumbent in an examination chair. There must be room to place the chair supine in case the patient has a vasovagal attack from instrumenting the nasal cavity. For right-handed surgeons, the surgeon will be to the right of the patient, and the video tower should be ergonomically placed to the left of the patient for comfortable viewing over a prolonged period of time. The assistant is best placed wherever they can most easily provide equipment to the surgeon while closely monitoring the patient (**Fig. 1**). The equipment needed on the assistant's tray depends on the procedure, but in general it can include a straight and curved suction, straight and angled forceps (either cutting or noncutting), cotton pledgets, and additional topical and local anesthetic. We also have powered instrumentation available in the office for procedural use. The senior author routinely uses pediatric endoscopes in the office to allow for easy instrumentation in an awake patient. A 30° rigid endoscope allows appropriate visualization into all sinuses. A 0° can be used as well, but may not provide appropriate visualization into the frontal recess/sinus, anterior or far lateral portions of the maxillary sinus, or inferior portions of the sphenoid sinus. Additional equipment requirements are discussed with each procedure.

In case of an emergency, the room should be set up to facilitate additional personnel. All individuals involved in the care of the patient should know the protocol

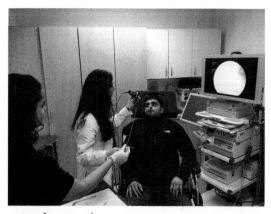

Fig. 1. Office room setup for procedures.

if an emergency arises. The room should be equipped with a blood pressure machine and continuous oxygen saturation monitoring. An automated external defibrillator and oxygen tank should be located nearby in case of an emergency. As in any procedure room or operating suite, a "crash cart" with appropriate medication to run a code (ie, epinephrine, atropine) should be available.

PATIENT SELECTION

Not all patients are comfortable undergoing procedures while awake, and it is important for the surgeon to gauge well in advance whether the patient is capable of tolerating the procedure. A thorough and honest discussion with the patient about the level of discomfort they may experience is paramount to selecting patients appropriately. If, despite your preoperative due diligence, it becomes apparent during a procedure that a patient cannot tolerate instrumentation regardless of a reasonable amount of local and/or regional anesthetic, the procedure can always be aborted and electively performed in the operating room at a later date. Procedures may be aborted owing to discomfort from poor access; therefore, it is important to recognize that simple and straightforward procedures performed in the operating room can become substantially more difficult in patients with a deviated septum or narrow nose. Consequently, in general, it is a contraindication to perform in-office procedures in patients who have demonstrated access issues on prior endoscopy. Other possible contraindications include allergy to local anesthetic, and if a patient has scarring from prior surgeries that does not allow for appropriate intranasal localization based on traditional endoscopic landmarks. Just as when operating in a traditional setting, after thorough discussion of the risks, benefits, and alternatives of a procedure, informed consent to perform the procedure should always be obtained.

Also, similarly to when proceeding with patients in the operating room, surgeons should ensure that patients are medically fit to undergo the procedure. Some comorbidities that would increase a patient's cardiovascular risk were they to undergo the stress of general anesthesia may show these patients to be better suited for an office procedure instead. In contrast, coagulopathies can be a relative contraindication to operating in an office setting where controlling blood loss is not as simple as cauterization; generally, the pain associated with thermal cauterization would be too great in an awake patient. Those who are taking medications such as aspirin or clopidogrel should stop their medications 7 to 10 days before the procedure. However, if patients have a history of coronary artery bypass, guidelines indicate they should continue with at least aspirin without interruption.[3] When taking patients off blood thinning agents, it is always prudent to discuss the potential cardiovascular risk of that action with their primary doctors or cardiologists. Nonsteroidal anti-inflammatory drugs should also be discontinued 7 days before the procedure. Regardless of whether the patient is inherently more likely to bleed or not, in any procedure where greater than minimal blood loss is expected, the controlled environment of the operating room is likely best to ensure control of the airway if compromise occurs.

Last, in our current health care system where insurance coverage is highly variable for particular procedures, and can differ depending on the location (operating room vs office) and the specific equipment or device being used, these logistical factors may sometimes also come into play in patient selection. If coverage is denied, like in any other circumstance where this happens, it then should lead to a conversation between the provider and patient based on the specific practice protocol that generally determines who would be responsible for the cost going uncovered by the insurance company. This is never a conversation that should be left for after the procedure is performed—cost should always be an upfront, completely transparent topic and the patient should never be left feeling surprised about this aspect of care.

INTRANASAL PREPARATION

The anesthetic component is arguably the most critical component in doing in-office procedures successfully. The degree of anesthesia varies depending on the procedure, but having patience and properly anesthetizing the nasal cavity allows the surgeon to best perform the procedure in a comfortable and cooperative patient.

There are many techniques for anesthetizing the nose both topically and with local injections. Our technique is to initially decongest and topically anesthetize with 4% lidocaine and 1% phenylephrine, then place pledgets or cotton swabs soaked in lidocaine and phenylephrine at the surgical site intranasally at the onset of the patient encounter for at least 5 to 10 minutes to allow maximal time for anesthesia and decongestion before beginning any form of instrumentation. Topical application of lidocaine and epinephrine allow for better visualization and, equally important, decongestion decreases inadvertent mucosal trauma and bleeding because there is more room for instrumentation. There are other topical agents available such as 4% cocaine and tetracaine. Cocaine was commonly used in the past because it acted as a topical anesthetic and vasoconstrictor simultaneously but a number of surgeons have strayed away from it owing to adverse cardiac effects such as severe bradycardia and ventricular ectopy. If cocaine is to be used, it is important to obtain a cardiac history before use. Tetracaine is a common alternative to lidocaine. Tetracaine acts longer and in combination with a vasoconstrictor provides comparable results to our use of lidocaine and phenylephrine. Areas of expected dissection can be further injected with 1% lidocaine and 1:100,000 epinephrine. Injection is optimally performed slowly with a small needle ($\leq$25 gauge). It is important to consider injecting areas that the scope or instruments may touch along the nasal cavity (ie, lateral nasal wall if performing a septoplasty with sharp spur) to limit patient discomfort owing to instrumentation. As always, one must withdraw before injection to prevent intravascular injection of local anesthetic.

If intravenous sedation is required to perform the procedure, appropriate staff and monitoring equipment are necessary in the office. Owing to limitations in monitoring after sedation, we prefer to perform only procedures requiring topical or injection anesthetic in our office setting.

OFFICE-BASED POLYPECTOMY
Indication

The incidence of symptomatic CRS with nasal polyps is 1% to 4%.[4] CRS with nasal polyps presents surgeons with a unique management opportunity compared with CRS without polyps. Patients with CRS with nasal polyps can present with symptoms including facial pain/pressure, nasal obstruction, anterior or posterior nasal discharge, and hyposmia.[5] Surgeons can provide dramatic symptomatic improvement, especially in those with previously operated sinuses, through an office-based polypectomy.

Patient Selection

Computed tomography (CT) imaging and endoscopy are necessary for determining if patients are candidates for office-based polypectomy. Additionally, an MRI should be ordered before the procedure (whether it is planned for the office or operating room) if there is any question at all that the polyp may instead be a meningoencephalocele or tumor. The most common presentation of patients who are good candidates for office-based polypectomy are those who have had previous sinus surgery and have open bony ostia and sinus cavities that are obstructed with polypoid soft tissue. CT should be used to delineate the extent of disease as well as to demonstrate any residual bony partitions remaining within the sinuses. The CT should also be reviewed as usual in a standardized fashion to assess for dangerous findings such as a dehiscent orbit and low-lying anterior ethmoid artery. Incomplete surgical dissection of multiple or thickened bony partitions may lead the surgeon to suggest a more comprehensive surgery under general anesthetic, depending on the goals of the procedure. However, even if it is decided that patients would benefit most from formal endoscopic surgery in the operating room, in those that have a long waiting period owing to centralized health care systems (ie, Canada, UK) or perhaps if comorbidities prevent them from undergoing general anesthetic after all, in-office removal of polyps from within the nasal cavity itself will certainly improve nasal obstruction, possibly enhance topical drug delivery, and improve their quality of life.

Procedure

Before and after surgical treatment, surgeons should also provide medical management of CRS with nasal polyps. Although this is not within the scope of this article, the longevity of success of office-based polypectomy depends on medical management.

Appropriate equipment is required to perform this procedure successfully in the office. The most common instrument used to remove polyps is the microdebrider. The ability to simultaneously suction and sharply cut polyps has revolutionized the treatment of CRS.[6,7] Electrically powered microdebriders frequently used in the operating rooms are commonly used in the clinic setting as well (**Fig. 2**), but other mechanical and suction-powered options have recently been made available and can be also be used with high efficacy (**Fig. 3**).[8] The use of coblation to remove nasal polyps has shown some promising results with respect to mucosal healing and decreased blood loss in human subjects, but has not been as adopted widely.[9–11]

The intranasal preparation has been mentioned and the surgical technique is similar to the approach in the operating room, except that the patient is sitting in a relatively upright chair, awake with local anesthesia alone. Hemostasis is improved through the avoidance of general anesthetics that cause vasodilation[12] and the position of the head being elevated.[13] Isolated polyps can be addressed with through-cutting instruments, but extensive polyps are addressed with powered

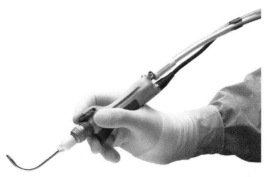

Fig. 2. Electrically powered microdebrider. (*Courtesy of* Medtronic, Minneapolis, MN; with permission. © Medtronic, Inc.)

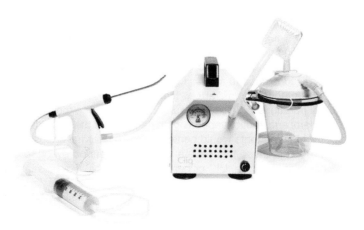

Fig. 3. Suction-powered microdebrider. (*Courtesy of* Laurimed, Redwood City, CA; with permission.)

instrumentation. Polyps are removed in an anterior to posterior and inferior to superior fashion. Removal of pedunculated nasal polyps should have minimal bleeding and cause minimal discomfort to patients. If bleeding does occur or the patient experiences discomfort, the use of pledgets soaked in 1% lidocaine with 1:1000 epinephrine will help with both visualization and pain control. The ethmoid and sphenoid sinuses are best addressed with straight instruments, and the maxillary and frontal sinuses with curved instruments.

Possible Complications

As noted, if a meningoencephaocele is not recognized before performing the procedure, it will result in a large cerebrospinal fluid leak. If this complication arises, it is absolutely necessary to be able to recognize it, move the procedure to the more controlled setting of an operating room, and repair it immediately. If a surgeon does not feel capable of repairing this themselves, they should refer the patient immediately to a surgeon with the expertise who can.

During the polypectomy, care should be taken when approaching the area of the sphenopalatine artery. If the vessel is inadvertently cut, direct cauterization over the mucosa can be performed, although this will likely be quite uncomfortable for the awake patient, or a nasal pack can be placed and the patient taken to the operating for a formal sphenopalatine artery cautery or ligation.

Finally, in patients with fulminant nasal polyposis, it is not uncommon to have erosion of the thin bones between the sinuses and important surrounding structures such as the orbit and intracranial cavity. Care must be taken when approaching these limits to ensure no damage to these structures is incurred, potentially leading to orbital hematoma, extraocular muscle damage, blindness, cerebrospinal fluid leak or worse. Although in-office navigation units are available, the experienced surgeon should be able to examine a CT scan preprocedurally and use that knowledge to identify the important landmarks endoscopically. The same risks that are discussed for sinus surgery in the operating room setting should be discussed for surgery in the office setting.

Postprocedure Considerations

Postprocedure considerations are similar to those with a recently patients with CRS with nasal polyps who undergo an operation in an operating room. Based on practice preferences, topical and/or oral steroids can be given to control the disease process. The senior author prescribes budesonide-impregnated saline irrigation after in-office polypectomies. Oral steroids are typically reserved for patients who have not had extensive cumulative dosing of steroids in the past and who have pervasive, debilitating disease still present.

IN-OFFICE TREATMENT OF MUCOCELES
Indication

Patients who have undergone prior sinus surgery will often present with mucocele formation, whether from scarring and entrapped secretions, or lateralization of turbinate remnants causing blocked cells to expand and press on surrounding structures. Mucoceles are among the simplest problems to address in the patient with refractory CRS, with appropriate surgical marsupialization often completely resolving symptomatology.

Procedure

Endoscopic drainage of mucoceles can be successfully done in the office setting.[14] The ability to perform the procedure primarily depends on the location and proximity to neoosteogenesis. The diagnosis of a mucocele is primarily made with a CT scan, but MRI can help to delineate the extent of the lesion if unclear on CT. The most common location of a mucocele is within the frontal sinus.[15] Good candidates for in-office procedures for frontal sinus mucoceles are previously operated patients with mucoceles presenting at the level of the frontal sinus ostia, or at least low enough to be easily accessed with endoscopic instrumentation. The primary goal of marsupialization of a mucocele can be achieved with the usual frontal instrumentation of Kerrison, Hoseman, and angled giraffe through-cuts in the office. The entire lining of the mucocele does not need to be removed, whether the procedure is performed in the office or operating room, as long as there is an adequate opening made to prevent reformation of the mucocele and there is no blockage of surrounding structures. In a similar fashion, mucoceles in the ethmoid, sphenoid, and maxillary sinuses in previously operated patients can be treated in the clinic. Patients can be given the surgeon's standard postoperative medications to help heal the diseased mucosa.

Possible Complications

As in all sinus procedures bleeding, is a potential complication. Commonly, mucosal bleeding slows with a topical vasoconstrictor, but larger vessels may be inadvertently encountered. A suction bovie should always be available. Quick recognition and management of arterial bleeds can still result in a good patient experience.

Understanding the surrounding anatomy will prevent inadvertent instrumentation into vital structures. With respect to mucoceles that extend intracranially, when there is a large dead space that will be left over after complete drainage of a mucocele and there is a chance for shifting of brain parenchyma into that space, it may be safest to address these types of mucoceles in a controlled operative setting instead of the office, and even plan to monitor them for some time postoperatively. Intracranial extension eroding the skull base can also put patients at risk for cerebrospinal fluid leaks if the anatomy is not well-understood and careful dissection is not carried out; therefore, these cases may be best managed in the operating room by surgeons less practiced in performing these procedures in the office.

IN-OFFICE SEPTOPLASTY
Indication

An endoscopic septoplasty can be performed while the patient is awake in a similar fashion to when in the operating room. The potential limitation is the management of the maxillary and palatine spine. The use and sound of heavier instrumentation can be disturbing for some patients if fully awake, and one may need to consider intravenous sedation. The optimal patient for an in-office septoplasty is one with an isolated spur or limited cartilaginous deflection where very focused and directed surgical manipulation can create a great improvement in the patient's quality of life.

Procedure

The patient's nose is initially decongested and topically anesthetized with 1% lidocaine with 1:1000 epinephrine. The septum is further injected with 1% lidocaine and 1:100,000 epinephrine. Injection sites can vary depending on the goal of the septoplasty. The incision site should be injected, especially if a hemitransfixion incision is considered. Broad-based mucosal flaps will be raised more facilely if one injects the entire length of the septum to help establish a dissection plane underneath the subperichondrial layer. The remaining aspects of the procedure are performed in similar fashion as in the operating room. In our practice, quilting sutures (dissolvable) are placed with no nasal packing or splints to reapproximate the elevated mucosa. This results in improved patient comfort after the procedure with no detrimental effect on the outcome of the septoplasty.

For the isolated spur, a Cottle elevator can be used to incise along the length of the apex of the spur in an anterior to posterior direction. Mucosa should be completely raised surrounding the spur, and then the Cottle or a Freer elevator can be used to carefully carve off or "pop out" the deflected portion of cartilage or bone. As long as there has been no damage to the opposite flap of mucosa, there is no need for any suturing or closure after this technique. If a through and through perforation is noted at the completion of the procedure, the repair can be carried out in the office setting as well. It is important to have all the usual suture material available in the operating room. Some surgeons also choose to place a grafting material between the 2 mucosal leaves being sewn back together, and if that is to be carried out, and this material should also be available in the office setting.

Possible Complications

As in the operating room, bleeding and septal perforation are the rare but most likely complications after a septoplasty. Ensuring patient comfort before beginning the dissection can be the most useful way to avoid either of these complications. A stationary patient will be less likely to have mucosal injury or increased bleeding. If bleeding is encountered, topical vasoconstrictors are first-line options, with cautery always available. If tears are made through the opposing mucosal flaps at the same location, then care should be taken to suture the mucosal surfaces together carefully, and in some cases placing synthetic grafts between the 2 surfaces is the best option to promote healing without persistent perforation.

IN-OFFICE MANAGEMENT OF STENOSIS AND SYNECHIAE
Indication

Patients who have previously undergone sinus surgery often continue to have sinonasal symptoms, either owing to incomplete or misdirected surgery or postoperative scarring. Endoscopy, and potentially a repeat CT scan, may reveal these issues to be the cause of symptoms in a previously operated patient. Patients may experience stenosis or synechiae formation after sinus surgery and patients' symptoms can often be optimized by addressing these issues in the clinic. If a surgeon sees the beginnings of scar formation early in the postoperative period, appropriate debridement at this time can prevent mature scar formation. However, if a patient has come to the clinic long after some prior procedure and mature scar formation already exists, this situation can also be easily addressed in the office setting.

Procedures

The most common procedures performed in the clinic address postoperative changes secondary to sinus surgery, to keep ostial outflow tracts patent and prevent or address mucus recirculation. The degree of the stenosis and location of the opening dictate how aggressively a surgeon must work to reestablish a patent sinus. It is important that the natural ostium is included in the opening of a patent sinus cavity. Balloon ostial dilation (described elsewhere in this paper) is a common technique used to address mild to moderate stenosis.[16] This option should only be considered if the natural ostium is already included in the opening of the sinus. For severely stenosed sinuses with bony regrowth or sinuses that do not include the natural ostia, they can be reopened and connected to the natural ostia with through-cutting instruments in the standard fashion, as in the operating room.

Recirculation of mucus secondary to iatrogenic synechiae can also be successfully managed in the office setting.[17] It is important to recognize in the office that adjacent openings within a patent sinus can result in recirculation and stasis of mucus, which in turn will cause persistent sinonasal symptoms (**Fig. 4**). Back-biting and through-cutting instruments can be used to create one common cavity. To prevent reformation of the synechiae, it is important not to strip the mucosa and avoid apposing raw mucosal surfaces. In general, there are no special postprocedure instructions required for these patients. If there is a strong chance of synechiae reforming, a silastic sheet or

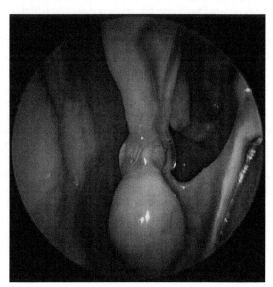

Fig. 4. Recirculation of mucus around basal lamella and vertical attachment of middle turbinate.

similar material may be used to separate the 2 raw surfaces. Consequently, the silastic requires in situ suturing or the placement of a suture that is taped to the cheek so it can be removed at a later date.

Possible Complications

Bleeding or damage to surrounding structures are always possible when instrumenting the sinuses, but are minimal when dealing with isolated synechiae or stenosis. The one major caution would be to ensure the frontal ostia that seems to be scarred down is definitively the true ostium of the sinus, or firm entrance with a balloon or seeker could inadvertently enter the eye or brain.

BALLOON DILATION

Balloon ostial dilation was initially coined "balloon sinuplasty" by Acclarent (Menlo Park, CA) in 2005,[17] but since their inception a number of similar devices have entered the market. The goal of balloon dilation is to dilate the sinus outflow paths without actually removing tissue from the sinus cavity. There are a number of safety and feasibility studies, most of which have been done when sinus dilation has been performed in the operating room,[18–20] with patency rate ranging from 85.1% to 91.6% depending on whether patency was determined endoscopically or radiologically, respectively.[20,21] A large retrospective review by Levine and colleagues[22] showed that 73.8% of 1036 patients maintained improved symptoms at a mean follow-up of 40.2 weeks. A multicenter prospective trial, specifically assessing outcomes of balloon dilation in the office, showed significant reduction of disease specific quality of life measures ($P<.0001$) at 1 year with significantly fewer acute sinus infections ($P<.0001$), less antibiotic use ($P<.0001$), and fewer physician-related visits ($P<.0001$). One patient underwent revision surgery with no reported device or procedure related adverse events.[23] A recent systematic review showed subanalysis of patients solely undergoing balloon dilation in the office setting having a significant reduction in the impact of disease-specific quality of life measures, but not as great as those receiving the treatment in the operating room. However, the review illustrates the need for unbiased research in this area further evaluating outcomes of balloon dilation in the office setting.[24]

The main criticism of this procedure is the lack of a true surgical control arm in these studies, as well as the relatively short-term follow-up studied thus far.

Indications

Most studies have used balloon dilation in conjunction with functional endoscopic sinus surgery. Therefore, it is difficult to determine the most appropriate patient that will benefit from balloon dilation alone. Contraindications for balloon ostial dilation include patients with primarily ethmoid disease, polyps, fungal disease or neoplasm. Although there may be no clear patient indication at this time, the senior author turns to balloons for previously operated and now mucosally stenosed sinuses, or in patients whom she cannot take to the operating room owing to patient preference or medical impediments. Surgeons who commonly use this tool have suggested possible indications to include CRS patients with limited disease involving the maxillary, frontal, or sphenoid sinus, or those who present with a previously unoperated sinus cavity with a new sinus infection; however, the senior author does not use the balloon for these purposes.

Procedure

Intranasal preparation is similar to that for the aforementioned procedures. Each device on the market includes a sinus guidewire, sinus delivery catheter, sinus balloon, and an inflation device (**Fig. 5**). Some devices have different tips with different angulations depending on the sinus being dilated or tips that can be angulated for any particular sinus. The guidewire is passed through the catheter, and the balloon is passed over the catheter using the Seldinger technique. Guidewires either use an optical fiber to correctly identify sinus cavity dilation or computer image guidance, which requires a navigation system. Just as in all endoscopic surgery, surgeons should have a comfort level with these techniques, but should not depend completely on either to confirm placement, and instead should use the usual endoscopic landmarks that confirm location. The balloon is advanced until it occupies the ostium, at which point it is inflated to the recommended pressure. Depending on the device, the balloon pressure will reach up to 12 atm. The balloon is brought to its recommended pressure, then back to 0 atm. The device is retracted partially, and then the balloon is reinflated. This may be repeated to ensure dilation of the entire drainage pathway.

Possible Complications

Balloon dilation seems to be fairly safe in the office setting. The reported major complication rate per sinus is calculated at 0.0035% in the operating room.[25] The US Food and Drug Administration (FDA) has reported 3 complications secondary to balloon dilation when performed in the operating room. Two involved penetration of the lamina papyracea resulting in pain, ecchymosis, and erythema. One patient had a cerebrospinal fluid leak in a hybrid case, but it is unclear whether the microdebrider or balloon caused the cerebrospinal fluid leak. Recent systematic review of balloon dilation in the office could not make conclusions on the safety of the procedure, but prior large studies have shown it to be safe in the office setting.[23,24]

Postprocedure Considerations

Medical therapy is continued after the procedure with either regular saline irrigations or budesonide-impregnated saline irrigations. Serial follow-up is required to determine if symptomatic relief and endoscopic patency persist. Recurrent stenosis after dilation attempts is usually an indication to go to the operating room for a larger, more definitive surgery.

STEROID-ELUTING STENTS

Steroid-eluting stents can be a viable option in scenarios that require a continued slow release of topical steroids in patients with nasal polyposis despite complete functional endoscopic sinus surgery. Steroid-eluting stents were initially placed intraoperatively within the open ethmoid cavity to preserve sinus patency and reduce medical and surgical interventions after surgery and showed promising results.[26–28] Subsequently,

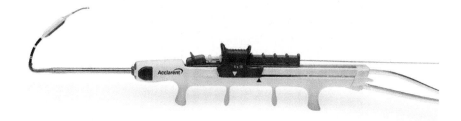

Fig. 5. Balloon sinuplasty device. (*Courtesy of* Acclarent, Irvine CA; with permission. © Acclarent, Inc. 2017.)

further studies showed the in-office placement of steroid-eluting stents into the open ethmoid cavity in postoperative patients was safe, feasible, and effective.[29,30] Despite these studies, the use of these stents in the office setting is not yet approved by the FDA at this time.

Patient Selection

There is no defined population that steroid-eluting stents are used for among patients with CRS, but the stent is used primarily for patients who would benefit from topical steroid delivery. The senior author typically places a steroid-eluting stent into the ethmoid cavity in patients with refractory CRS with nasal polyps who cannot tolerate oral steroid therapy, cannot tolerate or cannot obtain topical steroid irrigations, and those in whom she wishes to use the stenting nature of the device against a lateralizing turbinate. This practice is based on a recent study by Han and colleagues,[31] who performed a randomized, controlled, blinded study involving 100 patients with CRS with nasal polyps refractory to medical therapy and considered candidates for revision functional endoscopic sinus surgery. The study showed a symptomatic improvement and statistically significant reduction in polyp grade. These stents can also be used in patients directly after revision surgery in the office setting.

Procedure

The only implant that has FDA approval is a product called Propel Steroid-Releasing Implant (Intersect ENT, Palo Alto, CA; **Fig. 6**). It has 370 μg of mometasone furoate within its polylactide-co-glycolide polymer matrix allowing for the diffusion of the drug over time, and the implant is expected to dissolve within 30 days.[32] There are a number of other steroid-eluting stents are available, but only Propel is discussed because it is the only product with FDA approval (in the operating room).

These stents use a deploying mechanism with a push cock that places the stent within the sinus cavity. The standard size Propel stent can be maneuvered within the ethmoid cavity so that it does not cover the maxillary sinus ostia while providing drainage to the frontal recess. The Propel Mini has been constructed for the frontal sinuses for targeted therapy, but can also be placed in the posterior ethmoids in cases where direct steroid therapy is required in that cavity.

Patients are best seen around 1 month postoperatively for debridement of any remaining matrix material. The stent may be removed earlier if crusting on the stent impedes sinus drainage. This is easily performed in the office with the use of a grasper and suction.

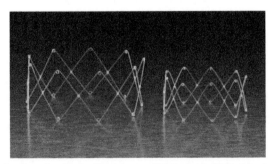

Fig. 6. Steroid-releasing implant. (*Courtesy of* Intersect ENT, Menlo Park, CA; with permission.)

Possible Complications

There have been minimal adverse effects reported in the trials using the Propel stent, which include infection, crusting, and granulation tissue formation.[32] These complications usually can be avoided with appropriate follow-up. With other sinus implants that are not FDA approved, major complications such as orbital violation resulting in severe orbital pain and permanently dilated pupil have been reported.[33]

Postprocedure Considerations

Patients should continue with saline irrigation. They may impregnate the solution with budesonide for additional steroid therapy, but the goal of placement would be for decreased need of other topical steroids. If patients are seen before the 30-day mark, the surgeon can leave the stent in place and have the patient return at the appropriate time for removal or may remove the stent early if it is believed to have served its purpose or seems to be causing too much crusting.

TOPICAL THERAPY APPLIED IN OFFICE

Despite complete surgery and maximal medical therapy, patients can continue to suffer from CRS. Despite low-level evidence, surgeons sometimes choose to try options that may work on a small percentage of patients. We discuss here a few therapies that have been used in the office setting and may provide an option for those who have exhausted all forms of conventional therapy in this challenging subset of patients.

Topical Antibiotic Irrigation

Patients are able to irrigate their sinonasal cavities at home with saline irrigation impregnated with culture-specific antibiotics, but there are instances when such irrigations may be beneficial in the clinic. The general goal of topical antibiotic therapy is to deliver high concentrations of antibiotics while limiting the systemic absorptions and associated side effects.[34] Unfortunately, there may be pockets of infection that at-home irrigations are not addressing and direct irrigation of topical antibiotics with the use of an endoscope may help to resolve the infection. Approximately 30% of cultures are positive for *Pseudomonas aeruginosa* or methicillin-resistant *Staphylococcus aureus* after functional endoscopic sinus surgery.[35] These infections can cause enough inflammation in small pockets of the sinuses to trigger persistent sinonasal symptoms that may benefit from topical antibiotics. Unfortunately, the optimal dosing and treatment duration is unknown. Therefore, patients need close follow-up to establish the optimum individualized regimen for possible repeat irrigation.

Topical Chemical Surfactant

In similar fashion to topical antibiotic therapy, baby shampoo can be added to a patient's own home saline irrigation, but in-office direct irrigation with an endoscope may help to address the direct source of biofilm if this is an underlying problem for the patient. Chiu and colleagues[36] showed that 1% baby shampoo nasal irrigations reduced thickened nasal secretions and postnasal drainage. However, more research regarding chemical surfactants is required with respect to safety. Recently, SinuSurf (NeilMed Pharmaceuticals, Santa Rosa, CA) showed potential clinical improvement, but 1 of its additives seemed to cause anosmia, resulting in the product being removed from the market.

Impregnated Topical Gel Therapy

The concern with impregnated saline irrigation with antibiotics or steroids is the questionability of its capacity to coat the diseased mucosa long enough to have a clinical effect. Alava and colleagues[37] used 2 to 10 mL of 1200 µg/5 mL of mometasone furoate gel in symptomatic patients after functional endoscopic sinus surgery and noted improvement in their symptoms and a reduction in the amount of topical and oral steroids used. In similar fashion, gels can be impregnated with antibiotics and can be considered for use in chronically infected sinuses. Compound pharmacies are required for these type of medications. Further research is required to determine the long-term efficacy of topical gel therapy, and they are not currently FDA approved for this clinical indication.

Photodynamic Therapy

Patients suffering from persistent biofilm may benefit from photodynamic therapy (PDT) in the office setting. In vitro studies have shown that photodynamic therapy reduced CRS polymicrobial biofilm by greater than 99.99% after a single treatment.[38] An in vivo study using 23 symptomatic patients with CRS after surgical showed objective and subjective improvement.[39] Unfortunately, there is still a paucity of literature in this area, despite data from a number of other fields in which photodynamic therapy is used with good supporting evidence.

SUMMARY

The office can be the optimal setting in which to treat patients with refractory CRS. Knowing the appropriate indications, proper patient selection, and availability of equipment and instrumentation necessary are all key components of a successful office procedure.

REFERENCES

1. Smith TL, Kern R, Palmer JN, et al. Medical therapy vs surgery for chronic rhinosinusitis: a prospective, multi-institutional study with 1-year follow-up. Int Forum Allergy Rhinol 2013;3(1):4–9.
2. Rudmik L, Smith TL, Mace JC, et al. Productivity costs decrease after endoscopic sinus surgery for refractory chronic rhinosinusitis. Laryngoscope 2016;126(3): 570–4.
3. Bell AD, Roussin A, Cartier R, et al. The use of anti-platelet therapy in the outpatient setting: Canadian Cardiovascular Society guidelines. Can J Cardiol 2011; 27(Suppl A):S1–59.
4. Larsen K, Tos M. The estimated incidence of symptomatic nasal polyps. Acta Otolaryngol 2002;122(2):179–82.
5. Rosenfeld RM, Piccirillo JF, Chandrasekhar SS, et al. Clinical practice guideline (update): adult sinusitis. Otolaryngol Head Neck Surg 2015;152(2 Suppl):S1–39.
6. Govindaraj S, Adappa ND, Kennedy DW. Endoscopic sinus surgery: evolution and technical innovations. J Laryngol Otol 2010;124(3):242–50.
7. Krouse JH, Christmas DA. Powered nasal polypectomy in the office setting. Ear Nose Throat J 1996;75(9):608–10. Available at: http://www.ncbi.nlm.nih.gov/pubmed/8870366. Accessed February 1, 2016.
8. Gan EC, Habib A-RR, Hathorn I, et al. The efficacy and safety of an office-based polypectomy with a vacuum-powered microdebrider. Int Forum Allergy Rhinol 2013;3(11):890–5.

9. Swibel Rosenthal LH, Benninger MS, Stone CH, et al. Wound healing in the rabbit paranasal sinuses after Coblation: evaluation for use in endoscopic sinus surgery. Am J Rhinol Allergy 2009;23(3):360–3.

10. Swibel-Rosenthal LH, Benninger MS, Stone CH, et al. Wound healing in the paranasal sinuses after coblation, part II: evaluation for endoscopic sinus surgery using a sheep model. Am J Rhinol Allergy 2010;24(6):464–6.

11. Eloy JA, Walker TJ, Casiano RR, et al. Effect of coblation polypectomy on estimated blood loss in endoscopic sinus surgery. Am J Rhinol Allergy 2009;23(5): 535–9.

12. Baker AR, Baker AB. Anaesthesia for endoscopic sinus surgery. Acta Anaesthesiol Scand 2010;54(7):795–803.

13. Hathorn IF, Habib A-RR, Manji J, et al. Comparing the reverse Trendelenburg and horizontal position for endoscopic sinus surgery: a randomized controlled trial. Otolaryngol Head Neck Surg 2013;148(2):308–13.

14. Barrow EM, DelGaudio JM. In-office drainage of sinus mucoceles: an alternative to operating-room drainage. Laryngoscope 2015;125(5):1043–7.

15. Scangas G, Gudis D, Kennedy DW. The natural history and clinical characteristics of paranasal sinus mucoceles: a clinical review. Int Forum Allergy Rhinol 2013;3(9):712–7.

16. Luong A, Batra PS, Fakhri S, et al. Balloon catheter dilatation for frontal sinus ostium stenosis in the office setting. Am J Rhinol 2008;22(6):621–4.

17. DelGaudio JM, Ochsner MC. Office surgery for paranasal sinus recirculation. Int Forum Allergy Rhinol 2015;5(4):326–8.

18. Brown CL, Bolger WE. Safety and feasibility of balloon catheter dilation of paranasal sinus ostia: a preliminary investigation. Ann Otol Rhinol Laryngol 2006; 115(4):293–9 [discussion: 300–1]. Available at: http://www.ncbi.nlm.nih.gov/pubmed/16676826. Accessed February 1, 2016.

19. Kuhn FA. An integrated approach to frontal sinus surgery. Otolaryngol Clin North Am 2006;39(3):437–61, viii.

20. Kuhn FA, Church CA, Goldberg AN, et al. Balloon catheter sinusotomy: one-year follow-up–outcomes and role in functional endoscopic sinus surgery. Otolaryngol Head Neck Surg 2008;139(3 Suppl 3):S27–37.

21. Weiss RL, Church CA, Kuhn FA, et al. Long-term outcome analysis of balloon catheter sinusotomy: two-year follow-up. Otolaryngol Head Neck Surg 2008; 139(3 Suppl 3):S38–46.

22. Levine HL, Sertich AP, Hoisington DR, et al. Multicenter registry of balloon catheter sinusotomy outcomes for 1,036 patients. Ann Otol Rhinol Laryngol 2008; 117(4):263–70. Available at: http://www.ncbi.nlm.nih.gov/pubmed/18478835. Accessed February 1, 2016.

23. Gould J, Alexander I, Tomkin E, et al. In-office, multisinus balloon dilation: 1-Year outcomes from a prospective, multicenter, open label trial. Am J Rhinol Allergy 2014;28(2):156–63.

24. Levy JM, Marino MJ, McCoul ED. Paranasal sinus balloon catheter dilation for treatment of chronic rhinosinusitis: a systematic review and meta-analysis. Otolaryngol Head Neck Surg 2016;154(1):33–40.

25. Melroy CT. The balloon dilating catheter as an instrument in sinus surgery. Otolaryngol Head Neck Surg 2008;139(3 Suppl 3):S23–6.

26. Forwith KD, Chandra RK, Yun PT, et al. ADVANCE: a multisite trial of bioabsorbable steroid-eluting sinus implants. Laryngoscope 2011;121(11):2473–80.

27. Marple BF, Smith TL, Han JK, et al. Advance II: a prospective, randomized study assessing safety and efficacy of bioabsorbable steroid-releasing sinus implants. Otolaryngol Head Neck Surg 2012;146(6):1004–11.
28. Han JK, Marple BF, Smith TL, et al. Effect of steroid-releasing sinus implants on postoperative medical and surgical interventions: an efficacy meta-analysis. Int Forum Allergy Rhinol 2012;2(4):271–9.
29. Matheny KE, Carter KB, Tseng EY, et al. Safety, feasibility, and efficacy of placement of steroid-eluting bioabsorbable sinus implants in the office setting: a prospective case series. Int Forum Allergy Rhinol 2014;4(10):808–15.
30. Lavigne F, Miller SK, Gould AR, et al. Steroid-eluting sinus implant for in-office treatment of recurrent nasal polyposis: a prospective, multicenter study. Int Forum Allergy Rhinol 2014;4(5):381–9.
31. Han JK, Forwith KD, Smith TL, et al. RESOLVE: a randomized, controlled, blinded study of bioabsorbable steroid-eluting sinus implants for in-office treatment of recurrent sinonasal polyposis. Int Forum Allergy Rhinol 2014;4(11):861–70.
32. Wei CC, Kennedy DW. Mometasone implant for chronic rhinosinusitis. Med Devices (Auckl) 2012;5:75–80.
33. Villari CR, Wojno TJ, Delgaudio JM. Case report of orbital violation with placement of ethmoid drug-eluting stent. Int Forum Allergy Rhinol 2012;2(1):89–92.
34. Leonard DW, Bolger WE. Topical antibiotic therapy for recalcitrant sinusitis. Laryngoscope 1999;109(4):668–70.
35. Chiu AG, Antunes MB, Palmer JN, et al. Evaluation of the in vivo efficacy of topical tobramycin against Pseudomonas sinonasal biofilms. J Antimicrob Chemother 2007;59(6):1130–4.
36. Chiu AG, Palmer JN, Woodworth BA, et al. Baby shampoo nasal irrigations for the symptomatic post-functional endoscopic sinus surgery patient. Am J Rhinol 2008;22(1):34–7.
37. Alava I, Isaacs S, Luong A, et al. Mometasone furoate gel: a novel in-office treatment of recalcitrant postoperative chronic rhinosinusitis. J Otolaryngol Head Neck Surg 2012;41(3):183–8. Available at: http://www.ncbi.nlm.nih.gov/pubmed/22762700. Accessed February 1, 2016.
38. Biel MA, Pedigo L, Gibbs A, et al. Photodynamic therapy of antibiotic-resistant biofilms in a maxillary sinus model. Int Forum Allergy Rhinol 2013;3(6):468–73.
39. Krespi YP, Kizhner V. Phototherapy for chronic rhinosinusitis. Lasers Surg Med 2011;43(3):187–91.

Topical Therapies for Refractory Chronic Rhinosinusitis

Akshay Sanan, MD, Mindy Rabinowitz, MD, Marc Rosen, MD,
Gurston Nyquist, MD*

KEYWORDS

- Topical therapy • Chronic rhinosinusitis • Anti-inflammatory • Antimicrobial
- Surfactant • Stents

KEY POINTS

- Chronic rhinosinusitis (CRS) is a common disease that has a substantive impact on quality of life. CRS treatments are aimed at reducing sinonasal inflammation, infection, and re-establishing mucociliary clearance.
- Sinus surgery is an effective adjunct for topical sinonasal drug delivery for patients with CRS.
- With a 5% to 10% failure rate from surgery, there is an additional subset of patients who are recalcitrant to conventional medical and surgical therapies, leading to alternative therapies centered on anti-infective and anti-inflammatory nasal irrigations.
- Topical therapies have become an integral component in the management plan for CRS.
- Although topical therapy is not a panacea, it can, because of its safety profile, be repeated and/or sustained over extended periods, thus avoiding the risks of prolonged oral corticosteroids, intravenous antibiotics, and/or repeat surgery.

OVERVIEW

Chronic rhinosinusitis (CRS) is a multifactorial disorder that is heterogeneous in presentation and clinical course. Treatment of CRS is based on several factors including the type of rhinosinusitis (acute, chronic, or fungal), presence of nasal polyposis, concurrent medical comorbidities, symptom severity, and response to previous medical treatments.[1] Medical treatment should be considered the cornerstone of disease treatment of CRS, with sinus surgery reserved for medical failures or patients' complications. However, with a 5% to 10% failure rate from surgery, there is an additional

Department of Otolaryngology – Head & Neck Surgery, Thomas Jefferson University Hospital, Philadelphia, PA, USA
* Corresponding author. Division of Endoscopic Sinus & Skull Base Surgery, Department of Otolaryngology – Head & Neck Surgery, 925 Chestnut Street, 7th Floor, Philadelphia, PA 19107.
E-mail address: Gurston.Nyquist@Jefferson.edu

Otolaryngol Clin N Am 50 (2017) 129–141
http://dx.doi.org/10.1016/j.otc.2016.08.011
0030-6665/17/© 2016 Elsevier Inc. All rights reserved.

subset of patients who are refractory to conventional medical and surgical therapies.[2] The focus of this article is on therapies centered on topical delivery and application for refractory CRS.

CRS has been simplified to two subgroups: CRS with nasal polyps (NP) and CRS without NP.[3] In the past, these two entities were considered to be a spectrum of one disease where CRS with NP was thought to be the end point of CRS. However, it has been shown that these two diseases have distinct differences and patients can respond differently to medical treatment.[3,4] This article mentions specific recommendations based on the CRS subgroup when possible.

Generally, the treatment of CRS is intended to reduce symptoms, improve quality of life, and prevent disease progression or recurrence. More specifically, topical therapies are aimed at reducing mucosal inflammation, reducing pathogenic bacterial burden and improving mucociliary clearance and sinonasal function. Clinicians often try to minimize systemic medical therapies and favor the use of topical therapies to focus drug delivery locally. Major factors that impact topical therapy success include the patient's anatomy and the dynamics of the delivery device. Advantages of topical medical therapy include direct delivery onto diseased tissue, potential for delivering higher local drug concentrations, and minimizing systemic absorption. Disadvantages of topical medical therapy include challenges with application technique; local adverse effects, such as epistaxis or patient discomfort; and variable sinus penetration. Because of the accessible nature of the sinonasal cavity, it is amenable to topical medical therapy and this has become an integral strategy in the management of refractory CRS.

Effective drug delivery to the involved tissue is a challenge that all topical drug therapies must overcome during the management of CRS. Endoscopic sinus surgery (ESS) is an important component in the management of medically refractory CRS, clinically and economically.[5,6] One major advantage of ESS is creating an open and accessible cavity. This has been demonstrated to optimize sinonasal penetration of topical medical therapy.[7] Potential topical sinonasal therapy strategies include topical saline irrigations, topical corticosteroids, topical antibiotics, topical antifungals, topical stents, and topical alternative medications.

METHODS OF DELIVERY

The main factors associated with particle penetration include the size of the sinus ostia, the size of the particle, and the flow rate (liters per minute) of the aerosol. Particles greater than 10 μm in size typically do not make it past the nasal cavity, and particles less than 5 μm enter the lungs.[8] Early studies estimated that the ideal particle size for maxillary sinus penetration is between 3 μm and 10 μm. Further studies concluded that smaller particle size, 45-degree insertion angle of the topical therapy, and higher flow rate (5 L/min compared with 1 L/min as demonstrated by Saijo and colleagues[9]) improved maxillary sinus penetration.[8]

Nasal sprays are a popular option for topical drug delivery because of their ease of use and diverse available formulations. Typical nasal sprays generate droplets of 50 μm to 100 μm in diameter and deliver 70 μL to 150 μL of drug per puff, at velocities of 7.5 L/min to 20 L/min.[10] However, a large fraction of the spray is deposited in the anterior nasal cavity without any paranasal sinus penetration. Also, half of the spray is cleared within 15 minutes from the nasal cavity, with minimal activity occurring at 6 hours.[10]

Nebulizers deliver medications in mist form and are commonly used for treating disease of the lower airway. Multiple nebulizers exist for topical sinonasal topical delivery. Some studies on pulsating aerosol nebulizers demonstrated increased deposition in the maxillary ostia, increased deposition in the posterior nasal cavity, and slower clearance time compared with the nasal pump sprays.[11] Although nebulizers represent a technologic advance compared with nasal pump sprays, the literature to support their efficacy is not definitive.[12]

TOPICAL SINONASAL SALINE

- Use high-volume, low-pressure sinonasal saline irrigations in addition to other topical therapies for CRS. Saline irrigation is well-tolerated without significant adverse effects. It is recommended as a beneficial treatment of CRS.

Saline irrigations and sprays are the most commonly used intervention for rhinitis and rhinosinusitis. Saline nasal irrigation has been recommended in the most recent clinical guidelines for CRS.[13] It is a common treatment adjunct in the management of CRS. Saline irrigation mechanically removes mucus, crusts, debris, and allergens from the sinonasal cavity, and potentially has the additional benefit of improving mucociliary clearance, ciliary beat frequency, and protecting the sinonasal mucosa.[14] The mechanical clearance of mucus by saline is thought to be the most important factor. Both hypertonic and isotonic saline have been shown to have a positive impact on mucociliary clearance time. There is substantial variability in the volume (low or high), pressure (low or high), and frequency (once daily to four times daily) of saline irrigation protocols. Large-volume, low-pressure nasal irrigation is more effective than saline sprays or nebulizers in penetrating the sinus ostia.[15] In multiple randomized trials, saline irrigation for CRS improved symptoms, quality of life, endoscopic examination findings, and was tolerated without any significant harmful effects.[9] The favorable safety profile, lack of systemic absorption risk, and good patient acceptance make it an appealing long-term topical therapy strategy.[16]

Daily hypertonic saline irrigation improved disease-specific symptom and health-related quality of life after 6 months.[17–21] Bachmann and colleagues[18] evaluated the effects of isotonic and hypertonic saline irrigations and demonstrated that both solutions improve sinonasal symptoms, with no significant differences between groups. Hypertonic preparations have been shown to elicit some pain and discomfort greater than 2.7%. At concentrations greater than 5.4%, patients experience nasal obstruction secondary to vasodilation and there is reduced airspace as measured by acoustic rhinomanometry.[22] Rabago and colleagues[17] randomized patients into two groups (hypertonic saline irrigations and no treatment) and demonstrated that daily hypertonic nasal saline irrigations significantly improved CRS health-related quality of life, symptoms scores, and decreased CRS medication usage. Pynnonen and colleagues[23] compared high-volume (240 mL), low-pressure isotonic saline irrigation with low-volume nasal saline spray and evaluated 20-item Sino-Nasal Outcomes Test (SNOT-20) and symptom scores at 2, 4, and 8 weeks posttreatment. Their study demonstrated that both groups had improvement in health-related quality of life at 8 weeks, but there was statistically significant long-term health-related quality of life and symptoms in patients using high-volume saline irrigations. This study focused on a community population of patients with sinonasal complaints and excluded patients with recent sinus surgery.

With adherence to therapy, side effects were minimal and included local irritation, nosebleeds, nasal burning, nausea, and headaches. In a follow-up study, patients reported reduced sinusitis symptoms and sinusitis-related medication use for an additional 12 months.[24] Another study found Dead Sea salt saline more beneficial compared with hypertonic saline for CRS symptoms.[25] There is substantial evidence to support the use of sinonasal saline irrigations in the management of CRS.[17–21] Because of the excellent safety profile of sinonasal saline irrigations, it is a great topical therapy option for patients with refractory CRS. Isotonic and hypertonic saline irrigations seem to provide similar outcomes, and high-volume, low-pressure saline irrigations are superior to low-volume nasal saline spray.

TOPICAL SINONASAL STEROIDS

Topical sinonasal steroid therapy can achieve local steroid effects while minimizing potential adverse effects associated with systemic steroid therapy (**Box 1**). Corticosteroids are potent medications that target the proinflammatory pathway. Because of the localized effects and excellent safety profile, topical sinonasal steroid therapy has become a common treatment option for CRS with and without nasal polyposis. Nasal corticosteroids have been shown to inhibit immediate and late-phase reactions to antigenic stimulation in patients with allergic rhinitis.[26] Generally, sinonasal steroids with low systemic bioavailability, such as mometasone furoate or fluticasone furoate, have not been associated with reduced bone growth or adrenal suppression, which was first noted with more systemically available sinonasal steroids, such as beclomethasone dipropionate.[27] However, high-dose dexamethasone nasal spray (0.132% aqueous nasal spray) given for at least 6 weeks does seem to have the potential to cause a decrease in serum cortisol levels.[28] There is also no clear evidence that the use of sinonasal corticosteroids correlates with systemic changes in bone mineral biology, cataracts, or glaucoma. In fact, Martino and colleagues[28] showed that a 6-week course of high-dose dexamethasone nasal spray (0.132% aqueous nasal spray) was not associated with ocular hypertension. Adverse effects of topical sinonasal steroids include epistaxis, headache, cough, nasal irritation, and nasal crusting. These happen in less than 5% of patients.[29,30] Rarely, septal perforations have been reported with sinonasal steroid use. Because of this, patients are instructed to direct the nasal spray toward the lateral nasal cavity wall instead of toward the septum.

There are several potential topical steroid solutions that are categorized into Food and Drug Administration (FDA)-approved and off-label use for sinonasal topical therapy. FDA-approved therapies apply to metered-dose topical steroid solutions and include mometasone furoate, fluticasone propionate, fluticasone furoate, budesonide, beclomethasone diproprionate, cicleosnide, flunisolide, and triamcinolone acetonide.

Box 1
Topical corticosteroids

Food and Drug Administration–Approved Topical Corticosteroids

- Topical corticosteroids are effective in CRS with and without polyps. They decrease polyp size in CRS with polyps. They help control symptoms in CRS without polyps. Topical corticosteroids are well-tolerated without significant adverse effects. It is recommended as a beneficial treatment of CRS.

"Off-Label" Use Topical Corticosteroids

- "Off-label" topical corticosteroids include the following: (1) budesonide nasal saline irrigations, (2) intranasal dexamethasone ophthalmic drops, (3) intranasal prednisolone ophthalmic drops, and (4) intranasal ciprofloxacin/dexamethasone otic drops. Further research is needed before making a definitive recommendation.

Off-label topical steroids lack FDA approval for nasal therapy. Although ample evidence exists on FDA-approved topical therapies, there is a growing body of literature for the off-label use of sinonasal steroid solutions. Advantages of off-label steroid solutions include delivery of the higher volume and higher concentrations of topical steroid to the sinonasal mucosa. However, the unknown risk of off-label topical sinonasal steroid use is the potential systemic absorption resulting in short- and long-term sequelae, which is yet to be determined.

Several studies have demonstrated the efficacy of intranasal steroids in the management of CRS with and without NP. These sprays are used most commonly in the management of symptoms associated with seasonal and perennial allergic rhinitis.[31] Guidelines recommend topical steroids as the first-line medication based on the results of several randomized controlled trials with fluticasone propionate, beclomethasone dipropionate, budesonide, or mometasone furoate.[32] Topical nasal steroids are effective for the treatment of CRS with polyposis and are often considered the first-line treatment option.[33] Nasal corticosteroids have also been shown to delay the recurrence of NP after surgery.[34]

Recent studies have demonstrated the efficacy of using budesonide respules for eosinophilic CRS or CRS with nasal polyposis. Budesonide respules are considered off-label use, because they are not FDA approved for nasal use. The respules are directly applied as nasal drops or as an addition to nasal irrigation. As described by the study authors, there is theoretically a higher concentration of steroids applied to the sinonasal mucosa with budesonide respules compared with traditional steroid sprays.[35] The intranasal clinical improvement in patients with nasal polyposis using budesonide rinses seems significant, especially in patients with eosinophilic chronic sinusitis with NP.[36] There is fear of systemic steroid side effects with off-label use of steroid solutions, but many studies have shown there is a lack of systemic effects. Bhalla and colleagues[37] studied the effect of off-label topical budesonide irrigations and demonstrated no significant adrenal suppression. Lastly, Welch and colleagues[38] demonstrated that twice-daily budesonide nasal irrigation following ESS did not alter the serum cortisol or 24-hour urine cortisol levels and concluded that high-volume delivery techniques, such as Neti pot, result in less than 5% of the solution remaining in the sinuses, and that the actual concentration of steroid the patient is exposed to is low and may be lower than traditional steroid nasal sprays.

Other off-label solutions include intranasal dexamethasone ophthalmic drops, prednisolone ophthalmic drops, and ciprofloxacin/dexamethasone otic drops. In contrast to the low systemic side-effect profile of budesonide rinses, studies demonstrate a decrease in serum cortisol levels after 6 weeks of intranasal dexamethasone spray.[28] DelGaudio and Wise[39] studied intranasal dexamethasone ophthalmic drops, prednisolone ophthalmic drops, and ciprofloxacin/dexamethasone otic drops and only 1 of 36 patients required medication discontinuation because of a decrease in morning cortisol level. Although there can be significant clinical improvement with the use of dexamethasone and prednisolone intranasal sprays for the treatment of nasal polyposis, these medications have a higher systemic side effect profile and impact the hypothalamic-pituitary-adrenal axis.

Nasal pump sprays, the most common delivery method of topical nasal corticosteroids, have almost no sinus penetration in nonoperated patients. Studies are needed to assess the long-term safety of off-label used nasal steroids. Finally, to optimize treatment with intranasal steroid sprays, patients should be educated on the delivery technique to maximize application to the sinonasal mucosa instead of simple nasal application.

TOPICAL SINONASAL ANTIBIOTICS

- Topical antibiotics are not first-line therapy for CRS. Stronger evidence exists for its use in patients with cystic fibrosis. It is recommended against use of topical antibiotics (spray and nebulizer) for CRS.

Topical antibiotics have emerged as adjunctive treatment of CRS because they offer the potential for high local concentration at the desired target site with minimization of systemic side effects.[40] The extent to which bacterial colonization, infection, and biofilms contribute to the pathophysiology of CRS is controversial. Systemic antibiotics are typically reserved for treatment of acute exacerbations of CRS. However, some evidence exists that long-term systemic macrolide therapy and doxycycline can improve subjective and objective outcomes while providing anti-inflammatory and prociliary benefits in addition to antimicrobial effects.[41,42] Systemic antibiotics do have potential side effects including cramping, diarrhea, increasing bacterial resistance, allergic reactions, and potential for organ toxicity.

Sykes and colleagues[43] evaluated dexamethasone/tramazoline and neomycin/dexamethasone compared with a placebo and used a four-times-daily spray technique. They demonstrated that both groups had symptomatic improvement compared with placebo. Desrosiers and Salas-Prato[44] evaluated a topical tobramycin-saline solution using a large-particle nebulizer compared with saline alone. Aerosolized forms of tobramycin were initially used in the treatment of pseudomonal pulmonary infections in patients with cystic fibrosis. After a 4-week treatment course, they demonstrated that both groups received clinical improvement, with no additional benefit derived from the topical tobramycin. Tobramycin nasal irrigations in patients with cystic fibrosis yielded reduction in revision sinus surgery and improved outcome scores.[44] Videler and colleagues[45] evaluated a Rhinoflow (Respironics, Inc., Cedar Grove, NJ) nebulizer of bacitracin/colimycin compared with placebo and they demonstrated clinical improvement in both groups with no additional benefit perceived by the topical antibiotic group. Topical high-volume mupirocin-saline irrigation has been studied as a potential therapeutic option for patients with *Staphylococcus aureus*, including methicillin-resistant *S aureus* culture-positive refractory CRS. Uren and colleagues[46] evaluated the effects of a twice-daily mupirocin saline irrigation for 3 weeks in patients with *S aureus*–positive refractory CRS. Their group demonstrated improved endoscopic and overall symptom scores with minimal adverse effects. Even though high-volume mupirocin saline irrigations have demonstrated promising results in *S aureus*–positive refractory CRS, reinfection is common. A growing concern is the development of mupirocin resistance, and mupirocin-resistant strains of methicillin-resistant *S aureus* may make the topical use of mupirocin obsolete in the future.

The current literature on topical antibiotics in the management of CRS is heterogeneous and limited by lack of prospective and randomized controlled trials. Thus, it is difficult to definitively support the use of topical antibiotics. More research is needed to evaluate the safety of topical antibiotic therapies and the potential risks of bacterial resistance and local and systemic adverse effects. Interestingly, Desroriers and Salas-Prato[44] noted a paradoxic increase in nasal congestion with nebulized tobramycin. The risk of bacterial resistance is a serious concern and needs to be thoroughly vetted before recommending topical antimicrobial therapy.

Given the low-level evidence, topical antibiotics should not be first-line management but may be attempted in patients refractory to the traditional topical steroids and oral antibiotics. Larger and better-designed randomized, double-blinded, placebo-controlled trials are required to more fully evaluate this modality of treatment. If the clinician uses topical antibiotic therapy, therapy should be guided by cultures and sensitivities.

TOPICAL SINONASAL ANTIFUNGALS

- There is no evidence to promote the use of topical antifungals for CRS. It is recommended against the use of topical antifungal therapy.

The significance of fungal infection on CRS has long been debated.[47] Two studies have demonstrated the low occurrence rate (1.6%–2.4%) of fungal organisms among patients with CRS.[48,49] In classically defined allergic fungal sinusitis, fungal elements are believed to underlie an IgE-mediated hypersensitivity that drives the eosinophilic inflammatory process. Antifungals have been suggested as systemic or topical preparations when fungus-related sinus inflammation is suspected. Because systemic antifungals have significant side effects that involve the liver and kidney, topical antifungals are more often advocated as a treatment modality for CRS. Ponikau and colleagues[50] performed a double-blinded, randomized control trial and showed that topical amphotericin B was associated with lower reoccurrence of NP, improvement in symptoms and computed tomography scans, and endoscopic scores. However, the results of Ponikau and colleagues[50] were limited to objective measures of endoscopy and computed tomography scan scores, with no significant difference in patient CRS health-related quality of life outcome scores. One study demonstrated when amphotericin B was included in the solution used for nasal irrigation, 39% of patients with CRS resolved their NP at the end of treatment.[51]

Given the preliminary data, future subsequent studies included a large number of randomized control trials evaluating topical antifungal therapy. These groups were not able to replicate Ponikau and colleagues' results and found no significant improvement or benefit in symptoms with topical antifungal therapy. For example, topical amphotericin B had no effect on inflammatory markers. Rather, the placebo group had higher levels of wound recovery.[52] One double-blinded, randomized control trial showed that antifungal therapy had no benefit over the control group and had higher adverse effects than the control trial.[53] Another double-blinded, randomized multicenter study demonstrated no significant differences in symptom scores between the patients with CRS who used topical amphotericin B and the placebo. Two meta-analyses also agreed that although topical antifungal therapy did show improvements in radiographic measurements, they did not significantly impact patient symptoms. Furthermore, patients had a higher rate of adverse effects compared with the placebo group.[54,55] The authors concluded there is no evidence to support the use of topical antifungal therapy for CRS and that antifungals not only lack evidence but have a preponderance of harm and are not recommended for topical therapy use. Side effects of topical antifungal therapy include nasal burning, skin irritation, epistaxis, and acute flare-ups of CRS.[56]

TOPICAL SINONASAL STENTS

- Topical stents are used in adjunct to other topical therapies for CRS. They are well tolerated without significant adverse effects. It is recommended as a beneficial adjunct for CRS.

Newer drug delivery devices via topical stents are addressing the shortcomings of nasal aerosol delivery. Stents allow for the slow release of topical drugs at targeted sites and have been used in the paranasal sinuses over the past decade. Early studies in animal models showed that drug-eluting stents have decreased granulation tissue without any epithelial damage, decreased postoperative stromal proliferation, and have negligible systemic absorption.[57,58] Most studies have focused on topical steroid stent use but some studies have also examined the role of antibiotic stents.[59,60]

The Relieva Stratus MicroFlow Spacer (Acclarent, Menlo Park, CA) is a drug-eluting stent that is temporarily implanted in the frontal or ethmoid sinus. It was introduced in 2009 and it provides local and targeted delivery of triamcinolone acetonide.[61,62] However, the Relieva Stratus was recently pulled off the market after a lawsuit was filed against Acclarent for promoting off-label use of the stent.[63] PROPEL sinus implant (Intersect ENT, Palo Alto, CA) was approved by the FDA in 2011 for topical steroid delivery in the paranasal sinus cavity (**Fig. 1**). The implant is a bioabsorbable implant that self-expands and releases mometasone furoate over 4 weeks.[64] Murr and colleagues[64] did a prospective double-blinded trial on the Propel sinus implant and noted significantly reduced inflammation and prevention of significant adhesions compared with the control implant in patients with CRS with polyposis. The Advance II trial by Marple and colleagues[65] was a prospective, randomized, controlled, double-blinded study that concluded the Propel sinus implant yielded decreased adhesions, decreased nasal polyposis, and decreased postoperative interventions with no observable ocular safety risk when compared with a nondrug releasing implant. Lastly, Rudmik and colleagues[66] demonstrated that an off-label drug-eluting middle meatal spacer of dexamethasone and Sinu-Foam (Arthrocare, Sunnyvale, CA) did not improve endoscopic outcomes in the early postoperative period when combined with postoperative saline irrigations and a short-course systemic steroids for patients with CRS without nasal polyposis. Drug-eluting stents are a promising new technology in the otolaryngologist's armamentarium for CRS. Future stent design should focus on larger steroid dose and/or longer duration of drug elution along with use of additional anti-inflammatory medications, such as antivascular endothelial growth factor.

OTHER TOPICAL SINONASAL THERAPIES

- Alternative topical therapies exist for CRS. However, data are sparse and not definitive. No recommendation is made for alternative topical therapy for CRS.

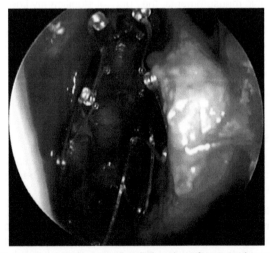

Fig. 1. The PROPEL mini implant is spring loaded and conforms to the patient's sinus anatomy on implantation. It is impregnated with mometasone furoate, which slowly releases over the course of 30 days.

Refractory CRS is a medically and surgically challenging subset of patients. Hence, creative alternatives have been explored. Topics to be discussed include surfactants, topical manuka, honey and topical xylitol.

A small prospective noncontrolled, nonblinded study of patients treated with twice-daily sinus irrigations with 1% baby shampoo in saline resulted in subjective improvement in SNOT-22 scores in 47% of heavily pretreated patients with CRS.[67] Baby shampoo is thought to act as a surfactant with the ability to thin mucus, disrupt microbial cell membranes, and potentially reduce biofilm formation. Surfactants are compounds that lower the surface tension of liquids and are thought to improve mucociliary clearance by reducing the adherence of mucus to the epithelial layer. Chiu and colleagues[68] followed up with a study that demonstrated baby shampoo irrigation resulted in a transient increase in ciliary beat frequency in murine nasal explants with no evidence of ciliary or epithelial toxicity. Isaacs and colleagues[69] studied mucociliary clearance time in patients using topical baby shampoo in saline compared with saline alone and found statistically significant increased mucociliary clearance time in the surfactant group. Surfactants were also thought to help decrease biofilm formation. Citric acid zwitterionic surfactant was noted to be highly effective in killing bacterial biofilms in animal studies.[70] However, because of its ciliotoxic properties, the reduction of cilia allowed biofilms to proliferate approximately 7 days after initial treatment in a rabbit model.[71] Clinically, patients have complained of foul taste, nasal burning, epistaxis, and headache. Future research with randomized, double-blinded, controlled trials is needed to determine the true impact of topical surfactants in CRS.

Manuka (*Leptospermum scoparium*) honey and the active component, methylglyoxal (MGO), have been described as a natural, inexpensive, and nontoxic topical therapy for CRS. These have been shown to possess antistaphylococcus and antipseudomonas biofilm properties in vitro.[72] Jervis-Bardy and coworkers[72] evaluated the antibiofilm properties of manuka honey and MGO-only solutions. MGO, a derivative from the manuka flower, is considered to be the main antimicrobial agent, with honey potentiating its effects through an unknown mechanism. They demonstrated that antibiofilm properties existed with both topical solutions. However, this study was limited by the fact it was an in vitro analysis. Future in vivo studies are required to determine the effects of manuka honey and MGO in patients with CRS.

Xylitol is a sugar alcohol that has gained prominence as a naturally occurring antibacterial agent. Weissman and colleagues[73] performed a randomized, double-blinded controlled trial to study if topical xylitol saline irrigations yielded significant improvement in patients with CRS compared with saline irrigations. Their study demonstrated a statistically significant improvement in SNOT-22 scores in the xylitol group. There was no difference in adverse effects between the two groups. The most common adverse effects were sweet taste of the xylitol solution. This study was limited by its small sample size of 20 patients. Future studies with larger patient populations are needed to examine this topical treatment.

SUMMARY

Topical therapy has become an important tool in the otolaryngologist's armamentarium for refractory CRS. Daily high-volume sinonasal saline irrigation and FDA-approved standard metered-dose topical nasal steroid therapy are supported by the most evidence. Nonstandard (off-label) topical sinonasal steroid therapies are a potential option for refractory CRS. Current evidence recommends against the use of topical antifungal therapy and topical antibiotic therapy delivered using spray and nebulized techniques in routine cases of CRS. There is insufficient evidence to provide clinical recommendations for alternative therapies, such as topical surfactant, manuka honey, or xylitol. Stents are a new modality with preliminary data showing they are an option when traditional treatment (oral antibiotics, saline, and steroid sprays) has failed. Further research with long-term effects and outcomes studies for refractory CRS are needed.

REFERENCES

1. Kennedy DW, Gwaltney JM, Jones JG. Medical management of sinusitis: educational goals and management guidelines. The International Conference on Sinus Disease. Ann Otol Rhinol Laryngol Suppl 1995;167:22–30.
2. Senior BA, Kennedy DW, Tanabodee J, et al. Long-term results of functional endoscopic sinus surgery. Laryngoscope 1998;108(2):151–7.
3. Meltzer EO, Hamilos DL, Hadley JA. Rhinosinusitis: establishing definitions for clinical research and patient care. Otolaryngol Head Neck Surg 2004;131(6 Suppl):S1–62.
4. Eloy P, Poirrier AL, De Dorlodot C, et al. Actual concepts in rhinosinusitis: a review of clinical presentations, inflammatory pathways, cytokine profiles, remodeling, and management. Curr Allergy Asthma Rep 2011;11(2):146–62.
5. Soler ZM, Wittenberg E, Schlosser RJ, et al. Health state utility values in patients undergoing endoscopic sinus surgery. Laryngoscope 2011;121:2672–8.
6. Bhattacharyya N, Orlandi RR, Grebner J, et al. Cost burden of chronic rhinosinusitis: a claims-based study. Otolaryngol Head Neck Surg 2011;144:440–5.
7. Harvey RJ, Goddard JC, Wise SK, et al. Effects of endoscopic sinus surgery and delivery device on cadaver sinus irrigation. Otolaryngol Head Neck Surg 2008; 139:137–42.
8. Laube BL. Devices for aerosol delivery to treat sinusitis. J Aerosol Med 2007; 20(Suppl 1):S5–17 [discussion: S17–8].
9. Saijo R, Majima Y, Hyo N, et al. Particle deposition of therapeutic aerosols in the nose and paranasal sinuses after transnasal sinus surgery: a cast model study. Am J Rhinol 2004;18(1):1–7.
10. Moller W, Lubbers C, Munzing W, et al. Pulsating airflow and drug delivery to paranasal sinuses. Curr Opin Otolaryngol Head Neck Surg 2011;19(1):48–53.
11. Moller W, Schuschnig U, Meyer G, et al. Ventilation and drug delivery to the paranasal sinuses: studies in a nasal cast using pulsating airflow. Rhinology 2008; 46(3):213–20.
12. Hwang PH, Woo RJ, Fong KJ. Intranasal deposition of nebulized saline: a radionuclide distribution study. Am J Rhinol 2006;20(3):255–61.
13. Rosenfeld RM, Andes D, Bhattacharyya N, et al. Clinical practice guideline: adult sinusitis 1. Otolaryngol Head Neck Surg 2007;137(Suppl 3):S1–3.
14. Harvey R, Hannan SA, Badia L, et al. Nasal saline irrigations for the symptoms of chronic rhinosinusitis. Cochrane Database Syst Rev 2007;(3):CD006394.
15. Wormald PK, Cain T, Oates L, et al. A comparative study of three methods of nasal irrigation. Laryngoscope 2004;114:2224–7.
16. Rabago D, Barrett B, Marchand L, et al. Qualitative aspects of nasal irrigation use by patients with chronic sinus disease in a multimethod study. Ann Fam Med 2006;4:295–301.
17. Rabago D, Zgierska A, Mundt M, et al. Efficacy of daily hypertonic saline nasal irrigation among patients with sinusitis: a randomized controlled trial. J Fam Pract 2002;51:1049–55.

18. Bachmann G, Hommel G, Michel O. Effect of irrigation of the nose with isotonic salt solution on adult patients with chronic paranasal sinus disease. Eur Arch Otorhinolaryngol 2000;257:537–41.

19. Heatley DG, McConnell KE, Kille TL, et al. Nasal irrigation for the alleviation of sinonasal symptoms. Otolaryngol Head Neck Surg 2001;125:44–8.

20. Pinto JM, Elwany S, Baroody FM, et al. Effects of saline sprays on symptoms after endoscopic sinus surgery. Am J Rhinol 2006;20:191–6.

21. Freeman SR, Sivayoham ES, Jepson K, et al. A preliminary randomised controlled trial evaluating the efficacy of saline douching following endoscopic sinus surgery. Clin Otolaryngol 2008;33:462–5.

22. Baraniuk JN, Ali M, Naranch K. Hypertonic saline nasal provocation and acoustic rhinometry. Clin Exp Allergy 2002;32(4):543–50.

23. Pynnonen MA, Mukerji SS, Kim HM, et al. Nasal saline for chronic sinonasal symptoms: a randomized controlled trial. Arch Otolaryngol Head Neck Surg 2007;133:1115–20.

24. Rabago D, Pasic T, Azierska A, et al. The efficacy of hypertonic saline nasal irrigation for chronic sinonasal symptoms. Otolaryngol Head Neck Surg 2005;133:3–8.

25. Friedman M, Vidyasagar R, Joseph N. A randomized, prospective, double-blinded study on the efficacy of dead sea salt nasal irrigations. Laryngoscope 2006;116:878–82.

26. Mabry RL. Pharmacotherapy of allergic rhinitis: corticosteroids. Otolaryngol Head Neck Surg 1995;113(1):120–5.

27. Holm AF, Fokkens WJ, Godthelp T, et al. A 1 year placebo-controlled study of intranasal fluticasone propionate aqueous nasal spray in patients with perennial allergic rhinitis: a safety and biopsy study. Clin Otolaryngol 1998;23(1):69–73.

28. Martino B, Church C, Seiberling K. Effect of intranasal dexamethasone on endogenous cortisol level and intraocular pressure. Int Forum Allergy Rhinol 2015;5(7):605–9.

29. Corren J. Intranasal corticosteroids for allergic rhinitis: how do different agents compare? J Allergy Clin Immunol 1999;104:S144–9.

30. Nasonex. Prod Inf. 2010. Available at: http://www.merck.com/product/usa/pi_circulars/n/nasonex/nasonex_pi.pdf. Accessed January 8, 2016.

31. Melvin TA, Patel AA. Pharmacotherapy for allergic rhinitis. Otolaryngol Clin North Am 2011;44(3):727–39.

32. Fokkens W, Lund V, Mullol J. On behalf of the European position paper on rhinosinusitis and nasal polyps group. Rhinol Suppl 2007;20:1–136.

33. Badia L, Lund V. Topical corticosteroids in nasal polyposis. Drugs 2001;51:573–8.

34. Stajme P, Olsson P, Alenius M. Use of mometasone furoate to prevent polyp relapse after endoscopic sinus surgery. Arch Otolaryngol Head Neck Surg 2009;135(3):296–302.

35. Steinke JW, Payne SC, Tessier ME, et al. Pilot study of budesonide inhalant suspension for chronic eosinophilic sinusitis. J Allergy Clin Immunol 2009;123:1352–4.

36. Jang DW, Lachanas VA, Segel J, et al. Budesonide nasal irrigations in the postoperative management of chronic rhinosinusitis. Int Forum Allergy Rhinol 2013;3(9):708–11.

37. Bhalla RK, Payton K, Wright ED. Safety of budesonide in saline sinonasal irrigations in the management of chronic rhinosinusitis with polyposis: lack of significant adrenal suppression. J Otolaryngol Head Neck Surg 2008;37:821–5.

38. Welch KC, Thaler ER, Doghramji LL, et al. The effects of serum and urinary cortisol levels of topical intranasal irrigations with budesonide added to saline in patients with recurrent polyposis after endoscopic sinus surgery. Am J Rhinol Allergy 2010;24:26–8.
39. DelGaudio JM, Wise SK. Topical steroid drops for the treatment of sinus ostia stenosis in the postoperative period. Am J Rhinol 2006;20:563–7.
40. Lim M, Citardi MJ, Leong JL. Topical antimicrobials in the management of chronic rhinosinusitis: a systematic review. Am J Rhinol 2008;22:381–9.
41. Soler ZM, Smith TL. What is the role of long-term macrolide therapy in the treatment of recalcitrant chronic rhinosinusitis? Laryngoscope 2009;119:2083–4.
42. Van Zele T, Gevaert P, Hotapples G, et al. Oral steroids and doxycycline: two different approaches to treat nasal polyps. J Allergy Clin Immunol 2010;125(5): 1069–76.
43. Sykes DA, Wilson R, Chan KL, et al. Relative importance of antibiotic and improved clearance in topical treatment of chronic mucopurulent rhinosinusitis. A controlled study. Lancet 1986;2:359–60.
44. Desrosiers MY, Salas-Prato M. Treatment of chronic 866. rhinosinusitis refractory to other treatments with topical antibiotic therapy delivered by means of a large-particle nebulizer: results of a controlled trial. Otolaryngol Head Neck Surg 2001; 125:265–9.
45. Videler WJ, van Drunen CM, Reitsma JB, et al. Nebulized bacitracin/colimycin: a treatment option in recalcitrant chronic rhinosinusitis with *Staphylococcus aureus*? A double-blind, randomized, placebo-controlled, cross-over pilot study. Rhinology 2008;46:92–8.
46. Uren B, Psaltis A, Wormald PJ. Nasal lavage with mupirocin for the treatment of surgically recalcitrant chronic rhinosinusitis. Laryngoscope 2008;118:1677–80.
47. Ebbens FA, Scadding GK, Badia L, et al. Amphotericin B nasal lavages: not a solution for patients with chronic rhinosinusitis. J Allergy Clin Immunol 2006;118: 1149–56.
48. Jennings BH, Andersson KE, Johansson SA. Assessment of systemic effects of inhaled glucocorticoids, the influence of the frequency of blood sampling technique on plasma cortisol and leucocytes. Eur J Clin Pharmacol 1990;39:127–31.
49. Mantovani K, Bisanha AA, Demarco RC, et al. Maxillary sinuses microbiology from patients with chronic rhinosinusitis. Braz J Otorhinolaryngol 2010;76:548–51.
50. Ponikau JU, Sherris DA, Kita H, et al. Intranasal antifungal treatment in 51 patients with chronic rhinosinusitis. J Allergy Clin Immunol 2002;110:862–6.
51. Ricchetti A, Landis BN, Maffioli A, et al. Effect of antifungal nasal lavage with amphotericin B on nasal polyposis. J Laryngol Otol 2002;116:261–3.
52. Ebbens FA, Georgalas C, Luiten S, et al. The effect of topical amphotericin B on inflammatory markers in patients with chronic rhinosinusitis: a multicenter randomized controlled study. Laryngoscope 2009;119:401–8.
53. Weschta M, Rimek D, Formanek M, et al. Topical antifungal treatment of chronic rhinosinusitis with nasal polyps: a randomized, double-blind clinical trial. J Allergy Clin Immunol 2004;113:1122–8.
54. Stankiewicz JA, Musgrave BK, Scianna JM. Nasal amphotericin irrigation in chronic rhinosinusitis. Curr Opin Otolaryngol Head Neck Surg 2008;16:44–6.
55. Isaacs S, Fakhri S, Luong A, et al. A meta-analysis of topical amphotericin B for the treatment of chronic rhinosinusitis. Int Forum Allergy Rhinol 2011;1:250–4.
56. Sacks PL, Harvey RJ, Rimmer J, et al. Topical and systemic antifungal therapy for the symptomatic treatment of chronic rhinosinusitis. Cochrane Database Syst Rev 2011;(8):CD008263.

57. Beule AG, Scharf C, Biebler KE, et al. Effects of topically applied dexamethasone on mucosal wound healing using a drug-releasing stent. Laryngoscope 2008; 118(11):2073–7.
58. Beule AG, Steinmeier E, Kaftan H, et al. Effects of a dexamethasone-releasing stent on osteoneogenesis in a rabbit model. Am J Rhinol Allergy 2009;23(4): 433–6.
59. Bleier BS, Kofonow JM, Hashmi N, et al. Antibiotic eluting chitosan glycerophosphate implant in the setting of acute bacterial sinusitis: a rabbit model. Am J Rhinol Allergy 2010;24(2):129–32.
60. Huvenne W, Zhang N, Tijsma E, et al. Pilot study using doxycycline-releasing stents to ameliorate postoperative healing quality after sinus surgery. Wound Repair Regen 2008;16(6):757–67.
61. Catalano PJ, Thong M, Weiss R, et al. The MicroFlow spacer: a drug-eluting stent for the ethmoid sinus. Indian J Otolaryngol Head Neck Surg 2011;63(3):279–84.
62. Taulu R, Numminen J, Bizaki A, et al. Image-guided, navigation-assisted Relieva Stratus MicroFlow Spacer insertion into the ethmoid sinus. Eur Arch Otorhinolaryngol 2015;272(9):2335–40.
63. J&J Hit with New Multimillion-Dollar Fraud Suit. 2016. Available at: http://www.qmed.com/mpmn/medtechpulse/jj-hit-new-multimillion-dollar-fraud-suit. Accessed January 31, 2016.
64. Murr AH, Smith TL, Hwang PH, et al. Safety and efficacy of a novel bioabsorbable, steroid- eluting sinus stent. Int Forum Allergy Rhinol 2011;1(1): 23–32.
65. Marple BF, Smith TL, Han JK, et al. Advance II: a prospective, randomized study assessing safety and efficacy of bioabsorbable steroid-releasing sinus implants. Otolaryngol Head Neck Surg 2012;146(6):1004–11.
66. Rudmik L, Mace J, Mechor B. Effect of a dexamethasone Sinu-Foam™ middle meatal spacer on endoscopic sinus surgery outcomes: a randomized, double-blind, placebo-controlled trial. Int Forum Allergy Rhinol 2012;2(3):248–51.
67. Chiu AG, Palmer JN, Woodworth BA, et al. Baby shampoo nasal irrigations for the symptomatic post-functional endoscopic sinus surgery patient. Am J Rhinol 2008;22(1):34–7.
68. Chiu AG, Chen B, Palmer JN, et al. Safety evaluation of sinus surfactant solution on respiratory cilia function. Int Forum Allergy Rhinol 2011;1(4):280–3.
69. Isaacs S, Fakhri S, Luong A, et al. The effect of dilute baby shampoo on nasal mucociliary clearance in healthy subjects. Am J Rhinol Allergy 2011;25:e27–9.
70. Desrosiers M, Myntti M, James G. Methods for removing bacterial biofilms: in vitro study using clinical chronic rhinosinusitis specimens. Am J Rhinol 2007;21(5): 527–32.
71. Tamashiro E, Banks CA, Chen B, et al. In vivo effects of citric acid/zwitterionic surfactant cleansing solution on rabbit sinus mucosa. Am J Rhinol Allergy 2009; 23(6):597–601.
72. Jervis-Bardy J, Foreman A, Bray S, et al. Methylglyoxal-infused honey mimics the anti-*Staphylococcus aureus* biofilm activity of manuka honey: potential implication in chronic rhinosinusitis. Laryngoscope 2011;121:1104–7.
73. Weissman JD, Fernandez F, Hwang PH. Xylitol nasal irrigation in the management of chronic rhinosinusitis: a pilot study. Laryngoscope 2011;121:2468–72.

Revision Functional Endoscopic Sinus Surgery

Corinna G. Levine, MD, MPH[a],*, Roy R. Casiano, MD[b]

KEYWORDS

- Refractory rhinosinusitis • Revision FESS • Polyps • Stenosis • Scarring
- Neo-osteogenesis • Chronic rhinosinusitis

KEY POINTS

- The causes of primary functional endoscopic sinus surgery (FESS) failure are usually multifactorial; all aspects of anatomic, patient disease, and postoperative care should be considered.
- Revision FESS requires a clear understanding of the anatomic sites contributing to recurrence. Systematic assessment is essential.
- Traditional anatomic landmarks are distorted or absent during revision FESS. Alternative anatomic landmarks, which are consistently present despite prior surgery, are used to maintain clear surgical orientation.
- Revision FESS must address all the anatomic sites that contribute to recurrence. Wide antrostomies permit intraoperative access to disease and facilitates postoperative care.
- Revision FESS is a viable treatment option for patients who fail primary FESS and maximal medical treatment for recurrent chronic rhinosinusitis and have possible outflow tract obstruction.

INTRODUCTION

In the mid 1980s, otolaryngologists began using functional endoscopic sinus surgery (FESS) to address refractory chronic rhinosinusitis (CRS) that failed to respond to medical treatment. FESS can provide short- and long-term improvement in disease symptoms and quality of life.[1–3] Approximately 250,000 patients undergo endoscopic sinus surgery in the United States alone[1,4] with general good success rates ranging from 67% to 98%.[5–10] However, approximately 10% to 15% of patients who have

No disclosures (C.G. Levine); Consultant for Medtronic, Olympus, Laurimed Inc (R.R. Casiano).
[a] Department of Otolaryngology, University of Miami, Miller School of Medicine, 1120 Northwest 14th Street, 5th Floor, Miami, FL 33136, USA; [b] American Rhinologic Society, Rhinology and Endoscopic Skull Base Program, Department of Otolaryngology, Head & Neck Surgery, University of Miami, Miller School of Medicine, Clinical Research Building, 5th Floor, 1120 Northwest 14th Street, Miami, FL 33136, USA
* Corresponding author.
E-mail address: Cxl861@miami.edu

Otolaryngol Clin N Am 50 (2017) 143–164
http://dx.doi.org/10.1016/j.otc.2016.08.012
0030-6665/17/© 2016 Elsevier Inc. All rights reserved.

sinus surgery will undergo revision surgery.[8,11,12] Multiple factors contribute to the need for revision surgery, including surgical technique, extent of disease, anatomic obstruction, and postoperative care.[11,13,14] The need for revision can be of particular concern in patients with CRS with nasal polyps who have been shown to have a high rate of regrowth.[15,16] This article reviews the main causes of primary FESS failure and discusses an approach to the medical and surgical treatment of recalcitrant CRS.

REASONS FOR FAILURE OF PRIMARY FUNCTIONAL ENDOSCOPIC SINUS SURGERY

When assessing patients who failed primary FESS, it is vital to determine the underlying cause(s) of persistent disease. Frequently, the cause is multifactorial and thus all contributing factors should be evaluated and addressed.

Anatomic, Mucosal, and Bony Factors

A number of studies evaluated the etiology of primary FESS failure and among the following causes anatomic factors are particularly common[13,14] (**Box 1**). *Middle turbinate lateralization* is cited as a common anatomic finding in 30% to 78% in those who fail FESS.[11,17–19]

Incomplete surgery

Multiple studies report incomplete surgical technique contributing to recurrent disease (**Fig. 1**): incomplete anterior or posterior ethmoidectomy in 31% to 74%, incomplete uncinectomy in 37%, and retained agger nasi cell in 13% to 49%[9,11,18,19] Additional findings included retained intersinus septations or intrasinus cells including frontal cells and Haller (infraorbital) cells.[18,19] These cells block the natural drainage pathways of the frontal, ethmoid, and even the sphenoid sinuses. Other issues include failure to locate and open the diseased sphenoid sinus, which can be mistaken for an Onodi (suprasphenoidal) cell.[17,20]

Ostium stenosis, scaring, and synechiae

Stenosis occurs when circular openings contract, preventing drainage. This can be exacerbated by the buildup of scar tissue in or near these openings, creating a thick band of tissue that obstructs the sinus and fails to respond to topical treatments. Scarring

---

Box 1
Anatomic factors contributing to recurrent chronic rhinosinusitis

Frontal sinus outflow stenosis

Incomplete anterior ethmoidectomy/agger nasi retention

Incomplete posterior ethmoidectomy

Middle turbinate lateralization

Retained uncinate

Missed ostium

Middle meatus stenosis

Maxillary recirculation

Sphenoid ostium stenosis

Synechia (in any sinus)

Neo-osteogenesis

Recurrent mucosal disease

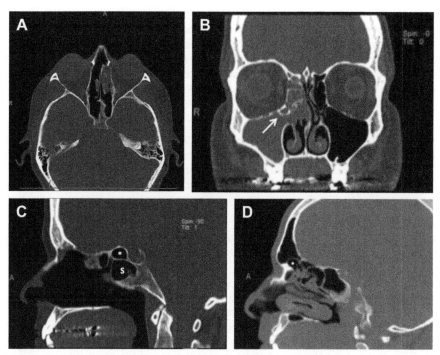

Fig. 1. Computed tomography scan findings of retained sinus cells after primary surgery. (*A*) Retained left ethmoid septations. (*B*) Haller cell in right maxillary sinus (*arrow*), ethmoid septation neo-osteogenesis. (*C*) Onodi cell overlying the sphenoid sinus (*asterisk*). S, sphenoid sinus. (*D*) Type 1 frontal cell (*asterisk*).

and stenosis of the maxillary ostium (**Fig. 2**) can be a common finding in revision FESS, reported in 27% to 39% of cases.[9,11] Similarly, 12% to 50% of revision FESS frontal outflow tracts had scaring and/or stenosis.[9,11,18] Although scaring and stenosis seemed to be less of an issue for the sphenoid sinus at 7%, this area is not as well-described.[11]

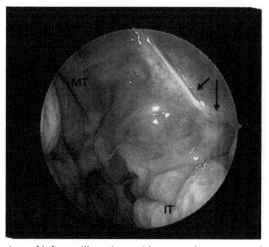

Fig. 2. Endoscopic view of left maxillary sinus with scar and contracture (*arrows*). C, choana; IT, inferior turbinate; MT, middle turbinate; S, septum.

Recirculation

A condition of sinus drainage obstruction where mucus is transferred out of the natural ostium, but reenters the sinus via the unconnected surgical sinusotomy. Parsons and colleagues in 1996[21] described in detail how failure to identify and connect the natural maxillary ostium to the surgical maxillary sinusotomy results in continued obstruction. Recirculation was documented in 4% to 15% of the subjects in several series of revision FESS subjects.[9,11]

Neo-osteogenesis

This is a feature of unclear etiology described in CRS and more frequently in recurrent CRS.[22] It may be associated with the degree of tissue eosinophilia[23] and was found in 36% to 53% of patients with CRS (using radiographic and pathologic criteria).[24] Neo-osteogenesis was thought to be a main finding contributing to recurrent CRS in multiple sinuses[18,19,25] (**Fig. 3**).

Recurrent mucosal disease

Return of mucosal thickening, and particularly polyps, was documented in many studies as a main factor in ostium obstruction in recalcitrant CRS[11,18,25] (**Fig. 4**).

Patient Disease

Patients with recalcitrant CRS disease and persistent symptoms after primary surgery often have recurrent mucosal disease that can be partly triggered by their underlying disease etiology. Although surgery reduces the disease burden, it often does not address the underlying etiology of disease. Studies document that patients with CRS and nasal polyps tend to have higher rates of recurrent disease.[15,16] In these patients, the approach to primary surgery technique (removal of the middle turbinate, wide osteotomies, etc) and postoperative management with frequent debridements, topical and oral medical therapy, and monitoring, are critical to minimize the propensity for recurrence. However, there are particular subsets of CRS patients for whom it is of paramount importance to consider the underlying etiology and pattern of disease, so that patients receive appropriate treatment to reduce recurrence.

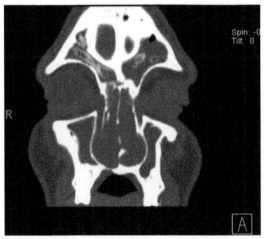

Fig. 3. Coronal computed tomography scan with neo-osteogeneic bone in frontal and ethmoid sinuses.

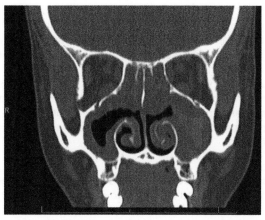

Fig. 4. Coronal computed tomography scan demonstrating a patient with a history of prior sinus surgery who had recurrent polypoid mucosal inflammation despite widely opened sinuses.

Allergic fungal sinusitis

Bent and Kuhn[26] developed 5 main diagnostic criteria for allergic fungal sinusitis: allergy to fungi, positive fungal stain of the sinus contents, nasal polyposis, characteristic findings on radiography, and production of eosinophilic mucin. The pathophysiology is not clearly understood, but is likely related to type 1 hypersensitivity to fungal antigens.[26–28] The characteristic thick obstructive mucin is not easily cleared, reduces sinus aeration, and can promote a fertile environment for inflammation and bacterial overgrowth.[29] Surgery is the mainstay of treatment[28] with wide sinusotomies facilitating postoperative debridements and topical therapy. However, there is an high rate of recurrent disease.[30–32] Thus, in addition to surgery, aggressive medical treatment with systemic and topical nasal steroids are necessary.[33]

In the initial postoperative period, the senior author combines monthly postoperative nasal endoscopies with or without debridements (after the initial postoperative visit at 7–10 days), along with nasal saline rinses, topical nasal steroids, and culture-directed topical and oral antibiotics. Cultures are collected intraoperatively. In patients who have remaining postoperative polypoid tissue, an oral steroid burst with 1 week of each 40 mg/d followed by 20 mg/d, is given with culture-directed oral antibiotics. Subsequent bacterial infections are treated with a steroid burst and culture-directed topical and oral antibiotics. Additionally, patients are evaluated and treated for significant environmental allergies.

Impaired secretion clearance

Patients with impaired ciliary clearance (ciliopathies: primary ciliary dyskinesia, Kartagener syndrome, etc[34]) or mucosal stasis (cystic fibrosis[35,36]) are prone to recurrent obstruction, infection, and mucosal inflammation after surgery. These patients require frequent debridements and wider sinusotomies, to permit in-office debridement and removal of secretions that the patient cannot clear by rinsing alone.

Biofilms

A biofilm is an organized matrix of bacterial microcolonies that can share plasmids, promoting antibiotic resistance, and permitting greater adhesion of the organisms to the mucosal surface.[37,38] Biofilms reduce susceptibility to antibiotics and lead to poorer quality of life, with more frequent postoperative infections.[39] Prince and colleagues[40] showed that patients who had prior sinus surgeries had a higher prevalence of biofilm-forming bacteria. The severity of disease and pattern of postoperative response may vary with the species of biofilm forming bacteria; *Staphylococcus aureus* is associated with worse postoperative disease.[41–43] There is a significant amount of research into biofilm eradication strategies. Foreman and colleagues[44] divided these strategies into 3 categories: topical antibiotics such as mupirocin and tobramycin; biofilm dispersal, including surfactant and enzymes; and physical removal with hydrodebridment.

Immune deficiencies
Patients with recurrent CRS seem to have an increased prevalence of immunoglobulin deficiencies, reported at 4% to 22%.[36,45–47] A metaanalysis by Schwitzguebel and colleagues[48] found the pooled prevalence of immunoglobulin (Ig)G, IgA, and IgM deficiencies was 13% in recurrent CRS patients. These patients require specific treatment to address their underlying immune system deficits. The senior author routinely orders a basic immune work-up including immunoglobulin levels (with IgG subtypes) in patients who present with a history of recurrent sinusitis and severe recurrent upper airway infections unresponsive to antibiotics or with symptoms out of proportion to endoscopic or radiographic findings.

Aspirin-exacerbated respiratory disease
Often presenting as Samter's triad with aspirin sensitivity, asthma, and nasal polyposis, attributed to manifestations of abnormal arachidonic acid metabolism. The inhibition of cyclooxygenase exacerbates the production of leukotrienes and mast cell degranulation.[49] The nasal polyps in these patients are often less responsive to standard medical or surgical treatment.[50] Mendelsohn and colleagues[16] found patients with Samter's triad were 2.7 times more likely to have recurrent disease and revision surgery than CRS patients. Multiple studies found a significant decrease in the number of revision sinus surgeries after aspirin desensitization therapy.[51]

Postoperative Care

There are no standardized protocols for postoperative care. Postoperatively, there is a propensity for sinonasal buildup of old blood, purulence, mucous, and/or unabsorbed packing, which form hard crusts on raw mucosal surfaces. This results in nasal obstruction, retained secretions, and reduced sinus aeration. The environment can lead to increased inflammation and scarring, and create a fertile breeding ground for bacteria.

Medical treatment
Nasal saline irrigations help to flush out and remove the postoperative buildup of loose crusts, while moisturizing the nasal airway. Several high-level studies found postoperative nasal saline rinses improve postoperative symptoms and endoscopic appearance.[52,53]

Topical antibiotics are useful in CRS[54] by reducing the need for repeat surgery, and improving postoperative symptoms and endoscopic findings. The literature on the use of postoperative oral antibiotics is mixed. Evidence does not support using short courses of antibiotic postoperatively, but some studies show that a longer course of antibiotics can improve endoscopic scores and crusting.[55] None of the studies used culture-directed antibiotics. The senior author routinely collects cultures (tissue or purulence) intraoperatively and places patients on 4 weeks of culture–directed oral and topical antibiotics postoperatively. No antibiotics are given before surgery to ensure representative culture data.

Topical steroids are useful for long-term maintenance and control of mucosal inflammation, particularly in patients with polyps. Cochrane reviews found that topical steroids improved symptom scores and had a greater proportion of responders in both polyp and nonpolyp CRS patients. Subgroup analysis indicated that sinus delivery methods (saline rinses) tended to be more successful than nasal delivery (nasal spray) methods in patients who underwent sinus surgery.[56,57] The senior author routinely places patients on postoperative long-term topical nasal steroids. Several nasal steroid sprays are currently available without a prescription and are traditionally well-tolerated and affordable, and have minimal side effects. In select refractory polyp cases, topical budesonide is a helpful adjunct.

Endoscopic debridements
Debridement improves postoperative endoscopic appearance and symptoms, and reduces the risk of synechiae development or middle turbinate lateralization.[55,58] The procedure involves removing sinonasal debris in the office, using a rigid endoscope and a variety of instruments, such as assorted suctions and forceps. The timing and the frequency of debridements varies widely, although it is generally accepted that debridements are necessary for 1 to 2 months postoperatively. The senior author performs debridements at 1 and 4 weeks postoperatively, and if necessary, monthly thereafter until the mucosal membranes start to normalize. Once patients improve, nasal endoscopies are spaced to 3 to 6 months for the first year, or more frequently if the patient experiences worsening symptoms. In these visits, meticulous removal of crusts, retained secretions, granulation tissue, and devitalized bone are performed. Scarring and synechiae are lysed with a through-cut forceps or endoscopic scissors. Developing infections or early recurrence of polypoid tissue are treated aggressively with culture-directed antibiotics, and oral and/or topical steroids. In-office polyp removal (using a microdebrider) is performed if polyps obstruct a major sinus outflow tract.

Allergy assessment and treatment
The exact role of allergy in CRS has not been determined fully. Even the association of allergy with CRS has conflicting reports in the literature.[59] There is some evidence to suggest that allergy may predispose patients to the development of CRS.[36] Tan and colleagues[60] suggest that allergy may play a role in the development of an impaired epithelial barrier and thus acts as a modifier of sinusitis. The senior author routinely refers patients with characteristic symptoms or recalcitrant disease for allergy evaluation and treatment.

TREATMENT OF RECALCITRANT SINUSITIS

Recurrent sinusitis is extremely challenging to treat. It is essential to reevaluate prior workups and treatments, and systematically approach additional treatment. Interventions should emphasize treating the patient and not the imaging studies. In particular, the focus is on maximizing quality-of-life outcomes.

Maximize Medical and Nonsurgical Treatments

Many patients who develop recurrent disease after primary surgical treatment respond to appropriate medical therapy, including a steroid burst for 2 to 3 weeks, and culture-directed antibiotics. In addition, it is important to review the role of maintenance treatment, with at least twice daily nasal saline rinses and topical steroids. Patient compliance is a critical factor influencing outcomes. Frequently, patients who have initial postoperative success will reduce or cease the use of maintenance treatments. The role of patient education about the chronicity of their disease, appropriate self-management, and maintenance treatments should not be forgotten.

Prior preoperative history, workup, and postoperative course are reviewed in detail to help the rhinologist identify gaps and assess for untreated underlying patient disease. Strong consideration is given to the patient disease states mentioned elsewhere in this article, as well as environmental changes, new exposures, and autoimmune disorders. If allergy assessment was not performed, this is completed before considering surgical intervention. Additional treatment options include immune modulators such as interleukin-5 inhibitors, leukotriene antagonists,[61] immunosuppressants such as methotrexate, and monoclonal anti-IgE therapy.[62,63] Collaboration with allergists, immunologists, pulmonologists, and infectious disease specialists may be necessary in particularly challenging patients.

In select patients with isolated polyp disease, in-office polypectomy can be considered, provided the patient does not have significant comorbidities or anticoagulant medications. The senior author performs these procedures using a microdebrider with topical anesthesia. Steroid-eluting stents are a relatively new option for patients with recurrent ethmoid polyposis, and small studies indicate improvement in short-term patient outcomes and polyp grade.[64]

Principles of Revision Surgery

In revision surgery, it is essential to develop a clear picture of the anatomic sites contributing to recurrence to create a well-defined plan for surgery. This begins with a thorough in-office endoscopic examination looking at the sites of disease, assessing the state of the mucosa, and documenting scarring and landmark distortion. A detailed thin-cut sinus computed tomography scan is performed with axial, coronal, and sagittal views, to allow a triplanar assessment of the postsurgical sinonasal cavities. A detailed evaluation includes at least the elements covered in **Box 2**. These

---

Box 2
Preoperative computed tomography checklist before revision endoscopic sinus surgery

Presence of each sinus with attention to frontal and sphenoid asymmetries

Septum position and perforations

Frontal sinus and frontal recess anatomy (agger, frontal cells)

Supraorbital ethmoid cells

Anterior ethmoid artery location

Location of inferior turbinate in relation to orbital floor

Presence of the middle turbinate

Location of uncinate attachment superiorly

Skull base slope anterior to posterior and Keros classification[66]

Dehiscences of bone around skull base, orbit, carotid, optic nerve

Sphenoid intersinus septum relationship to the carotid

Onodi (suprasphenoidal) cells

Haller (infraorbital) cells

items permit a thorough evaluation of the "danger" areas and set appropriate expectations for surgical intervention.[13,17,65]

Detailed preoperative counseling sets realistic expectations for patient outcomes. The surgeon reviews the areas of disease, the plan to address these areas, and how this surgery will be performed differently than the prior surgery. Although recent studies do not indicate differences in complication rate between primary and revision surgery,[66] the more complex nature of the surgery and the risks are covered in detail. The postoperative care plan is laid out in advance to permit the patient to ask questions and clarify expectations.

Patients are assessed for comorbidities that require preoperative optimization and clearance and counseled to avoid all nonessential anticoagulants (prescription, over the counter, and natural substances). Consideration is given to preoperative steroids in severe polyp cases to minimize inflammation and decrease intraoperative blood loss.[67]

Particular attention is paid to comorbidities that can be associated with higher rates of recurrence or worse outcomes. Smith and colleagues[68] found that aspirin sensitivity was predictive of poorer endoscopic and quality-of-life outcomes. Depression was predictive of poorer quality-of-life outcomes as well.

Landmarks and Surgical Approach

In revision surgery, the standard anatomic landmarks are often distorted or absent. To ensure clear orientation, consistent landmarks are used to navigate. This section presents a stepwise approach to landmark identification and revision sinus surgery used by the senior author (**Box 3**); this is described in similar fashion in several publications.[17,65,69]

Although rarely used by the senior author, many surgeons find that select use of intraoperative navigation can be helpful for confirming that areas of recurrent disease are addressed. However, using navigation is not a substitute for a clear understanding of the preoperative imaging. The surgeon should be prepared to operate without intraoperative navigation in the event of navigation failure or inaccuracy.

In cases where anatomic causes of failure are due to retained cells or structures, it is vital that revision surgery addresses these specific sites. In situations with scaring, contracture, synechiae, neo-osteogenesis, or recurrent polyp disease, the surgeon should plan to create wide unobstructed openings into the sinuses that will remain patent in the event of contracture or mucosal inflammation.

Box 3
Revision endoscopic sinus surgery anatomic landmarks
Nasal floor
Septum
Choanal arch
Nasolacrimal convexity
Posterior maxillary wall
Medial orbital floor
Lamina papyracea
Planum sphenoidale
Fovea ethmoidalis

Nasal landmarks

In the initial endoscopic evaluation, the nasal floor is visualized and followed posteriorly to the nasopharynx, where the choanal arch is identified. This aspect of the nasal cavity remains consistent over multiple surgeries and sets the anterior and posterior dimensions of the nasal airway. The nasal septum or remnant is seen medially.

The middle turbinate remnant is evaluated. If severely scarred, unstable, or involved in polyp disease, at least partial resection is performed to prevent lateralization or a focus of persistent obstructive sinus disease. Partial resection is associated with a longer interval until revision surgery is required.[70]

Maxillary antrostomy

The nasolacrimal arch formed by the posterior edge of the lacrimal bone that marks the lacrimal duct, can be identified in most revision cases. This convexity sets the anterior-most boundary of the maxillary cavity (**Fig. 5**). Inferiorly, the remnant of the inferior turbinate is identified. In revision cases, often the natural maxillary ostium or prior antrostomy is not visible. Thus, safe entry into the maxillary sinus is via the posterior fontanelle, providing the largest distance between the posterosuperiorly angled orbital floor and the inferior turbinate. This point, located above the posterior one-third of the inferior turbinate (**Fig. 6**), is entered with an angled probe or curette, incising the mucosa and minimizing the chance of elevating the maxillary sinus mucosa laterally. The probe is angled inferior and posterior away from the orbital floor. Working retrograde along the medial orbital floor (MOF), the fontanelle is removed and a wide antrostomy is created incorporating the natural ostium just behind the nasolacrimal convexity.

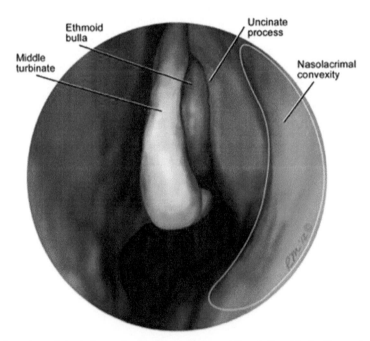

Fig. 5. Location of the left nasolacrimal convexity and its relationship to the uncinate process and middle turbinate. (*From* Casiano R. Endoscopic sinonasal dissection guide. New York: Thieme Medical Publishers, Inc; 2012; with permission.)

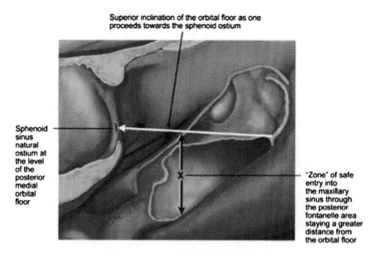

Fig. 6. The safest zone of entry into the left maxillary sinus posterior fontenelle above the posterior one-third of the inferior turbinate. This location has the greatest distance from the orbital floor (*x*). The *white line* demonstrates how the medial orbital floor sets the trajectory to the sphenoid sinus ostium. (*From* Casiano R. Endoscopic sinonasal dissection guide. New York: Thieme Medical Publishers, Inc; 2012; with permission.)

Common causes for persistent maxillary sinus disease are addressed, including scarring, residual uncinate, or a bridge of tissue creating recirculation (visualized with a 30° or 70° scope). When the ostium is identified, it is enlarged posteriorly and inferiorly including any accessory ostia, and removal of any Haller cells.[13,14,17,25] The superior border of the natural maxillary ostium is the junction with the MOF and inferior medial orbital wall. The resected edge of the posterior fontanelle creating the middle meatal antrostomy forms a ridge. This landmark helps to maintain the correct anterior–posterior trajectory when locating the sphenoid sinus (see **Fig. 6**). The antrostomy ridge has a horizontal component (horizontal border of the antrostomy), a transitional component, and a vertical component (**Fig. 7**), that help to define the location of the subsequent sinuses. Anterior ethmoid cells (starting with the ethmoid bulla inferiorly) are located medial to the horizontal ridge, the posterior ethmoid cells are entered through the coronal plane of the transitional ridge, and the sphenopalatine foramen is medial to the vertical ridge. The greater palatine nerve courses within the vertical ridge of the antrostomy and thus resection should not be flush with the posterior wall of the maxillary sinus. The coronal plane of the posterior wall of the maxillary sinus sets the approximate level of the sphenoid sinus anterior wall adjacent to the nasal septum.

Ethmoidectomy
The ethmoid bulla is often not visible or absent, or there may be significant neo-osteogenesis. The MOF is used to enter the inferior posterior ethmoid cells by visualizing a horizontal line from the posterior MOF to the septum (parallel to the nasal floor) and entering the posterior ethmoid through the midpoint of this line using a Cottle elevator or probe, which takes the surgeon through the horizontal basal lamella of the middle turbinate approximately 5 cm from the columella (**Fig. 8**). Once the lamina

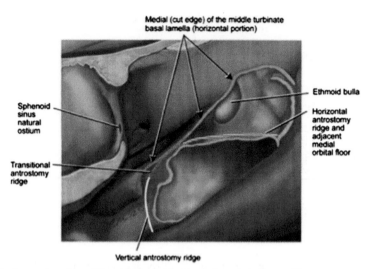

Fig. 7. Left nasal cavity with middle turbinate removed. Left maxillary antrostomy ridge zones: horizontal component, transitional component, and vertical component. The anterior ethmoid cells located medial to the horizontal ridge. Posterior ethmoid cells are entered through the plan of the transitional ridge. Sphenopalatine foramen is medial to the vertical ridge. (*From* Casiano R. Endoscopic sinonasal dissection guide. New York: Thieme Medical Publishers, Inc; 2012; with permission.)

papyracea is identified laterally within the posterior ethmoid sinus, the surgeon can work superiorly and anteriorly in a retrograde manner. Conversely, the sphenoid may be identified next (as described elsewhere in this article) and the resultant landmarks used to perform the ethmoidectomy retrograde. During ethmoidectomy the surgeon initially stays laterally along the skull base, parallel to the lamina, defining the thicker bone of the fovea ethmoidalis, and avoiding the medial ethmoid roof (adjacent to the cribriform plate). Once the ethmoid roof is well-identified, then the medial aspect of the skull base is defined, keeping in mind that the skull base will slope inferomedially.

The many aspects leading to recurrent ethmoid disease are addressed, including persistent agger nasi cells, unopened ethmoid cells (including supraorbital cells), scarring/synechiae, and neo-osteogenesis. Frequently, in the setting of neo-osteogenic bone, the microdebrider is ineffective, and potentially unsafe, to remove the thick bone. Instead, a frontal sinus probe or curette is used to carefully break up septations moving from posterior to anterior. Additionally, an up-angled non–through-cut forceps is used parallel to the medial orbital wall to safely remove the thickened bony septations from the lamina. The side of the forceps is used to palpate dehiscences in the lamina papyracea. Periodic palpation of the eye is a must to identify areas of dehiscence.

Sphenoidotomy

Identifying the sphenoid is a reliable way to set the posterior level of the skull base, which is also the inferior-most aspect of the skull base. The skull base projects superiorly, moving from posterior to anterior in the sagittal plane. In general, the natural ostium is 1.5 cm above the choanal arch and 7 cm from the columella although variability exists among patients. The natural os is about 1 cm superomedial to the

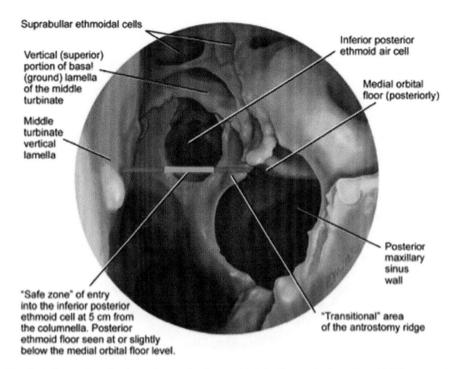

Suprabullar ethmoidal cells

Vertical (superior) portion of basal (ground) lamella of the middle turbinate

Middle turbinate vertical lamella

Inferior posterior ethmoid air cell

Medial orbital floor (posteriorly)

Posterior maxillary sinus wall

"Safe zone" of entry into the inferior posterior ethmoid cell at 5 cm from the columnella. Posterior ethmoid floor seen at or slightly below the medial orbital floor level.

"Transitional" area of the antrostomy ridge

Fig. 8. Left nasal cavity zone demonstrating entry into the posterior ethmoid. The central one-third of the line from the posterior medial orbital floor to the septum, parallel to the nasal floor, is a safe zone of entry into the inferior posterior ethmoid sinus cells. (*From* Casiano R. Endoscopic sinonasal dissection guide. New York: Thieme Medical Publishers, Inc; 2012; with permission.)

superior turbinate tail, but is often not visible in revision surgery. Thus, the MOF and posterior maxillary wall are used to identify the sphenoid by drawing a horizontal line from the posterior MOF to the septum (**Fig. 9**). The sphenoid is entered using a Cottle elevator, in the medial aspect of this line adjacent to the septum, placing the surgeon in the middle one-third of the sphenoid with most of the sphenoid sinus inferiorly. Entering medially protects the laterally located carotid. The superior border of the sphenoid makes up the planum sphenoidale located above the sella convexity. The posterior wall of the sphenoid (clivus) is approximately 9 cm from the columella (**Fig. 10**).

The ostium is widely opened to permit topical medication treatment and postoperative observation. The main causes for persistent sphenoid disease are addressed, including scarring, thick neo-osteogenic bone, failure to open the sphenoid os (mistaking the Onodi cell for the sphenoid), and recirculation (not including the natural sphenoid os in the sinusotomy), as with transethmoidal approaches.[17]

Frontal sinusotomy

Once a complete ethmoidectomy is performed, removing the agger nasi and opening of the suprabullar/supraorbital cells, then the frontal infundibulum may be easy to locate (**Fig. 11**). However, in revision cases it is common for scarring, polyps, and neo-osteogenesis to obscure this area. A 30°, 45°, or 70° scope is used to view the

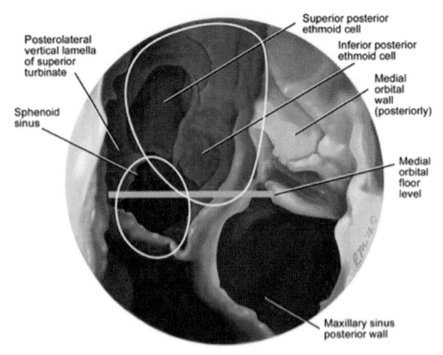

Fig. 9. The left nasal cavity demonstrating the relationship of the sphenoid to the maxillary and posterior ethmoid sinuses. Safest entry into the sphenoid sinus is located on the medial aspect of the line from the posterior medial orbital floor to the septum, parallel to the nasal floor. Entry in the middle one-third of the sphenoid and protects lateral structures. (*From* Casiano R. Endoscopic sinonasal dissection guide. New York: Thieme Medical Publishers, Inc; 2012; with permission.)

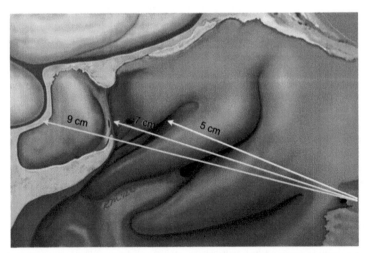

Fig. 10. A sagittal view of the left nasal cavity marking the distances from the columella to the superior turbinate (5 cm), the sphenoid ostium (7 cm), and the posterior sphenoid wall (9 cm).

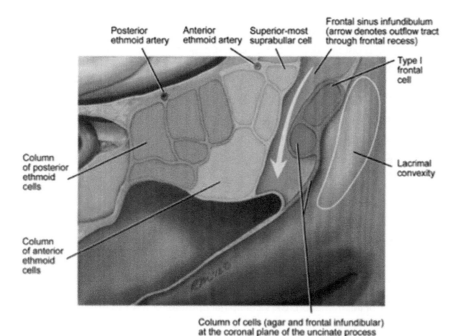

Fig. 11. Left frontal outflow tract demonstrating relationship to the nasolacrimal convexity, the anterior ethmoid, the suprabullar cells, agger nasi, and frontal cells. (*From* Casiano R. Endoscopic sinonasal dissection guide. New York: Thieme Medical Publishers, Inc; 2012; with permission.)

area of the frontal infundibulum. A series of landmarks can be used to locate the frontal sinus infundibulum:

- Nasolacrimal convexity defines the trajectory to enter the frontal sinus.
- A line from the anterior border of the natural maxillary ostium, posterior and parallel to the nasolacrimal duct, represents the coronal plane of the frontal sinus infundibulum. This is also the coronal plane of the uncinate process and agar nasi cell.
- The anterior ethmoid artery is approximately 1 cm posterior to the ostium, running along the posterior septation of the suprabullar cell, even when the cell extends supraorbitally.[71] This cell lies in the coronal plane of the ethmoid bulla.
- Anterior attachment of the middle turbinate is 5 to 10 mm anterior to the posterior wall of the frontal infundibulum.

The senior author advocates for entry into the frontal infundibulum with a frontal sinus probe using minimal pressure. The probe is directed slightly laterally into the frontal sinus, confirming with transillumination once opened. It is important not to confuse supraorbital ethmoid cells with the frontal sinus. Residual septations are taken down carefully with a probe or frontal sinus curette in an inferior direction, with the goal of preserving mucosa.[72] However, in the presence of neo-osteogenesis or severe polyp disease, the latter is not possible. It is essential to know the frontal sinus anatomy from the computed tomography and address any frontal cells because they are found in up to one-third of patients undergoing FESS.[73,74]

The anatomic causes for recurrent frontal disease are addressed. If this is the first time the frontal is fully opened, with all frontal cells removed, and the disease is addressed with a patent wide opening (Draf I), then no further intervention is necessary. However, if the opening is narrow, there is neo-osteogenesis, or there is a propensity for scarring and recurrent mucosal disease, then a more involved procedure is necessary (described elsewhere in this article).

Advanced Procedures to Address Specific Issues in Severe Recurrent Disease

Maxillary disease inaccessible with a wide middle meatal antrostomy

- Extended maxillary sinusotomy combines a wide middle meatal antrostomy with an inferior meatal antrostomy leaving the inferior turbinate attached anteriorly and posteriorly (**Fig. 12**).[75] If this is insufficient to access all aspects of maxillary sinus disease then a medial maxillectomy ("mega-antrostomy") or modified Denker procedure may be necessary (addressed elsewhere in this issue).

Insufficient frontal sinus opening achieved by Draf I frontal sinusotomy

- Draf IIa: A narrow frontal infundibulum is selectively enlarged in the anterior and/or medial direction permitting good visualization of frontal disease, access to frontal cells, postoperative aeration, and access to topical therapies, even in the event of inflammation. Cervical spinal curettes or a 40 to 60° cutting burr is used to remove bone, creating a large opening through which instrumentation and scopes can easily pass.
- Draf IIb: Extending the medial frontal infundibulum to the nasal septum by removing the anterior quarter of the middle turbinate vertical lamella, which makes up the medial wall of the frontal infundibulum. Bone is removed with a

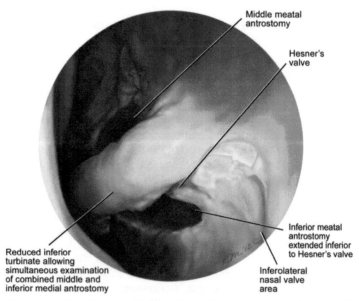

Fig. 12. Left nasal cavity demonstrating a wide middle meatal antrostomy combined with an inferior meatal antrostomy with inferior turbinate left in place, attached anteriorly and posteriorly. (*From* Casiano R. Endoscopic sinonasal dissection guide. New York: Thieme Medical Publishers, Inc; 2012; with permission.)

Frontal sinus

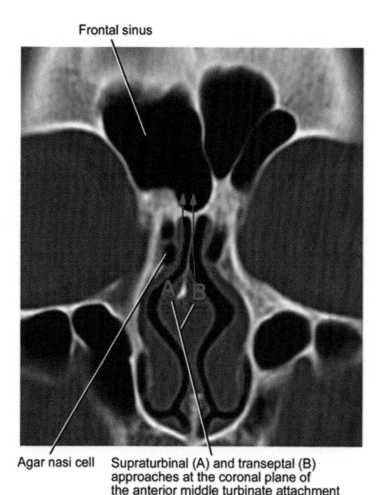

Agar nasi cell   Supraturbinal (A) and transeptal (B)
approaches at the coronal plane of
the anterior middle turbinate attachment

Fig. 13. Coronal sinus computed tomography scan with *arrows* demonstrating methods of alternative medial entry into the frontal sinus performed in the coronal plane of the anterior attachment of the middle turbinate. *Line A*, supraturbinal entry point; *line B*, transeptal entry point. (*From* Casiano R. Endoscopic sinonasal dissection guide. New York: Thieme Medical Publishers, Inc; 2012; with permission.)

cervical spine curette or 40 to 60° cutting burr, until reaching the junction of the nasal septum (superior perpendicular plate of the ethmoid) with the frontal inter-sinus septum. The posterior wall mucosa of the infundibulum is preserved, mini-mizing circumferential scar and contracture. This procedure improves access to medial and lateral frontal sinus disease. However, if appropriate access is not achieved, then a Draf III may be necessary (see elsewhere in this issue).

Neo-osteogenesis of the frontal prevents location of the infundibulum

- In rare cases of extremely severe neo-osteogenesis, the frontal is inaccessible via the laterally located frontal recess and infundibulum. A more midline approach into the frontal sinus may be indicated (transeptal or supraturbinal approach at coronal plane of the anterior attachment of the middle turbinate). In these cases drilling directly into the medial frontal sinus, bypassing the ethmoids, is an option **(Fig. 13)**.[76,77]

- Frontal sinus trephination and other external incisions can be combined with these endoscopic procedures to aid in location, and removal of disease, from the frontal sinus.[78]

REVISION SINUS SURGERY OUTCOMES

Revision FESS improves outcomes in patients that fail maximum medical therapy and prior sinus surgery for CRS. Lee and colleagues[79] compared surgical outcomes between primary and revision FESS for CRS with nasal polyps and found similar objective and subjective outcomes after surgery. Similarly, McMains and Kountakis[80] analyzed 125 patients requiring revision surgery after failing primary surgery and maximal medical treatment. At 2 years postoperatively, there was retained improvement in quality of life and endoscopic score with an overall failure rate of 8%,[80] which is similar to that of primary CRS FESS surgery. Litvack and colleagues'[81] prospective comparison of primary and revision FESS also found similar results. Taken together, studies indicate that revision FESS is a viable treatment option for patients who fail primary sinus surgery and maximal medical treatment for recurrent CRS.

REFERENCES

1. Soler ZM, Mace J, Smith TL. Symptom-based presentation of chronic rhinosinusitis and symptom-specific outcomes after endoscopic sinus surgery. Am J Rhinol 2008;22(3):297–301.
2. Damm M, Quante G, Jungehuelsing M, et al. Impact of functional endoscopic sinus surgery on symptoms and quality of life in chronic rhinosinusitis. Laryngoscope 2002;112(2):310–5.
3. Soler ZM, Smith TL. Quality-of-life outcomes after endoscopic sinus surgery: how long is long enough? Otolaryngol Head Neck Surg 2010;143(5):621–5.
4. Osguthorpe JD. Surgical outcomes in rhinosinusitis: what we know. Otolaryngol Head Neck Surg 1999;120(4):451–3.
5. King JM, Caldarelli DD, Pigato JB. A review of revision functional endoscopic sinus surgery. Laryngoscope 1994;104(4):404–8.
6. Schaefer SD, Manning S, Close LG. Endoscopic paranasal sinus surgery: indications and considerations. Laryngoscope 1989;99(1):1–5.
7. Lazar RH, Younis RT, Long TE, et al. Revision functional endonasal sinus surgery. Ear Nose Throat J 1992;71(3):131–3.
8. Smith LF, Brindley PC. Indications, evaluation, complications, and results of functional endoscopic sinus surgery in 200 patients. Otolaryngol Head Neck Surg 1993;108(6):688–96.
9. Ramadan HH. Surgical causes of failure in endoscopic sinus surgery. Laryngoscope 1999;109(1):27–9.
10. Senior BA, Kennedy DW, Tanabodee J, et al. Long-term results of functional endoscopic sinus surgery. Laryngoscope 1998;108(2):151–7.
11. Musy PY, Kountakis SE. Anatomic findings in patients undergoing revision endoscopic sinus surgery. Am J Otolaryngol 2004;25(6):418–22.
12. Chandra RK, Palmer JN, Tangsujarittham T, et al. Factors associated with failure of frontal sinusotomy in the early follow-up period. Otolaryngol Head Neck Surg 2004;131(4):514–8.

13. Sillers M, Lay K. Principles of revision functional endoscopic sinus surgery. Operative Techniques in Otolaryngology 2016;17(1):6–12. Available at: http://www.optecoto.com/article/S1043-1810(05)00117-X/abstract.

14. Lee JM, Chiu AG. Role of maximal endoscopic sinus surgery techniques in chronic rhinosinusitis. Otolaryngol Clin North Am 2010;43(3):579–89, ix.

15. Wynn R, Har-El G. Recurrence rates after endoscopic sinus surgery for massive sinus polyposis. Laryngoscope 2004;114(5):811–3.

16. Mendelsohn D, Jeremic G, Wright ED, et al. Revision rates after endoscopic sinus surgery: a recurrence analysis. Ann Otol Rhinol Laryngol 2011;120(3):162–6.

17. Stankiewicz JA, Donzelli JJ, Chow JM. Failures of functional endoscopic sinus surgery and their surgical correction. Operative Techniques in Otolaryngology 1996; 7(3):297–304. Available at: http://www.optecoto.com/action/showMultipleAbstracts.

18. Otto KJ, DelGaudio JM. Operative findings in the frontal recess at time of revision surgery. Am J Otolaryngol 2010;31(3):175–80.

19. Chiu AG, Vaughan WC. Revision endoscopic frontal sinus surgery with surgical navigation. Otolaryngol Head Neck Surg 2004;130(3):312–8.

20. Metson R, Gliklich RE. Endoscopic treatment of sphenoid sinusitis. Otolaryngol Head Neck Surg 1996;114(6):736–44.

21. Parsons DS, Stivers FE, Talbot AR. The missed ostium sequence and the surgical approach to revision functional endoscopic sinus surgery. Otolaryngol Clin North Am 1996;29(1):169–83.

22. Telmesani LM, Al-Shawarby M. Osteitis in chronic rhinosinusitis with nasal polyps: a comparative study between primary and recurrent cases. Eur Arch Otorhinolaryngol 2010;267(5):721–4.

23. Sacks PL, Snidvongs K, Rom D, et al. The impact of neo-osteogenesis on disease control in chronic rhinosinusitis after primary surgery. Int Forum Allergy Rhinol 2013;3(10):823–7.

24. Lee JT, Kennedy DW, Palmer JN, et al. The incidence of concurrent osteitis in patients with chronic rhinosinusitis: a clinicopathological study. Am J Rhinol 2006; 20(3):278–82.

25. Richtsmeier WJ. Top 10 reasons for endoscopic maxillary sinus surgery failure. Laryngoscope 2001;111(11 Pt 1):1952–6.

26. Bent JP 3rd, Kuhn FA. Diagnosis of allergic fungal sinusitis. Otolaryngol Head Neck Surg 1994;111(5):580–8.

27. Collins M, Nair S, Smith W, et al. Role of local immunoglobulin E production in the pathophysiology of noninvasive fungal sinusitis. Laryngoscope 2004;114(7): 1242–6.

28. Ryan MW, Marple BF. Allergic fungal rhinosinusitis: diagnosis and management. Curr Opin Otolaryngol Head Neck Surg 2007;15(1):18–22.

29. Schubert MS. Allergic fungal sinusitis: pathogenesis and management strategies. Drugs 2004;64(4):363–74.

30. Kuhn FA, Javer AR. Allergic fungal sinusitis: a four-year follow-up. Am J Rhinol 2000;14(3):149–56.

31. Kupferberg SB, Bent JP 3rd, Kuhn FA. Prognosis for allergic fungal sinusitis. Otolaryngol Head Neck Surg 1997;117(1):35–41.

32. Schubert MS, Goetz DW. Evaluation and treatment of allergic fungal sinusitis. II. Treatment and follow-up. J Allergy Clin Immunol 1998;102(3):395–402.

33. Gan EC, Thamboo A, Rudmik L, et al. Medical management of allergic fungal rhinosinusitis following endoscopic sinus surgery: an evidence-based review and recommendations. Int Forum Allergy Rhinol 2014;4(9):702–15.

34. Leigh MW, Zariwala MA, Knowles MR. Primary ciliary dyskinesia: improving the diagnostic approach. Curr Opin Pediatr 2009;21(3):320–5.

35. Kang SH, Dalcin Pde T, Piltcher OB, et al. Chronic rhinosinusitis and nasal polyposis in cystic fibrosis: update on diagnosis and treatment. J Bras Pneumol 2015; 41(1):65–76.

36. Ryan MW, Brooks EG. Rhinosinusitis and comorbidities. Curr Allergy Asthma Rep 2010;10(3):188–93.

37. Hunsaker DH, Leid JG. The relationship of biofilms to chronic rhinosinusitis. Curr Opin Otolaryngol Head Neck Surg 2008;16(3):237–41.

38. Mah TF, O'Toole GA. Mechanisms of biofilm resistance to antimicrobial agents. Trends Microbiol 2001;9(1):34–9.

39. Singhal D, Psaltis AJ, Foreman A, et al. The impact of biofilms on outcomes after endoscopic sinus surgery. Am J Rhinol Allergy 2010;24(3):169–74.

40. Prince AA, Steiger JD, Khalid AN, et al. Prevalence of biofilm-forming bacteria in chronic rhinosinusitis. Am J Rhinol 2008;22(3):239–45.

41. Singhal D, Foreman A, Jervis-Bardy J, et al. Staphylococcus aureus biofilms: nemesis of endoscopic sinus surgery. Laryngoscope 2011;121(7):1578–83.

42. Bendouah Z, Barbeau J, Hamad WA, et al. Biofilm formation by Staphylococcus aureus and Pseudomonas aeruginosa is associated with an unfavorable evolution after surgery for chronic sinusitis and nasal polyposis. Otolaryngol Head Neck Surg 2006;134(6):991–6.

43. Foreman A, Wormald PJ. Different biofilms, different disease? A clinical outcomes study. Laryngoscope 2010;120(8):1701–6.

44. Foreman A, Jervis-Bardy J, Wormald PJ. Do biofilms contribute to the initiation and recalcitrance of chronic rhinosinusitis? Laryngoscope 2011;121(5):1085–91.

45. Batra PS, Tong L, Citardi MJ. Analysis of comorbidities and objective parameters in refractory chronic rhinosinusitis. Laryngoscope 2013;123(Suppl 7):S1–11.

46. Vanlerberghe L, Joniau S, Jorissen M. The prevalence of humoral immunodeficiency in refractory rhinosinusitis: a retrospective analysis. B-ENT 2006;2(4): 161–6.

47. Chee L, Graham SM, Carothers DG, et al. Immune dysfunction in refractory sinusitis in a tertiary care setting. Laryngoscope 2001;111(2):233–5.

48. Schwitzguebel AJ, Jandus P, Lacroix JS, et al. Immunoglobulin deficiency in patients with chronic rhinosinusitis: systematic review of the literature and meta-analysis. J Allergy Clin Immunol 2015;136(6):1523–31.

49. White AA, Stevenson DD. Aspirin-exacerbated respiratory disease: update on pathogenesis and desensitization. Semin Respir Crit Care Med 2012;33(6): 588–94.

50. Rotenberg BW, Zhang I, Arra I, et al. Postoperative care for Samter's triad patients undergoing endoscopic sinus surgery: a double-blinded, randomized controlled trial. Laryngoscope 2011;121(12):2702–5.

51. Xu JJ, Sowerby L, Rotenberg BW. Aspirin desensitization for aspirin-exacerbated respiratory disease (Samter's Triad): a systematic review of the literature. Int Forum Allergy Rhinol 2013;3(11):915–20.

52. Fooanant S, Chaiyasate S, Roongrotwattanasiri K. Comparison on the efficacy of dexpanthenol in sea water and saline in postoperative endoscopic sinus surgery. J Med Assoc Thai 2008;91(10):1558–63.

53. Freeman SR, Sivayoham ES, Jepson K, et al. A preliminary randomised controlled trial evaluating the efficacy of saline douching following endoscopic sinus surgery. Clin Otolaryngol 2008;33(5):462–5.

54. Lim M, Citardi MJ, Leong JL. Topical antimicrobials in the management of chronic rhinosinusitis: a systematic review. Am J Rhinol 2008;22(4):381–9.

55. Rudmik L, Soler ZM, Orlandi RR, et al. Early postoperative care following endoscopic sinus surgery: an evidence-based review with recommendations. Int Forum Allergy Rhinol 2011;1(6):417–30.

56. Snidvongs K, Kalish L, Sacks R, et al. Topical steroid for chronic rhinosinusitis without polyps. Cochrane Database Syst Rev 2011;(8):CD009274.

57. Kalish L, Snidvongs K, Sivasubramaniam R, et al. Topical steroids for nasal polyps. Cochrane Database Syst Rev 2012;(12):CD006549.

58. Rudmik L, Smith TL. Evidence-based practice: postoperative care in endoscopic sinus surgery. Otolaryngol Clin North Am 2012;45(5):1019–32.

59. Wilson KF, McMains KC, Orlandi RR. The association between allergy and chronic rhinosinusitis with and without nasal polyps: an evidence-based review with recommendations. Int Forum Allergy Rhinol 2014;4(2):93–103.

60. Tan BK, Zirkle W, Chandra RK, et al. Atopic profile of patients failing medical therapy for chronic rhinosinusitis. Int Forum Allergy Rhinol 2011;1(2):88–94.

61. Stewart RA, Ram B, Hamilton G, et al. Montelukast as an adjunct to oral and inhaled steroid therapy in chronic nasal polyposis. Otolaryngol Head Neck Surg 2008;139(5):682–7.

62. Pinto JM, Mehta N, DiTineo M, et al. A randomized, double-blind, placebo-controlled trial of anti-IgE for chronic rhinosinusitis. Rhinology 2010;48(3):318–24.

63. Piromchai P, Kasemsiri P, Laohasiriwong S, et al. Chronic rhinosinusitis and emerging treatment options. Int J Gen Med 2013;6:453–64.

64. Lavigne F, Miller SK, Gould AR, et al. Steroid-eluting sinus implant for in-office treatment of recurrent nasal polyposis: a prospective, multicenter study. Int Forum Allergy Rhinol 2014;4(5):381–9.

65. Lieberman S. Anatomical landmarks in revision sinus surgery and advanced nasal polyposis. Operative Techniques in Otolaryngology- Head and Neck Surgery 2014;25(2):149–55.

66. Krings JG, Kallogjeri D, Wineland A, et al. Complications of primary and revision functional endoscopic sinus surgery for chronic rhinosinusitis. Laryngoscope 2014;124(4):838–45.

67. Ecevit MC, Erdag TK, Dogan E, et al. Effect of steroids for nasal polyposis surgery: a placebo-controlled, randomized, double-blind study. Laryngoscope 2015;125(9):2041–5.

68. Smith TL, Mendolia-Loffredo S, Loehrl TA, et al. Predictive factors and outcomes in endoscopic sinus surgery for chronic rhinosinusitis. Laryngoscope 2005; 115(12):2199–205.

69. May M, Schaitkin B, Kay SL. Revision endoscopic sinus surgery: six friendly surgical landmarks. Laryngoscope 1994;104(6 Pt 1):766–7.

70. Wu AW, Ting JY, Platt MP, et al. Factors affecting time to revision sinus surgery for nasal polyps: a 25-year experience. Laryngoscope 2014;124(1):29–33.

71. Jang DW, Lachanas VA, White LC, et al. Supraorbital ethmoid cell: a consistent landmark for endoscopic identification of the anterior ethmoidal artery. Otolaryngol Head Neck Surg 2014;151(6):1073–7.

72. Casiano R. Endoscopic sinonasal dissection guide. New York: Thieme Medical Publishers, Inc; 2012.

73. Meyer TK, Kocak M, Smith MM, et al. Coronal computed tomography analysis of frontal cells. Am J Rhinol 2003;17(3):163–8.

74. DelGaudio JM, Hudgins PA, Venkatraman G, et al. Multiplanar computed tomographic analysis of frontal recess cells: effect on frontal isthmus size and frontal sinusitis. Arch Otolaryngol Head Neck Surg 2005;131(3):230–5.

75. Rodriguez MJ, Sargi Z, Casiano RR. Extended maxillary sinusotomy in isolated refractory maxillary sinus disease. Otolaryngol Head Neck Surg 2007;137(3): 508–10.

76. Lanza DC, McLaughlin RB Jr, Hwang PH. The five year experience with endoscopic trans-septal frontal sinusotomy. Otolaryngol Clin North Am 2001;34(1): 139–52.

77. McLaughlin RB, Hwang PH, Lanza DC. Endoscopic trans-septal frontal sinusotomy: the rationale and results of an alternative technique. Am J Rhinol 1999; 13(4):279–87.

78. Bent JP 3rd, Spears RA, Kuhn FA, et al. Combined endoscopic intranasal and external frontal sinusotomy. Am J Rhinol 1997;11(5):349–54.

79. Lee JY, Lee SW, Lee JD. Comparison of the surgical outcome between primary and revision endoscopic sinus surgery for chronic rhinosinusitis with nasal polyposis. Am J Otolaryngol 2008;29(6):379–84.

80. McMains KC, Kountakis SE. Revision functional endoscopic sinus surgery: objective and subjective surgical outcomes. Am J Rhinol 2005;19(4):344–7.

81. Litvack JR, Griest S, James KE, et al. Endoscopic and quality-of-life outcomes after revision endoscopic sinus surgery. Laryngoscope 2007;117(12):2233–8.

Extended Endoscopic and Open Sinus Surgery for Refractory Chronic Rhinosinusitis

Jean Anderson Eloy, MD[a,b,c,d,]*, Emily Marchiano, MD[a], Alejandro Vázquez, MD[a]

KEYWORDS

- Endoscopic sinus surgery • Extended maxillary antrostomy
- Endoscopic modified medial maxillectomy • Nasalization
- Extended sphenoid sinusotomy • Extended frontal sinusotomy
- Modified Lothrop procedure • Modification of Lothrop procedure

KEY POINTS

- Chronic recalcitrant maxillary sinusitis may require extended sinus surgery for adequate management, including the endoscopic maxillary mega-antrostomy and the endoscopic modified medial maxillectomy. The sublabial anterior maxillotomy is an external approach that can also be used in these patients.
- Revision total ethmoidectomy should be considered in refractory chronic rhinosinusitis with the goals of resection of all remaining ethmoid partitions, removal of all osteitic bone, and potential ethmoidal mucosal stripping (nasalization) to prevent recurrence.
- Chronic recalcitrant sphenoid sinusitis may require an extended sphenoid sinusotomy with creation of a single, large common cavity. This decreases the potential for scarring and obstruction and provides a large pathway for application of topical medications.

Continued

Financial Disclosures: None.

Conflicts of Interest: None.

[a] Department of Otolaryngology – Head and Neck Surgery, Rutgers New Jersey Medical School, Newark, NJ, USA; [b] Center for Skull Base and Pituitary Surgery, Neurological Institute of New Jersey, Rutgers New Jersey Medical School, Newark, NJ, USA; [c] Department of Neurological Surgery, Rutgers New Jersey Medical School, Newark, NJ, USA; [d] Department of Ophthalmology and Visual Science, Rutgers New Jersey Medical School, 90 Bergen Street, Suite 8100, Newark, NJ 07103, USA

* Corresponding author. Rhinology and Sinus Surgery, Otolaryngology Research, Endoscopic Skull Base Surgery Program, Department of Otolaryngology–Head and Neck Surgery, Neurological Institute of New Jersey, Rutgers New Jersey Medical School, 90 Bergen Street, Suite 8100, Newark, NJ 07103.

E-mail address: jean.anderson.eloy@gmail.com

Continued

- A variety of extended endoscopic endonasal and open frontal sinus procedures can be used in the management of refractory chronic frontal sinusitis. The goal of these endoscopic procedures is to create a patent nasofrontal outflow tract (frontal sinus drainage pathway) as an egress pathway and to provide access for application of adequate topical medications. The external approaches can be used to preserve frontal sinus function or to obliterate the frontal sinus. Cranialization of the frontal sinus represents the final remedy in treatment of recalcitrant frontal sinusitis.

Abbreviations	
AMT	Appropriate medical therapy
BCD	Balloon catheter dilation
CSF	Cerebrospinal fluid
EMMA	Endoscopic maxillary mega-antrostomy
ESS	Endoscopic sinus surgery
IGS	Image-guidance surgery
MCLP	Modified central-Lothrop procedure
MHLP	Modified hemi-Lothrop procedure
MLP	Modified Lothrop procedure
MMLP	Modified mini-Lothrop procedure
MSLP	Modified subtotal-Lothrop procedure

 Video content accompanies this article at http://www.oto.theclinics.com.

INTRODUCTION

Over the past 3 decades, the management of patients with chronic rhinosinusitis (CRS) has evolved from significantly invasive procedures to minimally invasive mucosal-preserving options. Currently, the overwhelming majority of patients with CRS can be treated effectively with appropriate medical therapy (AMT). For patients who failed AMT, the next option is surgical intervention. Initial surgical treatment usually involves endoscopic sinus surgery (ESS) with maximal mucosal preservation; this can be achieved using balloon dilation technology or functional ESS. In cases of failed initial surgical treatment, revision ESS using more aggressive techniques is often undertaken. Nonetheless, a subgroup of patients will go on to fail revision treatment with traditional ESS techniques. In these situations, more advanced surgical procedures may be necessary for extirpation of the disease process.[1] In this article, the authors describe advanced surgical techniques used for the maxillary, ethmoid, sphenoid, and frontal sinuses in patients with refractory CRS who have failed AMT and traditional ESS techniques.

EXTENDED MAXILLARY SINUS PROCEDURES

In his 1675 volume *Dissertationes anatomico-pathologicae*, the renowned anatomist Antonio Molinetti reports a case of maxillary sinusitis that was successfully treated via trephination through the anterior maxillary sinus wall.[2] More than 2 centuries later, 3 surgeons would independently publish descriptions of a technique that became the standard for the next one hundred years: George Caldwell (in 1893), Scanes Spicer (in

1894), and Henry Luc (in 1897) each described the creation of a temporary opening through the canine fossa and a simultaneous counter-opening in the inferior meatus.[3] This procedure came to be known as the Caldwell-Luc operation.

In the latter part of the twentieth century, advances in the understanding of maxillary sinus physiology, as well as the advent of new surgical technologies, would eventually lead to the development of so-called functional ESS.

Today, the initial management of chronic maxillary sinusitis is nonsurgical; surgery is reserved for cases whereby AMT has failed to achieve disease resolution. When an intervention is warranted, 2 major options exist: either balloon catheter dilation (BCD) or endoscopic endonasal maxillary antrostomy. BCD is an endoscopic procedure in which the sinus ostium is identified, cannulated with a balloon catheter, and dilated. Endoscopic maxillary antrostomy entails resection of the uncinate process followed by widening of the maxillary sinus ostium. In both cases, the goal is to establish patency of the maxillary sinus by widening its natural aperture, which should preserve the native mechanism of mucus egress (hence the designation of "functional" surgery).

Despite its high success rate, maxillary antrostomy failure is not uncommon.[4] In a study of patients undergoing revision ESS, for instance, middle meatal antrostomy stenosis was found in 39% of cases.[5] Multiple factors have been implicated in the development of persistent (or recalcitrant) maxillary sinusitis, including impaired mucociliary clearance (eg, in cystic fibrosis or primary ciliary dyskinesia), biofilm formation, and previous endoscopic or open surgery.[6]

Endoscopic Maxillary Mega-Antrostomy

In 2008, Cho and Hwang[7] described their experience with a less extensive form of salvage surgery: the endoscopic maxillary mega-antrostomy (EMMA). EMMA entails a partial inferior turbinectomy (ie, with preservation of at least its anterior one-third) and widening of the maxillary antrostomy down to the level of the nasal cavity floor (Video 1). This configuration allows for gravity-assisted drainage of a sinus in which mucociliary clearance has been rendered ineffective. It also facilitates irrigation, topical medication delivery, and access for in-office surveillance. In a follow-up to the aforementioned 2008 study, the original 28-patient cohort reported either complete/significant improvement (72.4%) or partial improvement (27.6%) after a mean follow-up period of 6.9 years.[8]

Endoscopic Modified Medial Maxillectomy

Although sometimes conflated in the literature, EMMA must be differentiated from the endoscopic modified medial maxillectomy (EMMM), an extended procedure that was originally conceived for the management of benign sinonasal neoplasms. In contrast to EMMA, EMMM entails a complete inferior turbinectomy and widening of the antrostomy to its anatomic limits: inferiorly, to the level of nasal cavity floor; superiorly, to the medial orbital floor; posteriorly, to the posterior wall of the maxillary sinus; and anteriorly, to the nasolacrimal duct. EMMM allows ample access to the maxillary sinus, including difficult-to-reach areas such as the lateral recesses, the posterior aspect of the anterior maxillary sinus wall, and the floor of the maxillary sinus (Video 2). In essence, in recalcitrant maxillary sinusitis, the indications for EMMM and EMMA are the same. The preservation of normal tissue that EMMA provides is desirable, but not always feasible. Moreover, in EMMM, widening of the antrostomy anteriorly may place the nasolacrimal duct at risk of injury.[6] During the EMMM for chronic recurrent sinusitis, auto-obliteration of the sinus may be the goal. In this situation, a decision can be made to completely eradicate the maxillary sinus mucosa and trigger the natural obliteration of the sinus (**Fig. 1**).

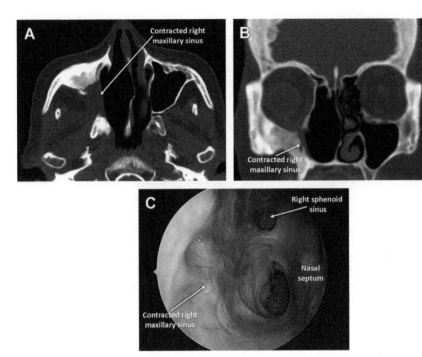

Fig. 1. Axial (*A*) and coronal (*B*) CT scans of the paranasal sinuses depicting the contraction/auto-obliteration of the maxillary sinus 1 year following a right EMMM. (*C*) In-office endoscopic image of the same patient approximately 1 year after the surgery.

Endoscopic-Assisted Sublabial Anterior Maxillotomy

After the introduction of ESS, the Caldwell-Luc operation remained an option for surgically refractory maxillary sinusitis. Sublabial maxillotomy is performed rarely these days for inflammatory disease; however, endoscopic-assisted sublabial anterior maxillotomy remains an option for disease that is otherwise difficult to reach endonasally (**Fig. 2**).

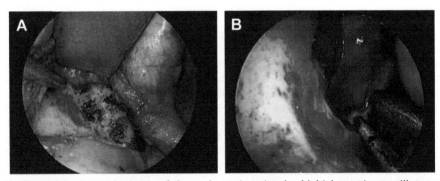

Fig. 2. Intraoperative depiction of the endoscopic-assisted sublabial anterior maxillotomy. (*A*) Left anterior maxillary wall after elevation of the soft tissue coverage in the subperiosteal plane. (*B*) Endoscopic view after bone removal. Note that a Kerrison rongeur or high-speed drill (depicted) can be used for bone removal.

Inferior Meatal Antrostomy

Widespread understanding of paranasal sinus physiology has caused another technique, the inferior meatal antrostomy, to fall out of favor. Hence, although the inferior meatal antrostomy provides a pathway for egress of maxillary sinus contents, this opening does not incorporate the natural ostium of the maxillary sinus where the mucociliary flow of this sinus converges. Consequently, there is a belief that this procedure could lead to mucous recirculation and prevent eradication of the disease process. Nevertheless, some have argued for its role in managing postoperative mucoceles, stating that it is effective and "easier to perform" than middle meatal antrostomy.[9] This procedure can be performed alone, or in combination with a middle meatal antrostomy (**Fig. 3**). The inferior meatal antrostomy (similar to the EMMA and the EMMM) can be useful in cases of improper mucociliary clearance due to ciliary dysfunction such as *primary ciliary dyskinesia*[10–12] (also known as Kartagener syndrome or immotile ciliary syndrome), or abnormally viscous mucous secretions, as seen in patients with *cystic fibrosis*.[12–14]

EXTENDED ETHMOID SINUS PROCEDURES

CRS often involves the ethmoid sinuses. When surgery is indicated, the standard contemporary approach is an endoscopic resection of the affected compartments

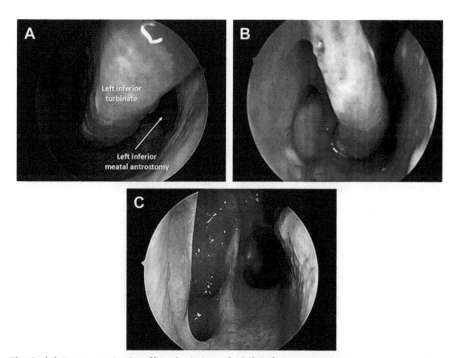

Fig. 3. (*A*) Postoperative in-office depiction of a left inferior meatal antrostomy in a patient who initially failed endoscopic maxillary antrostomy through the middle meatus. (*B*) Postoperative in-office depiction of a different patient who failed a right inferior meatal antrostomy. The patient continues to have purulent discharge despite the inferior meatal antrostomy. (*C*) In-office endoscopic view showing resolution of the disease process after a right EMMM.

(ie, the anterior ethmoid sinus and/or the posterior ethmoid sinus, which lies beyond the basal lamella). The principle of mucosal preservation applies: diseased tissue is removed and sinus patency is established, but healthy-appearing mucosa is spared whenever and wherever it is feasible. The preservation of healthy-appearing mucosa should, in theory, result in better postoperative function. However, this may not always hold true. There are situations in which a minimalist approach may in fact yield inferior postoperative outcomes.

Complete Total Ethmoidectomy with Mucosal Stripping

One such example is CRS with extensive polyposis. In 1997, Jankowski and colleagues[15] presented results of a retrospective study comparing conventional ethmoidectomy to a procedure termed nasalization (**Fig. 4**). Nasalization, or radical ethmoidectomy, is defined by the investigators as the act of "systematically removing all the bony lamellae and mucosa within the [ethmoid] labyrinth, with large [maxillary] antrostomy, sphenoidotomy, frontotomy, and middle turbinectomy." In this study, patients who underwent nasalization showed superior improvement in nasal symptoms relative to those who underwent more limited ethmoidectomy. Olfactory improvement remained stable for 3 years in the nasalization group and worsened after 2 years in the ethmoidectomy group. In a 2006 follow-up to this study, Jankowski and colleagues[16] found nasalization to be superior in terms of overall symptoms (as assessed by a questionnaire), endoscopic appearance of the mucosa, appearance on computed

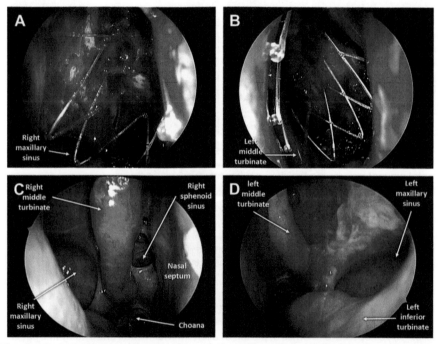

Fig. 4. Intraoperative endoscopic view of the right (*A*) and left (*B*) ethmoid cavities following a nasalization procedure or radical ethmoidectomy with steroid eluting implant in place. In this case, the middle turbinates were preserved. Note the demucosalization of the ethmoid labyrinth. Postoperative endoscopic image of the right (*C*) and left (*D*) ethmoid cavities after nasalization.

tomography, and total recurrence rate (22.7% in the nasalization group vs 58.3% in the traditional ethmoidectomy group).

External Frontoethmoidectomy

The external frontoethmoidectomy has been largely supplanted by ESS. In the management of ethmoid sinusitis, its role is essentially limited to the management of complications, as in the case where an anterior ethmoid artery ligation is necessary or for the management of an orbital abscess (the latter more commonly in the setting of acute rhinosinusitis).[17] A detailed discussion of this procedure in the context of external frontal sinus surgery can be found below.

EXTENDED SPHENOID SINUS PROCEDURES

In the setting of inflammatory disease, the sphenoid sinus is accessed surgically via one of 2 routes: the transnasal (or direct) route and the transethmoidal route. The latter technique is usually used when inflammatory disease also involves the posterior ethmoid sinuses. Similar to the Draf classification for frontal sinus surgery, a classification scheme has been proposed for sphenoid sinus surgery. According to Simmen and Jones, a type I sphenoidotomy entails identification of the ostium without further intervention; a type II sphenoidotomy entails enlargement of the ostium upward to the level of the cranial base, and inferiorly to one-half of the sinus height; and a type III sphenoidotomy involves widening the ostium to its most lateral extent.[18]

In general, more extensive sphenoid sinus surgery is reserved for cases wherein the disease process is extensive or previous surgery has failed. In some cases, a bilateral extended sphenoidotomy is necessary. In this procedure, the posterior aspect of the nasal septum is resected, along with the sphenoid rostrum, the intersinus septum, and other intrasphenoid partitions (Video 3), creating a common cavity with a broad drainage pathway. It also allows access to the lateral recesses of this sinus for removal, for instance, of large mucoceles, fungus balls, or extensive polyposis. The resulting cavity is essentially identical to that which is created by endoscopic transsphenoidal pituitary surgery, for which positive sinonasal outcomes have been widely reported.[1,19–21]

EXTENDED FRONTAL SINUS PROCEDURES

In patients with chronic frontal sinusitis that have failed AMT, management consists of frontal sinusotomy via either BCD or other limited frontal sinusotomy such a Draf I or Draf IIA. However, in cases of recalcitrant frontal sinusitis or recurrent disease after a previous frontal sinus procedure, a variety of extended endoscopic endonasal and open frontal sinus procedures can be used. The objective of the endoscopic procedures is the creation of a patent nasofrontal outflow tract (frontal sinus outflow pathway) and to provide access for application of topical medications. These endoscopic frontal sinus procedures include the Draf IIB, the modified Lothrop procedure (MLP), and 4 modifications of the MLP. The external approaches can be used to preserve frontal sinus function as well as for frontal sinus obliteration. These external approaches are the frontal sinus trephine procedure, the external frontoethmoidectomy, and the frontal sinus osteoplastic flap with or without obliteration.

EXTENDED ENDOSCOPIC FRONTAL SINUS APPROACHES
Draf IIB

A Draf IIB procedure may be viewed as the least extensive extended endoscopic frontal sinusotomy. This procedure has previously been described in the literature as a Nasofrontal approach type III, or Eloy type IIB[22] procedure. In this type of frontal sinusotomy, the frontal sinus outflow tract is enlarged by resecting the frontal sinus floor from the nasal septum medially to the ipsilateral lamina papyracea laterally (Video 4). After this procedure, unilateral maximal opening of the frontal sinus outflow tract is achieved. This procedure is indicated primarily after failure of Draf I or Draf IIA procedures, or in primary refractory frontal sinusotomy cases with difficult anatomy. In a recent retrospective chart review, Turner and colleagues[23] found this procedure to be most commonly used in revision cases of chronic frontal sinusitis secondary to lateralized middle turbinate remnant, frontal sinus mucocele, or postoperative synechiae.[23] The long-term patency of the created frontal sinusotomy in this cohort of patients was found to be greater than 90% after a mean follow-up of 16.2 months.

Modified Lothrop Procedure

The MLP (also termed an endoscopic modified Lothrop procedure, Draf III, nasofrontal approach type IV, or Eloy type III[22] procedure) consists of bilateral removal of the floor of the frontal sinus from one lamina papyracea to the contralateral lamina papyracea. In this procedure, a superior septectomy, intersinus septectomy, and resection of other frontal sinus partitions are also performed. By creating contiguous bilateral enlargement of the frontal sinus drainage pathway, this procedure provides the largest frontal sinus opening achievable (Video 5). This procedure can be used after failure of Draf I, Draf IIA, or Draf IIB procedures, or in primary refractory frontal sinusotomy cases with challenging anatomy. In 1998, Casiano and Livingston[24] reported the University of Miami's initial experience with the MLP in 21 patients. In that study, they found an overall patency rate of 90% after a mean follow-up of 6.5 months.[24] In 2006, Banhiran and colleagues[25] reported the University of Miami's experience using the MLP with stenting using a silastic sheet in 72 patients. The investigators could endoscopically visualize a common ostium in 94% of the cases (61.1% patent and 33.3% stenotic) after a mean follow-up of 22 months.[25] In a recent (2014) retrospective cohort study by Naidoo and colleagues[26] that included 229 patients undergoing MLP with a mean follow-up of 45.0 months, the investigators achieved a success rate of 95% with no further surgery being required. This same group of investigators later analyzed the failure rate of revision MLP and found it to be 21%.[27] They also noted that intraoperative purulence at the initial MLP, more than 5 previous sinus surgery, and aspirin-exacerbated respiratory disease increased the risk of failure.[27] In a 2003 systematic review on the MLP, Scott and colleagues[28] found that the evidence base for MLP was inadequate to assess its safety and efficacy. In 2009, Anderson and Sindwani[29] performed a systematic review and meta-analysis to assess the safety and efficacy of the MLP in 612 patients that met the inclusion criteria for their study. The investigators reported frontal sinus patency or partial stenosis in 95.9% of the patients at last follow-up. They found a rate of minor and major complications of less than 1% and 4%, respectively.[29]

Modified Lothrop Procedure Modifications

Recently, several modifications to the MLP have been described for select cases in order to address specific anatomic and pathologic challenges of frontal sinus disease while decreasing morbidity. These modifications include the modified hemi-Lothrop procedure (MHLP), the modified mini-Lothrop procedure (MMLP), the modified subtotal-Lothrop procedure (MSLP), and the modified central-Lothrop procedure (MCLP).[22]

Modified hemi-Lothrop procedure

The MHLP (also termed Eloy type IIC[22] procedure) is a technique described to increase access to the far lateral frontal sinus recess (supraorbital extension) or a supraorbital ethmoid cell.[30–32] In this procedure, a superior septectomy is added to an ipsilateral Draf IIB. This superior septectomy opening permits insertion of the endoscope and instruments via the contralateral nasal cavity, therefore providing greater access and visualization of the lateral frontal sinus recess of the affected ipsilateral frontal sinus or supraorbital ethmoid (**Fig. 5**). In this procedure, binostril and bimanual instrumentation can be performed for better disease eradication. Unlike in the MLP, the contralateral frontal sinus floor, recess, and frontal intersinus septum are preserved. The contralateral middle turbinate is also left untouched. This procedure has only been recently described, and data on its long-term efficacy are scarce. In a 2012 technique paper involving 15 patients (14 of which had CRS), a 100% success rate was reported for the MHLP after a mean follow-up of 18.2 months.[30]

Modified mini-Lothrop procedure

In some cases of chronic refractory frontal sinusotomy, the ipsilateral frontal sinus may not be safely accessible through the same side due to the disease process. These situations may include cases of prior iatrogenic or traumatic scarring, prior medial orbital wall decompression causing marked intraorbital contents obstructing the ipsilateral frontal sinus outflow tract, complex anatomic topography, severe frontal sinus recess stenosis, or severe osteoneogenesis. The MMLP (also termed Eloy type IID[22] procedure) addresses this issue. In this procedure, resection of the contralateral frontal sinus floor (Draf IIB) is coupled to a frontal intersinus septectomy (**Fig. 6**).[33,34] A complete intersinus septectomy is preferable in this situation, because this created opening becomes the drainage pathway for the contralateral diseased frontal sinus. Unlike in the MLP, the ipsilateral frontal sinus floor, recess, and most to all of the superior nasal septum are left undissected. The ipsilateral middle turbinate is also left untouched. Similar to the MHLP, information on the long-term efficacy of this procedure is limited. In a 2012 technique paper with 4 patients undergoing MMLP, a patent frontal sinus drainage pathway was maintained after a mean follow-up of 21 months.[34]

Modified subtotal-Lothrop procedure

In some cases of recalcitrant frontal sinusitis, an MSLP may be indicated. The MSLP (also termed Eloy type IIE[22] procedure) was described for the treatment of recalcitrant

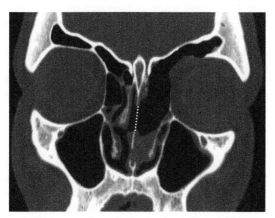

Fig. 5. Coronal computed tomography scan in a patient after a left MHLP (Eloy IIC). Note the superior septectomy window (*broken line*) used for contralateral access.

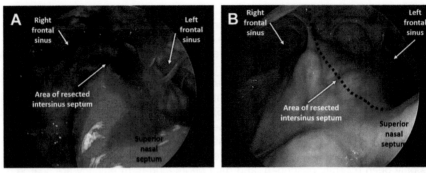

Fig. 6. Intraoperative (*A*) and in-office postoperative (*B*) images in a patient after a MMLP (Eloy IID).

bilateral frontal sinus disease and ipsilateral anterior skull base lesion resection, with an emphasis on preserving as much of the normal sinonasal architecture as possible.[35,36] In this procedure, removal of the frontal sinus floor unilaterally (Draf IIB) is performed with the addition of a superior septectomy and an intersinus septectomy (Video 6). This type of resection permits access and visualization of the ipsilateral and contralateral frontal sinus and binostril and bimanual frontal sinus manipulation. In this technique, the contralateral frontal sinus recess and contralateral middle turbinate are left untouched. As with MHLP and MMLP, the long-term efficacy of the MSLP has not been reported. In a recent retrospective review of 8 patients undergoing this procedure for tumor resection, a patent frontal sinus drainage pathway was achieved in all patients after a mean follow-up of 18.6 months.[36]

Modified central-Lothrop procedure

An additional modification of the MLP is the MCLP (also termed Eloy type IIF[22] procedure). The MCLP has only been very recently described.[22] During an MCLP, the bilateral medial frontal sinus floor is resected, and a superior septectomy and intersinus septectomy are added (Video 7). This technique provides access and visualization to both frontal sinuses with the added benefit of binostril and bimanual instrumentation. The MCLP can be used for recalcitrant frontal sinus disease located near the midline, including isolated disease/mucocele in a frontal intersinus cell, disease in a type IV frontal sinus cell located near the midline, or a central neoplastic process or skull base defect. The frontal sinus recesses and middle turbinates are left untouched. The MCLP may result in scarring and subsequent obstruction of the created central opening. Nonetheless, given that both frontal sinus outflow tracts would remain patent and a contiguous frontal sinus is created, there should be 2 egress pathways for any trapped frontal sinus contents to escape. Currently, long-term follow-up on this technique is not available.

EXTERNAL FRONTAL SINUS APPROACHES

The recent advances in endoscopic visualization and instrumentation have significantly decreased the need for external approaches to the frontal sinus. Nonetheless, in cases of recalcitrant chronic frontal sinusitis, these external procedures can still be used alone or in conjunction with endoscopic endonasal frontal sinus approaches. These external approaches include the frontal sinus trephination, the external frontoethmoidectomy, and frontal sinus osteoplastic flap with or without obliteration.

Indications for these procedures include disease involving the far lateral region of the frontal sinus, disease in a type 4 (intrasinus) frontal cell, osteomyelitis, and previous trauma.

Frontal Sinus Trephine

The first case of frontal sinus trephination may be credited to Alexander Ogstun[37] in 1884. In this case, an opening was created in the anterior table of the frontal sinus to evacuate purulent discharge; the nasofrontal outflow tract was then dilated and curetted to create a drainage route into the nasal cavity. Ogston[38] also described stenting of the created endonasal tract to prevent stenosis. In 1896, Luc described a similar procedure in the French literature without knowledge of Ogston's previous description. This procedure became known as the Ogston-Luc technique.

Frontal sinus trephination is a safe procedure; complications are relatively uncommon. Nowadays, this procedure exists mainly in the form of a mini-trephination enhanced by the use of an endoscope, which provides improved visualization and facilitates instrumentation through the trephine. In its current form, frontal sinus trephination is performed through a 0.5- to 1.5-cm incision placed under the medial one-third of the eyebrow (**Fig. 7**). The periosteum in this area is elevated, and an opening is made at the junction of the medial and superior orbital walls near the anterior border of the supraorbital ridge. The frontal sinus is drained, and the frontal sinus recess is opened. After evacuation of the disease process, a rubber catheter drain can be left in place for drainage and irrigation of the frontal sinus. The incision is subsequently closed in layers. The risk of a visible scar represents a potential disadvantage, but this can be minimized by limiting the trephine to 0.5 cm or less.[39,40] Paresthesias due to supratrochlear or supraorbital nerve injury, orbital injury, and injury to intracranial structures are potential but avoidable complications. A large series of patients who underwent trephination found a small risk of facial cellulitis (2.1%–4.5%); cerebrospinal fluid leak and orbital complications were rare.[41–44] Current indications for frontal sinus trephination include complicated acute frontal sinusitis, complicated chronic frontal sinusitis or frontal osteomyelitis, frontal sinusitis with difficult anatomic variants such as type III and IV frontal cells, and far lateral frontal sinus disease. This

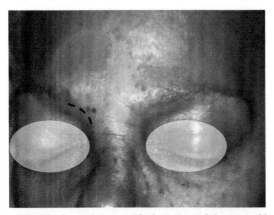

Fig. 7. Transilluminated right frontal sinus with depiction of the typical location of the skin incision (*black broken curve*) for the frontal sinus trephine procedure. Note that this incision can also be placed in the middle or lateral inferior border of the eyebrow based on the specific location of the frontal sinus abnormality and may also vary in length.

procedure can also be used in a variety of noninflammatory frontal sinus disorders that are beyond the scope of this article.

In a 2009 retrospective chart review, Seiberling and colleagues[43] described their experience in 188 mini-trephination procedures performed during 80 MLPs and 108 other frontal sinusotomies. The investigators found a 92% patency rate at an average follow-up of 25.5 months with 12 complications, the most common one being infection of the trephine site. Indications for the trephination in this study included difficulty in finding the frontal recess, severe edema/polyps, obstructing frontal cells (type III or IV frontal cells and intersinus septum cell), need for dissection assistance during an MLP, and need for postoperative irrigation.[43]

External Frontoethmoidectomy

The external frontoethmoidectomy (also termed a Lynch procedure) has been credited to Lynch, who in 1921 reported his results in 15 operations in the United States.[45] Around the same time, Howarth described a procedure similar to Lynch's in more than 200 cases in England.[46] However, the first description of this procedure was by Jansen in 1902, and Ritter in 1911, who reported a transorbital approach to the frontal sinus through resection of the ethmoid sinuses, and the creation of a contiguous space into the nasal cavity. Although this procedure is currently rarely used, the external frontoethmoidectomy is still being performed in some parts of the world for select but limited frontal, ethmoid, orbital, and skull base disease with or without endoscopic assistance. In its present form, the procedure involves a curvilinear incision made from beneath the medial aspect of the eyebrow to a point just below the medial canthus (**Fig. 8**). The periosteum is elevated, and the 2 limbs of the medial canthal ligament are detached from the anterior and posterior lacrimal crests. The lacrimal sac is lateralized from its fossa; the frontoethmoidal suture line is exposed, and the anterior and posterior ethmoid arteries are identified and coagulated with bipolar cautery. The bony medial orbital wall and the ethmoid sinus are subsequently removed. The floor of the frontal sinus is then resected to create a common cavity with the ethmoid sinus and nasal cavity. Some of the potential complications associated with this approach include nasofrontal outflow tract fibrosis and osteoneogenesis, lacrimal system injury, hematomas through avulsion of the anterior ethmoid artery, optic nerve injury and visual loss if dissection is carried out too far posterior, and intracranial injury.

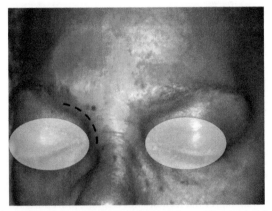

Fig. 8. Transilluminated right frontal sinus with depiction of the typical location of the skin incision (*black broken curve*) for the external frontoethmoidectomy.

Frontal Sinus Osteoplastic Flap with or Without Obliteration

The first reports of the osteoplastic flap were in the German literature by Schonborn in 1894[47] and Brieger in 1895.[48] This procedure was later popularized in Latin America by Bergara,[49] Bergara and Itoiz,[50] and Tato and colleagues.[51] Goodale and Montgomery[52–57] are credited for the popularization of this technique in the United States in the 1950s and 1960s. The use of frontal sinus osteoplastic flap with or without obliteration for recalcitrant frontal sinus disease has decreased significantly with the advent and expansion of endoscopic techniques. However, this procedure (and its variations) remains a key asset in the rhinologist's armamentarium and is a feasible option for the most severe and recalcitrant cases of frontal sinusitis. Some of the indications for these procedures include chronic recalcitrant frontal sinusitis after failure of endoscopic or open procedures, frontal sinus mucoceles, osteomyelitis, some cases of allergic frontal sinusitis, and so forth.

This procedure usually entails a bicoronal incision behind the hairline or across the vertex of the head (or infrequently may be performed directly through an eyebrow incision). The skin is then incised down to the pericranium, and dissection in the subgaleal plane is undertaken (**Fig. 9**A). Laterally, care should be taken to avoid injuring the frontal branch of the facial nerve by dissecting deeper than the temporoparietal fascia (ie, dissection should be in the areolar tissue over the superficial or deep temporalis fascia). Identification and preservation of the supratrochlear and supraorbital nerves are

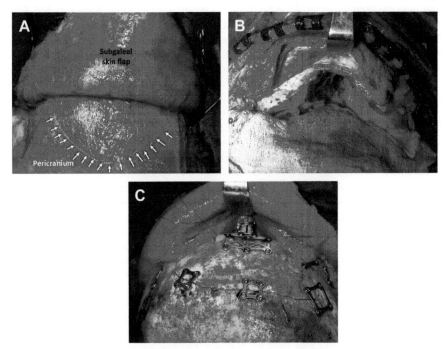

Fig. 9. (*A*) A bicoronal approach to the frontal sinus with elevation of the skin flap in the subgaleal layer. The pericranium is left attached to the anterior table of the frontal sinus. Arrows depict the location of the bone cut. (*B*) After resection of the anterior table of the frontal sinus. In this case, the bone flap is removed as a free bone flap that is not hinged on the pericranium. (*C*) Replacement of the bone flap that was previously removed using titanium plates.

subsequently undertaken to prevent postoperative anesthesia of the forehead. At this point, image guidance or a 6-foot Caldwell view radiograph can be used to delineate the borders of the frontal sinus. The periosteum is then incised along the marked border of the frontal sinus (see **Fig. 9**A), and the bone sectioned with an oscillating saw. Currently, an inferiorly based bone flap is most commonly used; however, a superiorly based bone flap has also been described. Beveling of the bone cut is useful to prevent penetration of the posterior table of the sinus. The bone flap is subsequently elevated, and the contents of the sinus evacuated. An attempt is then made to completely eradicate the frontal sinus mucosa using a high-speed diamond drill with or without microscopic assistance in order to prevent the potential for delayed mucocele formation, which has been reported to occur up to decades after osteoplastic flaps.[40] The frontal sinus may then be obliterated using a variety of materials, including autologous fat or muscle, or nonautologous materials. The nasofrontal outflow tracts are obstructed and separated from the frontal sinus if obliteration is the goal. Numerous variations of this procedure have previously been described in the literature. In some descriptions of the procedure, the mucosal surface of the sinus is removed without packing it with any obliterative material, instead relying on natural obliteration. If a decision is made not to obliterate the sinus, the nasofrontal outflow tracts are widely opened and may be combined into a contiguous opening as would be obtained with an MLP.

In some variations of external frontal sinus approaches that do not involve a pedicled bone flap hinged on the pericranium, the pericranial flap is elevated as a separate layer, and the anterior table of the frontal sinus is removed as a free bone flap (**Fig. 9**B). This bone flap is later replaced at the end of the procedure using a plating system (**Fig. 9**C). In yet another variation, the entire scalp flap is elevated as a single unit underneath the pericranium, followed by the free anterior table of the frontal sinus as described just above. One advantage for keeping the bone flap pedicled on the pericranium may be a decrease in the potential for necrosis of the anterior table of the frontal sinus.

Frontal Sinus Cranialization

In the most severe cases of refractory frontal sinusitis that have failed traditional endoscopic and open approaches, or in cases of osteomyelitis of the posterior table of the frontal sinus, cranialization of this sinus is viewed by most as the final step in management. Although typically performed by a neurologic surgeon, a discussion on extended frontal sinus surgery would not be complete without inclusion of this procedure. Cranialization of the frontal sinus was initially described by Donald and Bernstein in 1978 in 2 patients with penetrating frontal sinus injuries with intracranial penetration.[58] In the current form of this procedure, a bicoronal incision is made to approach the frontal sinus; the posterior table of the frontal sinus is resected, and any remnant frontal sinus mucosa is judiciously removed (using a high-speed diamond drill) to prevent the later development of intracranial mucocele. The nasofrontal outflow tracts are then obstructed with a vascularized strip of pericranium or temporalis muscle with or without the addition of fibrin glue. After this procedure, a frontal sinus no longer exists. In 2001, Ameline and colleagues[59] described 19 patients undergoing frontal sinus cranialization between 1984 and 1997 for "tumors, osteitis, traumatisms, and benign tumors or mucoceles" and noted no disease recurrence after a median follow-up of 29 months. The investigators concluded that cranialization of the frontal sinus harbored good results, with low morbidity in selected cases. In 2012, van Dijk and colleagues[60] reported on 15 patients with refractory chronic frontal sinusitis treated by cranialization of the frontal sinus at the University Medical Center Groningen in the

Netherlands from 1989 to 2008. The investigators found resolution of the signs and symptoms of CRS in all the patients with only 2 serious complications and better quality of life after a mean follow-up of 6.5 years.[60] They concluded that this procedure deserved consideration as the final remedy for refractory chronic frontal sinusitis when other options have failed.

SUMMARY

The primary treatment of CRS is AMT. Patients who fail AMT usually necessitate surgical intervention. Initial surgical management is typically performed through ESS with mucosal preservation, which can be achieved using BCD or functional ESS. In cases of failed initial surgical treatment, revision ESS is often undertaken. However, despite AMT and revision ESS, a subgroup of patients has refractory CRS that have failed the traditional ESS techniques. In these situations, more advanced surgical procedures (endoscopic or open) may be necessary for extirpation of the disease process. For the maxillary sinus, this can be achieved through procedures such as EMMA, EMMM, endoscopic-assisted sublabial anterior antrostomy, or inferior meatal antrostomy. For the ethmoid sinus, complete mucosal stripping or nasalization may be useful. Extended sphenoid sinusotomy through combining of the 2 sphenoid cavities into one contiguous space with or without mucosal removal can help with difficult recalcitrant sphenoid sinusitis. A variety of advanced endoscopic and open procedures can be performed for recalcitrant frontal sinus disease. The endoscopic procedures include the Draf IIB, the MLP, and the MLP's recently described variations (MHLP, MMLP, MSLP, MCLP), whereas the external approaches include the frontal sinus trephine, the external frontoethmoidectomy (rarely used today), the osteoplastic flap with or without obliteration, and frontal sinus cranialization.

SUPPLEMENTARY DATA

Supplementary data related to this article can be found at http://dx.doi.org/10.1016/j.otc.2016.08.013.

REFERENCES

1. Casiano RR, Herzallah IR, Anstead A, et al. Advanced endoscopic sinonasal dissection. In: Casiano RR, editor. Endoscopic sinonasal dissection guide. New York: Thieme Medical Publishers Inc; 2012. p. 59–99.
2. Guerini V, Association ND. A history of dentistry from the most ancient times until the end of the eighteenth century. Lea & Febiger; 1909.
3. The journal of laryngology, rhinology, and otology. Adlard & Son and West Newman, Limited; 1898.
4. Kennedy DW, Zinreich SJ, Shaalan H, et al. Endoscopic middle meatal antrostomy: theory, technique, and patency. Laryngoscope 1987;97:1–9.
5. Musy PY, Kountakis SE. Anatomic findings in patients undergoing revision endoscopic sinus surgery. Am J Otolaryngol 2004;25:418–22.
6. Konstantinidis I, Constantinidis J. Medial maxillectomy in recalcitrant sinusitis: when, why and how? Curr Opin Otolaryngol Head Neck Surg 2014;22:68–74.
7. Cho DY, Hwang PH. Results of endoscopic maxillary mega-antrostomy in recalcitrant maxillary sinusitis. Am J Rhinol 2008;22:658–62.
8. Costa ML, Psaltis AJ, Nayak JV, et al. Long-term outcomes of endoscopic maxillary mega-antrostomy for refractory chronic maxillary sinusitis. Int Forum Allergy Rhinol 2015;5:60–5.

9. Lee JY, Baek BJ, Byun JY, et al. Long-term efficacy of inferior meatal antrostomy for treatment of postoperative maxillary mucoceles. Am J Otolaryngol 2014;35:727–30.

10. Popatia R, Haver K, Casey A. Primary ciliary dyskinesia: an update on new diagnostic modalities and review of the literature. Pediatr Allergy Immunol Pulmonol 2014;27:51–9.

11. Noone PG, Leigh MW, Sannuti A, et al. Primary ciliary dyskinesia: diagnostic and phenotypic features. Am J Respir Crit Care Med 2004;169:459–67.

12. Carniol ET, Svider PF, Vázquez A, et al. Epidemiology and pathophysiology of chronic rhinosinusitis. In: Batra SP, Han KJ, editors. Practical medical and surgical management of chronic rhinosinusitis. Cham (Switzerland): Springer International Publishing; 2015. p. 3–18.

13. Egan M. Cystic fibrosis [Chapter 395]. In: Kliegman EA, editor. Nelson textbook of pediatrics. 19th edition. Philadelphia: Elsevier Saunders; 2011. p. 1481–96.

14. Chaaban MR, Kejner A, Rowe SM, et al. Cystic fibrosis chronic rhinosinusitis: a comprehensive review. Am J Rhinol Allergy 2013;27:387–95.

15. Jankowski R, Pigret D, Decroocq F. Comparison of functional results after ethmoidectomy and nasalization for diffuse and severe nasal polyposis. Acta Otolaryngol 1997;117:601–8.

16. Jankowski R, Pigret D, Decroocq F, et al. Comparison of radical (nasalisation) and functional ethmoidectomy in patients with severe sinonasal polyposis. A retrospective study. Rev Laryngol Otol Rhinol (Bord) 2006;127:131–40.

17. Kennedy DW, Bolger WE, Zinreich SJ. Diseases of the sinuses: diagnosis and management. Hamilton (ON): B.C. Decker; 2001.

18. Simmen D, Jones N. Manual of endoscopic sinus surgery and its extended applications. Germany: Thieme; 2005.

19. Carrau RL, Jho HD, Ko Y. Transnasal-transsphenoidal endoscopic surgery of the pituitary gland. Laryngoscope 1996;106:914–8.

20. Sethi DS, Pillay PK. Endoscopic management of lesions of the sella turcica. J Laryngol Otol 1995;109:956–62.

21. Aust MR, McCaffrey TV, Atkinson J. Transnasal endoscopic approach to the sella turcica. Am J Rhinol 1998;12:283–7.

22. Eloy JA, Vazquez A, Liu JK, et al. Endoscopic approaches to the frontal sinus: modifications of the existing techniques and proposed classification. Otolaryngol Clin North Am 2016;49(4):1007–18.

23. Turner JH, Vaezeafshar R, Hwang PH. Indications and outcomes for Draf IIB frontal sinus surgery. Am J Rhinol Allergy 2016;30:70–3.

24. Casiano RR, Livingston JA. Endoscopic Lothrop procedure: the University of Miami experience. Am J Rhinol 1998;12:335–9.

25. Banhiran W, Sargi Z, Collins W, et al. Long-term effect of stenting after an endoscopic modified Lothrop procedure. Am J Rhinol 2006;20:595–9.

26. Naidoo Y, Bassiouni A, Keen M, et al. Long-term outcomes for the endoscopic modified Lothrop/Draf III procedure: a 10-year review. Laryngoscope 2014; 124:43–9.

27. Morrissey DK, Bassiouni A, Psaltis AJ, et al. Outcomes of revision endoscopic modified Lothrop procedure. Int Forum Allergy Rhinol 2016;6(5):518–22.

28. Scott NA, Wormald P, Close D, et al. Endoscopic modified Lothrop procedure for the treatment of chronic frontal sinusitis: a systematic review. Otolaryngol Head Neck Surg 2003;129:427–38.

29. Anderson P, Sindwani R. Safety and efficacy of the endoscopic modified Lothrop procedure: a systematic review and meta-analysis. Laryngoscope 2009;119: 1828–33.

30. Eloy JA, Kuperan AB, Friedel ME, et al. Modified hemi-Lothrop procedure for su-praorbital frontal sinus access: a case series. Otolaryngol Head Neck Surg 2012; 147:167–9.
31. Eloy JA, Friedel ME, Murray KP, et al. Modified hemi-Lothrop procedure for supra-orbital frontal sinus access: a cadaveric feasibility study. Otolaryngol Head Neck Surg 2011;145:489–93.
32. Friedel ME, Li S, Langer PD, et al. Modified hemi-Lothrop procedure for supraor-bital ethmoid lesion access. Laryngoscope 2012;122:442–4.
33. Eloy JA, Friedel ME, Kuperan AB, et al. Modified mini-Lothrop/extended Draf IIb procedure for contralateral frontal sinus disease: a cadaveric feasibility study. Otolaryngol Head Neck Surg 2012;146:165–8.
34. Eloy JA, Friedel ME, Kuperan AB, et al. Modified mini-Lothrop/extended Draf IIB procedure for contralateral frontal sinus disease: a case series. Int Forum Allergy Rhinol 2012;2:321–4.
35. Eloy JA, Liu JK, Choudhry OJ, et al. Modified subtotal Lothrop procedure for extended frontal sinus and anterior skull base access: a cadaveric feasibility study with clinical correlates. J Neurol Surg B Skull Base 2013;74:130–5.
36. Eloy JA, Mady LJ, Kanumuri VV, et al. Modified subtotal-Lothrop procedure for extended frontal sinus and anterior skull-base access: a case series. Int Forum Allergy Rhinol 2014;4:517–22.
37. Ogston A. Trephining the frontal sinus for catarrhal diseases. Men Chron Man-chester 1884;1:235.
38. Luc H. Traitement des sinuses fontales suppurees chroniques par l'ouverture largesse de la paroi antérieure du sinus et le drainage par la voie nasale. Arch Int Laryngol 1896;9.
39. Bent JP 3rd, Spears RA, Kuhn FA, et al. Combined endoscopic intranasal and external frontal sinusotomy. Am J Rhinol 1997;11:349–54.
40. Schneider JS, Day A, Clavena M, et al. Early practice: external sinus surgery and procedures and complications. Otolaryngol Clin North Am 2015;48(5):839–50.
41. Batra PS, Citardi MJ, Lanza DC. Combined endoscopic trephination and endo-scopic frontal sinusotomy for management of complex frontal sinus pathology. Am J Rhinol 2005;19:435–41.
42. Patel AB, Cain RB, Lal D. Contemporary applications of frontal sinus trephination: a systematic review of the literature. Laryngoscope 2015;125(9):2046–53.
43. Seiberling K, Jardeleza C, Wormald PJ. Minitrephination of the frontal sinus: indi-cations and uses in today's era of sinus surgery. Am J Rhinol Allergy 2009;23: 229–31.
44. Walgama E, Ahn C, Batra PS. Surgical management of frontal sinus inverted pap-illoma: a systematic review. Laryngoscope 2012;122:1205–9.
45. Lynch RC. The technique of a radical frontal sinus operation which has given me the best results. (original communications are received with the understanding) that they are contributed exclusively to the laryngoscope.). Laryngoscope 1921;31:1–5.
46. Howarth WG. Operations on the frontal sinus. J Laryngol Otol 1921;36:417–21.
47. Wilkop A. Ein beitrag zur casuistik der erkrankungen des sinus frontalis. Wurz-burg (Germany): F. Frome; 1894.
48. Brieger. Uber chronische eiterungen des nebenhohlen er nase. Arch Ohren Na-sen Kehlkopfheilkd 1895;39:213.
49. Bergara R. Osteoplastic operation on the large frontal sinus in chronic suppura-tive sinusitis; end results. Trans Am Acad Ophthalmol Otolaryngol 1947;51:643–7.

50. Bergara AR, Itoiz AO. Present state of the surgical treatment of chronic frontal sinusitis. AMA Arch Otolaryngol 1955;61:616–28.
51. Tato JM, Sibbald DW, Bergaglio OE. Surgical treatment of the frontal sinus by the external route. Laryngoscope 1954;64:504–21.
52. Goodale RL, Montgomery WW. Experiences with the osteoplastic anterior wall approach to the frontal sinus; case histories and recommendations. AMA Arch Otolaryngol 1958;68:271–83.
53. Goodale RL, Montgomery WW. Anterior osteoplastic frontal sinus operation. Five years' experience. Trans Am Laryngol Assoc 1961;82:175–99.
54. Goodale RL, Montgomery WW. Anterior osteoplastic frontal sinus operation. Five years' experience. Ann Otol Rhinol Laryngol 1961;70:860–80.
55. Goodale RL, Montgomery WW. Technical advances in osteoplastic frontal sinusectomy. Arch Otolaryngol 1964;79:522–9.
56. Zonis RD, Montgomery WW, Goodale RL. Frontal sinus disease: 100 cases treated by osteoplastic operation. Laryngoscope 1966;76:1816–25.
57. Montgomery WW. Osteoplastic frontal sinus operation: coronal incision. Ann Otol Rhinol Laryngol 1965;74:821–30.
58. Donald PJ, Bernstein L. Compound frontal sinus injuries with intracranial penetration. Laryngoscope 1978;88:225–32.
59. Ameline E, Wagner I, Delbove H, et al. Cranialization of the frontal sinus. Ann Otolaryngol Chir Cervicofac 2001;118:352–8 [in French].
60. van Dijk JM, Wagemakers M, Korsten-Meijer AG, et al. Cranialization of the frontal sinus–the final remedy for refractory chronic frontal sinusitis. J Neurosurg 2012; 116:531–5.

A Practical Approach to Refractory Chronic Rhinosinusitis

Edward D. McCoul, MD, MPH[a], Abtin Tabaee, MD[b],*

KEYWORDS

- Chronic rhinosinusitis • Nasal polyps • Sinus surgery • Topical therapy

KEY POINTS

- A multidisciplinary and broad approach is required in the diagnostic evaluation of refractory CRS encompassing patient, environmental, and disease-related factors.
- Treatment of refractory CRSwP requires complete polyp removal and establishment of wide sinus openings to facilitate the postoperative delivery of topical corticosteroids.
- Treatment of refractory nonpolypoid CRS involves surgery to maximize sinus ventilation and drainage, using systemic or topical antibiotics or other adjunctive agents to minimize symptoms.
- A variety of emerging diagnostic and treatment pathways will likely improve management of CRS in the near future.

INTRODUCTION

As the understanding of chronic rhinosinusitis (CRS) has evolved from a monomorphic "infection" to a group of distinct inflammatory entities[1,2] so too has the approach to clinical evaluation and treatment. The need for an individualized approach to diagnosing and managing the possible variables that may have initiated the condition or spurred its persistence is becoming increasingly evident. This is especially true for individuals with refractory CRS. To elucidate the underlying pathophysiologic factors involved in a given patient, a list of several potential host and initiating events may be identified. Additionally, in patients with refractory CRS, the disease course itself

Disclosure Statement: There are no commercial or financial grant/assistance associated with this publication. Dr E.D. McCoul is a consultant for Acclarent. Dr A. Tabaee is on the scientific advisory board of Spirox.

[a] Department of Otorhinolaryngology, Ochsner Clinic Foundation, 1514 Jefferson Hwy, CT-4, New Orleans, LA 70121, USA; [b] Department of Otolaryngology, Weill Cornell Medicine, 1305 York Avenue, 5th Floor, New York, NY 10021, USA
* Corresponding author.
E-mail address: atabaee@hotmail.com

Otolaryngol Clin N Am 50 (2017) 183–198
http://dx.doi.org/10.1016/j.otc.2016.08.014
0030-6665/17/© 2016 Elsevier Inc. All rights reserved.

Abbreviations	
AERD	Aspirin-exacerbated respiratory disease
CF	Cystic fibrosis
CRS	Chronic rhinosinusitis
CRSwP	Chronic rhinosinusitis with polyposis

may compound the primary infection and contribute to perpetuation of inflammatory injury. Given this dynamic interplay between patient and disease variables, continued investigation and re-diagnosis of the relevant contributing factors is necessary throughout the lifespan of CRS. This article provides a practical approach to diagnostic evaluation and treatment considerations in refractory CRS. Integral to this discussion is an understanding of emerging concepts and future directions.

DIAGNOSTIC EVALUATION OF REFRACTORY CHRONIC RHINOSINUSITIS
General Principles

The approach to the clinical assessment of a patient with refractory CRS differs from that of routine CRS in several ways. The patient's prior history including disease course and treatment response is typically extensive. Additionally, the various etiologic issues may have evolved throughout the CRS history resulting in the emergence of CRS-related factors that may not have been initially present. Examples of this include osteitic bony changes and biofilm-producing bacteria. Therefore, a broad and comprehensive approach to diagnosis is imperative.

Patient History

Obtaining a complete medical history of a patient with refractory CRS is often time-consuming and complex. Symptom review encompasses the common sinonasal and related symptoms including nasal congestion, rhinorrhea or postnasal drip, facial pressure or pain, and disturbance in sense of smell or taste. Otologic, pulmonary, and general symptoms (fatigue, malaise, sleep disturbance) may also be present. Severity, duration, change over time, variability, associated modifying factors, and treatment response are assessed. A variety of sinonasal and general quality-of-life measures have been well described and are commonly used in clinical research. Although their role as a diagnostic tool and as an assessment of severity compared with a "normal" population have not been well defined, these tools are sensitive to change in symptom severity in a given individual and therefore have utility to establish a baseline quality-of-life score that can be followed during the course of the disease. The commonly used 22-item Sinonasal Outcome Test addresses multiple domains of sinonasal quality of life including rhinologic symptoms, extranasal rhinologic symptoms, ear/facial symptoms, psychological dysfunction, and sleep dysfunction.[3,4] The following past medical history should be carefully reviewed including the primary medical record whenever possible in addition to the patient's narrative report:

- Prior treatment modalities including a list of medications and surgical interventions with dates, durations, compliance, tolerance, and symptom response.
- Prior objective tests including laboratory tests, imaging studies, pathology results, and culture results. For imaging studies, the radiologist report and actual images should be reviewed.
- The medical records of prior treating otolaryngologists and associated medical specialties. Because most patients with refractory CRS have a prior history of sinus surgery, this also includes prior surgical reports.

Clinical Examination

Clinical evaluation of patients with refractory CRS encompasses routine otolaryngologic examination and a detailed endoscopy of the sinonasal cavity. Inspection of the ear, pharynx, and larynx and auscultation of the chest may elucidate extranasal manifestations of CRS given the common occurrence of multisystem dysfunction. Anterior rhinoscopy is performed to examine the position of the nasal septum, inflammatory changes of the inferior turbinate, patency of the nasal airway, and possible inflammatory changes of the nasal mucosa. Nasal endoscopy is performed systematically to examine the nasal cavity; middle meatal structures; sphenoethmoid recess; nasopharynx; and, in postoperative patients, the paranasal sinus cavities. A combination of flexible and rigid endoscopes (straight and angled) is used for a complete examination. Endoscopy allows for visualization of inflammatory changes and outflow tract patency and, when performed on subsequent occasions, fluctuations in disease severity. Debridement, management of postoperative synechia and stenosis, and obtaining mucopurulent secretions for culture are also integral to the care of patients with CRS. Future applications of nasal endoscopy may include attainment of material for additional diagnostic tests (eg, biofilm, microbiome). Finally, multiple reporting measures and grading systems have been described for nasal endoscopy.[5,6] These measures are largely used in clinical research without a well-defined role in routine patient care. To date, the ability to correlate nasal endoscopy findings to patient symptom scores remains limited, as does the interrater agreement of nasal endoscopy interpretation.[7,8] A greater degree of nasal endoscopy standardization is necessary.

Imaging

The role of imaging in patients with refractory CRS is multifold and is divided into structural and disease-related findings. Non-contrast computed tomography with fine cuts through the paranasal sinuses with bony windowing is the standard protocol for sinusitis evaluation. Soft tissue windowing can help differentiate various opacification patterns (eg, fungal findings). A systematic approach is used and includes triplanar radiographic evaluation of sinonasal anatomy, presence of anatomic variants, and patency of outflow tracts. In patients with a prior history of sinus surgery, postsurgical changes are also reviewed including patency of surgical sinusotomies, position and integrity of the middle turbinate, and completeness of the surgical changes. Disease assessment includes the extent, pattern, and severity of inflammatory changes, and presence of pathognomonic sinusitis variants (eg, allergic fungal sinusitis, odontogenic infection, osteitis) (**Fig. 1**). Review of prior studies is useful in determining the evolution of the inflammatory changes. MRI is considered in patients with complex soft tissue pathology and in patients with extension of inflammatory changes beyond the paranasal sinuses (eg, orbit and skull base). Various radiographic grading scores, including the Lund-Mackay scale,[9] are available and are routinely reported in clinical research. Additional assessment of sinus opacification relative to sinus pneumatization may improve the accuracy of radiographic scoring.[10] However, correlation of radiographic severity with patient symptom scores and the utility of these measures for clinical care are limited.

Microbiology

The role of pathogenic bacteria and fungi varies and may include acting as the primary initiating or perpetuating disease factor in certain CRS subtypes. Alternatively, pathogenic organisms may have no significant role, or a limited role, in other CRS

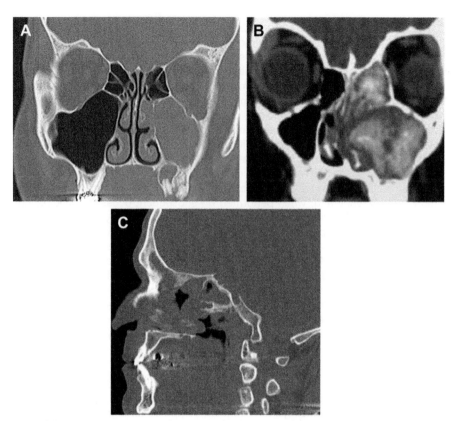

Fig. 1. (*A*) Noncontrast computed tomography (CT) sinus, bone window, coronal view of a patient with odontogenic sinusitis demonstrating disproportionate and asymmetric left maxillary sinus and infundibular opacification and associated periapical cyst from an infected maxillary molar. (*B*) Noncontrast CT sinus, soft tissue window, coronal view of a patient with allergic fungal sinusitis demonstrating asymmetric, expansile, heterogeneous inflammatory changes. (*C*) Noncontrast CT sinus, bone window, sagittal view of a patient with refractory CRS with osteitis changes of the superior ethmoid, frontal recess, and frontal sinus.

phenotypes including various polypoid variants. The interpretation of microbiologic data is based on the broader clinical, radiographic, and if available, pathology findings. In refractory CRS patients with presumed infectious component, cultures of mucopurulent secretions obtained with endoscopic visualization allow for specific assessment of speciation, antibiotic sensitivity, and directed medical therapy. Additionally, identification of specific bacterial pathogens may suggest the presence of biofilm and superantigens. Repeat cultures following treatment and throughout acute flare-ups are also useful given the fluctuations in the paranasal sinus microbiology.

Pathology

The histopathologic findings in most patients with CRS undergoing surgery are reported as nonspecific inflammatory changes. In patients with polypoid CRS, a more specific inflammatory pattern including eosinophilic tissue changes or allergic fungal sinusitis changes may be noted. Quantification of tissue eosinophilia may hold prognostic information, although this has not been fully defined.[11] Other specific CRS variants including osteitis, fungal CRS subtypes, and odontogenic CRS may be discernable on pathology. In these types of cases, direct communication with the pathologist regarding clinical considerations facilitates diagnosis. It is likely that a greater degree of sophistication in histopathologic analysis in the future will convey more specific diagnostic information in patients with CRS.

Host, Environmental, and Disease Cofactors

As reviewed in **Table 1**, there is an ever-expanding list of host, environmental, and disease-related factors. Although some of these pathophysiologic factors have a specific clinical phenotypic presentation and associated diagnostic test, several have an incompletely understood impact and several lack a clinically available diagnostic test. In many instances, meaningful feedback regarding the active pathophysiologic factors is attained from assessment of treatment response. It is likely that several cofactors may exist in a patient with CRS, especially refractory disease, including patient, environmental, and disease factors. The decision to pursue an extensive multidisciplinary evaluation and specialized testing for possible cofactors is individualized and may be especially indicated in patients with a suggestive clinical presentation and in patients with refractory disease.

Chronic Rhinosinusitis Phenotypes

CRS is increasingly understood as a group of inflammatory disorders each with unique pathophysiologic factors and phenotypes.[1,2] As the ability to subclassify CRS expands, an individualized approach to diagnosis is becoming increasingly possible. CRS classification is based on several different variables. Summating these variables for a given patient creates a deeper description of the specific CRS subtype. To date, although treatment options remain limited and applied similarly across multiple different phenotypes, more precise treatment pathways will likely be described based on specific disease factors in an algorithmic manner. The different variables used to classify CRS are reviewed in **Table 2**.

Future Considerations in Diagnosis

The current tools available including clinical evaluation, imaging, microbiology, and pathology provide limited perspectives on the underlying nature of the inflammatory changes. Several emerging concepts in CRS pathophysiology do not have clinically available tests including microbiome, genetics, and biofilms. As the role of these factors becomes better defined, the need for diagnosing these variables in clinical practice will be paramount. Improved and more detailed classification of CRS phenotypes will allow for a more tailored approach to treatment. This may include selective, targeted therapy; earlier interventions (including surgery) using evidence-based algorithms; and more cost-effective use of diagnostic and treatment modalities. The summation of these pathways will result in improved treatment outcomes and safety.

PRINCIPLES OF TREATMENT OF REFRACTORY CHRONIC RHINOSINUSITIS
Assumptions of Treatment

The approach to treatment of refractory CRS often involves multiple modalities and occasionally the participation of other medical specialists. In all cases, communication between the patient and physician is essential to establish reasonable expectations for treatment. A cornerstone of this process involves educating the patient that CRS is a chronic condition without a specific cure in most cases. Despite this, treatments are available to ameliorate symptoms and minimize impact on quality of life. A second

Table 1
Known etiologic disease factors and associated diagnostic tests

Disease Factor	Diagnostic Test
Patient host factor	
Anatomic variants, structural outflow tract obstruction	Nasal endoscopy, computed tomography scan
Primary immune deficiency	Total immunoglobulin levels, immunoglobulin subclass levels, specific antibody deficiency (*Streptococcus pneumonia*), complete blood count
Primary ciliary dysmotility	Ciliary morphology, ciliary beat frequency testing, genetic testing
Cystic fibrosis	Sweat chloride testing, genetic testing
Gastroesophageal reflux	Esophagogastroduodenoscopy, dual pH probe, treatment trial with medical therapy
Genetic predisposition	Family history, no commercially available test
Primary vasculitis/autoimmune disorder	Rheumatology evaluation, serology, tissue biopsies
Environmental factors	
Allergic rhinitis	Allergy testing (skin prick, radioallergosorbent test), treatment trial with medical therapy, nasal mucous IgE (not commercially available)
Toxin exposure	Patient history of occupational exposures, tobacco exposure, illicit drug use, intranasal medication use
Microbiologic factors	
Pathogenic microbiology	Middle meatus/sphenoethmoid/paranasal sinus cavity culture with endoscopic visualization when off antibiotics Include aerobe, anaerobe, fungus, and acid-fast bacillus testing
Biofilm	No commercially available test, more likely with specific bacteria (*Staphylococcus aureus*, *Pseudomonas aeruginosa*), treatment trial with topical surfactant therapy
Superantigen	No commercially available test, more likely with specific bacteria (*S aureus*)
Fungal infection subtypes (fungus ball, allergic fungal sinusitis, chronic invasive fungal sinusitis, granulomatous fungal sinusitis)	Patient factors (immune status), radiographic and nasal endoscopy findings, pathology and culture results
Specific infection/inflammatory patterns	
Odontogenic infection	Typical inflammatory radiographic pattern (unilateral, disproportionate involvement of maxillary sinus), radiographic evidence of odontogenic pathology, dental evaluation

(continued on next page)

Table 1 *(continued)*	
Disease Factor	**Diagnostic Test**
Chronic sinusitis with osteitis	Radiographic evidence of osteitis, more common in postoperative patients
Aspirin exacerbated respiratory disease (Samter triad)	Severe refractory polypoid CRS, known history of asthma and aspirin (nonsteroidal anti-inflammatory) reaction
Allergic fungal sinusitis	Characteristic imaging findings, presence of allergic mucin, presence of noninvasive fungal elements, atopy to fungi, polypoid CRS, minor Bent-Kuhn criteria[51]
Disruption of the normal sinonasal microbiome	No clinically available test

important concept is the shared role of medical and surgical therapy in the long-term management of CRS. Unlike other conditions where surgical treatment results in a definitive cure, the role of surgery in CRS is often aimed at facilitating the effectiveness of medical therapy. This may be accomplished by reducing disease burden, evacuating infectious agents, or providing exposure of sinus mucosa to topical agents. A third component of patient education, to introduce a note of optimism, acknowledges that this is an area of active research and the future holds promise for new treatments for refractory CRS.

The exact meaning of "refractory" remains incompletely defined, although for the purposes of this discussion several assumptions are implied. Individuals with refractory CRS are assumed to have been treated with one or more courses of conventional, broad-spectrum antibiotics from the penicillin, cephalosporin, or fluoroquinolone classes, in addition to either systemic or topical intranasal corticosteroids. The patient with refractory CRS is also assumed to have undergone conventional endoscopic sinus

Table 2 Factors used to classify variants of chronic rhinosinusitis	
Disease Factor	**Examples of Variants**
Time frame	• Acute (<1 mo of symptoms) • Subacute (1–3 mo of symptoms) • Chronic (>3 mo of symptoms)
Microbiology	• Specific microbiology culture patterns • Microbiome characterization (not currently available)
Pattern of inflammatory response	• With vs without polyposis • Th1 neutrophilic vs Th2 eosinophilic • Atopic vs nonatopic • Specific, well-described CRS variants (eg, aspirin-exacerbated respiratory disease, allergic fungal sinusitis)
Presence of identifiable initiating event	History of known events (eg, odontogenic infection, initial upper respiratory tract infection event)
Presence of identifiable host predisposition	See **Table 1** (eg, known immune dysregulation, ciliary dysfunction, obstructive anatomy)

surgery including ethmoidectomy and maxillary antrostomy. Individuals who continue to manifest symptoms of CRS despite these interventions may be subject to additional management as outlined next.

Treatment of Chronic Rhinosinusitis with Polyposis

Nonsurgical treatment

Most nasal polyps in the western hemisphere demonstrate an eosinophilic cellular profile. Because of this, the cornerstone of medical therapy involves systemic corticosteroids, which downregulate inflammatory cytokines and induce eosinophil apoptosis.[12–15] Prolonged use of systemic corticosteroids is not advised because of the multitude of potentially serious adverse effects. Topical nasal corticosteroids provide a valuable alternative with a more favorable safety profile and are recommended in nearly all cases of chronic rhinosinusitis with polyposis (CRSwP). Topical steroids decrease polyp size and impede polyp recurrence after surgery.[16] Most commercially available intranasal steroids are limited by a delivery device that produces a linear spray that does not effectively enter the frontal, sphenoid, or maxillary sinuses. As an alternative, other topical preparations, such as budesonide respules, can be applied as off-label therapy. Such preparations can be diluted in a large-volume sinus rinse, which has the dual effect of mechanically displacing mucus and infective agents while delivering the steroid into the peripheral sinuses. In cases of isolated frontal sinus polyposis, the undiluted medication may be instilled via gravity in a head-hanging position.[17]

Although primarily an inflammatory disease, CRSwP may be impacted by certain bacteria, particularly *Staphylococcus aureus*, as a cofactor in driving the inflammatory process.[18] Tetracycline class antibiotics, such as doxycycline, may prove useful in treating CRSwP through their ability to reduce bacterial load and downregulate certain inflammatory mediators.[19,20] The optimal duration of therapy remains undetermined, although courses of several weeks or longer have been used. Other antibiotics, such as those aimed at *Streptococcus pneumoniae* or *Haemophilus influenza*, may play a role if sinonasal purulence or symptoms of acute rhinosinusitis are present, which may be superimposed on CRSwP. However, these antibiotics are not likely to have a role in the long-term management of this disease.

Because CRSwP often coexists with atopy, comanagement of allergic disease is recommended. If an individual demonstrates significant sensitivity to one or more environmental antigens, immunotherapy may be considered to reduce the overall inflammatory load.[21] Comorbid asthma is also common in CRSwP, and should be managed in conjunction with a pulmonologist or other clinician with expertise in asthma management. Omalizumab is a monoclonal anti-IgE antibody that may reduce atopic inflammation in severely affected individuals, including sinonasal symptoms.[22,23] Other immunotherapeutic agents, such as anti-interleukin antibodies, are currently under investigation.

Surgical treatment

Surgical management of CRSwP represents an opportunity to optimize management by simultaneously reducing disease burden and enabling the delivery of topical postoperative medications to a maximum mucosal surface area. In the patient who has previously had sinus surgery, the surgeon should identify areas where failure to open all ethmoid cells or incomplete removal of bony partitions has resulted in unexposed recesses where inflammation can persist. This commonly occurs in the ethmoid labyrinth, frontoethmoidal recess, or sphenoethmoidal recess. The anterior and inferior surfaces of the maxillary sinus lumen also are subject to limited visibility and may result in residual polypoid disease. Residual uncinate tissue is also commonly encountered at the time of revision surgery. Surgical therapy should be as thorough as possible to avoid residual disease and provide an optimal baseline for postoperative medical therapy.

Removal of polyps should be as complete as possible without damaging the underlying periosteum or stripping of uninvolved mucosa. Doing so may result in the long-term development of a fibrotic, dysfunctional sinus without the ability for adequate mucociliary clearance. Conversely, merely "plucking" polyps from the nasal cavity without removing their site of origin within the sinus lumen is unlikely to prove adequate. Preservation of the structural integrity of the middle turbinate is preferable, with removal of polypoid tissue while preserving bony attachment points, although in severe cases bony attenuation may lead to a destabilized turbinate that may require resection to avoid postoperative lateralization. Application of a steroid-eluting stent at the conclusion of surgery may facilitate healing and slow the recurrence of polypoid inflammation.[24]

Beyond establishing ventilation of the involved sinuses, the surgeon should aim to create an opening into the different sinuses large enough to facilitate postoperative topical therapy. This may include wide maxillary antrostomy, transethmoidal sphenoidotomy, and extended frontal sinusotomy. In cases of multiple revision surgery, a modified Lothrop (Draf 3) procedure should be considered for severe frontal pathology. However, the indication for this procedure for inflammatory CRS remains incompletely defined. Balloon dilation in most patients with refractory CRSwP is not recommended because this is unlikely to produce a large enough opening for topical medication, and does not permit removal of inflammatory tissue.

In cases of ethmoid polyp recurrence in the setting of prior complete ethmoidectomy, in-office polypectomy may be a viable option. In addition, steroid-eluting stents and other steroid-impregnated materials may be considered for application in the office setting. These adjuncts are currently not Food and Drug Administration approved, but may become a standard part of the treatment of CRSwP in the future. The treatment options for CRSwP are summarized in **Table 3**.

Treatment of Nonpolypoid Chronic Rhinosinusitis

Nonsurgical treatment

Nonpolypoid CRS typically involves a noneosinophilic inflammatory profile and is associated with bacterial infection.[25] Because of this, corticosteroids may be less effective in management compared with CRSwP. However, unlike acute rhinosinusitis, the most common bacterial agents include *S aureus* and gram-negative bacilli,

Table 3 Treatment options for CRSwP with polyposis	
Nonsurgical Treatments	**Surgical Treatments**
Systemic corticosteroids	Revision ethmoidectomy
Topical steroids (low-volume spray, high-volume irrigation, concentrated drops)	Wide maxillary antrostomy
	Wide sphenoidotomy
Oral doxycycline	Extended frontal sinusotomy (Draf 2A, 2B, modified Lothrop)
Oral antibiotics for superimposed acute sinusitis	Polypectomy (in the setting of adequate prior ethmoidectomy)
Allergy management	Steroid-eluting implant
Asthma management	
Immunomodulators (emerging)	

such as *Pseudomonas aeruginosa*, and are often polymicrobial. Therefore, narrow-spectrum penicillins and cephalosporins are less likely to control the disease. Broad-spectrum aminopenicillins, third-generation cephalosporins, and respiratory fluoroquinolones may be required, the selection of which should be directed by endoscopically guided sinus culture. The increased prevalence of community-acquired methicillin-resistant *S aureus* poses an additional challenge, and may necessitate the use of other oral or intravenous antibiotic agents.[26]

Macrolides, such as clarithromycin and roxithromycin, may be useful in the management of nonpolypoid CRS. In addition to the bacteriostatic effect, macrolides exert an anti-inflammatory effect when given over a prolonged course.[27,28] The recommended dose is usually lower than the therapeutic dose for acute infections, and may require 3 months or longer of continuous therapy.[29] Macrolide therapy is most likely to be beneficial in individuals without atopy and without elevated IgE.[27]

Biofilms play an important role in an unknown but likely sizable number of cases of nonpolypoid CRS. Unlike planktonic infections, biofilms confer resistance to traditional systemic antibiotics. This has been established elsewhere in middle ear disease, where ototopical antibiotic preparations are preferred when a nonintact tympanic membrane is present. By the same principle, topical application of antibiotics to sinuses involved with biofilms may provide more potent drug delivery with fewer adverse effects compared with systemic antibiotics, although this modality remains unproven. The selection of antibiotic agent should be directed by sinus culture obtained under endoscopic visualization, and the principles of responsible antibiotic stewardship apply as with all antimicrobials. Available options include aminoglycosides, clindamycin, fluoroquinolones, vancomycin, and mupirocin.

Treatments aimed at mechanically disrupting biofilm membranes may have a role in the treatment of CRS. Topical saline irrigations may physically displace mucus and inflammatory elements, and are recommended preoperatively and postoperatively.[30] Hypertonic saline may be more effective than isotonic saline in disrupting molecular bonds. Several types of surfactant agents have been introduced, but no optimal agent has been identified. A nonirritating detergent, such as baby shampoo, may be a low-cost adjunct to other topical therapies.[31] Other topical therapies, such as manuka honey, and photodynamic therapy remain experimental.[32,33]

Surgical treatment

In contrast to CRSwP, a primary goal surgical management in nonpolypoid CRS is ensuring sinus ventilation rather than debulking of mucosal disease. Individuals who have previously undergone sinus surgery may demonstrate scar tissue or restenosis of previously opened sinus ostia. Fibrotic soft tissue bands and septations are often treated by lysis with conventional cutting instruments. Hypertrophic bony remodeling and osteitis may also be present as a nidus of inflammation. Hyperostosis may occur in any sinus, particularly the ethmoid labyrinth and frontal recess, which should be removed to optimize outcomes.[34] Drilling with a high-speed bur may be required. Stenosis of previously opened maxillary, frontal, or sphenoid sinuses may be treated with balloon catheter dilation, especially in cases where stenosis is limited to a single sinus. Balloon dilation may be offered either in the operating room or in the office setting under local anesthetic, with the latter preferred for individuals with medical comorbidities that would increase the risk of general anesthetic. Similarly, the avoidance of tissue incisions by a dilation procedure may be valuable in the anticoagulated patient who cannot safely discontinue their anticoagulation therapy.

The maxillary sinus often plays a major role in the symptomatology of nonpolypoid CRS, with the gravity-dependent portions of the antrum serving as a reservoir for mucus stasis and inflammation. A surgical remedy for this condition entails a modified medial maxillectomy with removal of the medial wall of the sinus along with a portion of inferior turbinate.[35,36] The resulting "mega-antrostomy" allows the two-fold purpose of improving gravity-dependent drainage of maxillary sinus contents while facilitating entry of postoperative topical medication. The sphenoid sinus may play a similar role as a reservoir for dysfunctional mucus clearance, which may be addressed by widely opening the sinus along the sphenoid rostrum laterally to the orbit and inferiorly to the choana.[37]

Extended frontal sinus procedures may be considered in cases of frontal sinus disease previously treated with Draf 1 or Draf 2A procedures in whom the turbinate has lateralized, those with postoperative synechiae or osteitis, or in whom a mucocele has formed.[38] A Draf 2B sinusotomy provides a wide unilateral opening, whereas a Draf 3 or one of the variations on a modified Lothrop procedure may be used to treat bilateral disease. Inert silastic or steroid-eluting stents may be beneficial in maintaining patency during the postoperative period.[39,40] The treatment options for nonpolypoid CRS are summarized in **Table 4**.

Treatment of Chronic Rhinosinusitis in Cystic Fibrosis

Nonsurgical treatment

The clinical manifestations of CRS in patients with cystic fibrosis (CF) show considerable variation because of the heterogenous underlying genetic mutations among individuals with the disease. Nonetheless, a uniform characteristic of CF is the presence of abnormally viscous mucus within the sinonasal tract and the lower airways. Nasal saline irrigation provides mechanical displacement of secretions, which may partially mitigate the abnormal mucociliary clearance present in these sinuses. Topical dornase alfa is useful in attenuating the viscosity of the mucus, which is abundant in extracellular deoxyribonucleotides.[41] Topical and systemic corticosteroids may be beneficial in individuals with nasal polyposis, although the neutrophilic character of these polyps may make them less responsive than polyposis in other forms of CRS.

The sinuses of individuals with CF are routinely colonized with pathogenic bacteria, most typically S aureus and P aeruginosa. This flora is believed to create a source of bronchopulmonary infection, which is a major cause of morbidity and hospitalization. Broad-spectrum oral or intravenous antibiotics are often required to control acute infectious exacerbations. Topical antibiotics may be used to treat the sinuses when acute inflammation is not present, with the goal of reducing bacterial load through increased potency at the mucosal surface. As with other cases of refractory CRS, endoscopically directed cultures should be used to guide therapy.

Table 4 Treatment options for nonpolypoid CRS	
Nonsurgical Treatments	**Surgical Treatments**
Topical or systemic corticosteroids	Removal of fibrotic tissue
Oral macrolide antibiotics	Removal of osteitic bone
Other culture-directed oral antibiotics	Dilation of stenotic sinus ostia (maxillary, frontal, sphenoid)
Culture-directed topical antibiotics	Revision ethmoidectomy
Saline irrigation	Modified medial maxillectomy (mega-antrostomy)
Surfactants (eg, baby shampoo)	Extended frontal sinusotomy

Individuals with CF require lifelong coordination of care among otolaryngologists, pulmonologists, and gastroenterologists, among others, to optimize longevity and quality of life. In patients with pulmonary failure, lung transplant is a life-saving intervention, albeit with the attendant risks of lifelong pharmacologic immunosuppression. Systemic treatments, such as ivacaftor, which target specific abnormal proteins on the surface of affected cells, have recently introduced the possibility of true disease-modifying interventions. Further study is needed to determine the effect of these medications on sinonasal disease.

Surgical treatment

As with other types of CRS, sinus surgery in CF has the potential to improve quality of life by reducing disease burden and sinonasal symptoms.[42] Surgery plays a role in removing obstructive polyps and lysing adhesions and other sequellae of chronic inflammation. An important component of surgical treatment of CF is the removal of retained secretions and infective matter within the sinuses, with subsequent lavage. Despite the potential benefits to sinonasal health, the effect on lower airway disease remains undetermined.[43] Because of dysfunctional mucociliary clearance, the maxillary sinuses may benefit from a modified medial maxillectomy, or mega-antrostomy, to maximize the degree of gravity-dependent drainage and facilitate the optimal penetration of topical irrigations and antibiotics postoperatively. A common characteristic of CF is marked hypoplasia of the frontal and sphenoid sinuses, which may obviate extensive surgery in those areas.[44] Nonetheless, all pneumatized areas should be explored during surgery to avoid leaving residual disease.

The optimal timing of sinus surgery with regard to lung transplantation remains undetermined. Prophylactic surgery may be beneficial in decreasing bacterial colonization and subsequent bronchopulmonary infections, although the effect on post-transplant survival is unclear.[45–47] Moreover, undergoing general anesthesia before transplant may increase the risk of intraoperative and postoperative complications, which underscores the need for communication between the otolaryngologist and the transplant care team, among others.

Treatment of Aspirin-Exacerbated Respiratory Disease

Nonsurgical treatment

Because aspirin-exacerbated respiratory disease (AERD) results from a defined disorder of arachidonic acid metabolism, it may be considered a prototype for disease-specific modifying interventions for refractory CRS. Zileuton has been used as a lipoxygenase inhibitor to decrease production of cysteinyl leukotrienes, which underlie the disease process. This medication may help with disease control, although the benefit on CRS in unclear, and monitoring of hepatic function is necessary.[48] Leukotriene receptor antagonists, such as montelukast, are more widely used, although their benefit in AERD remains to be studied.

As with other forms of CRSwP, topical and systemic corticosteroids play a major role in reducing mucosal inflammation and decreasing polyp size. Oral doxycycline may be considered as an adjunct to corticosteroids for the purpose of reducing staphylococcal-related inflammation.[19] Comorbid asthma should be managed by a pulmonologist or other qualified specialist.

Aspirin desensitization has a role in refractory AERD, with benefit for upper and lower airway disease.[49] This treatment must be initiated by an allergist with the relevant expertise, and requires careful titration and monitoring until complete desensitization is achieved. This option is typically reserved for refractory cases, because it entails lifelong maintenance of anticoagulation with the attendant risks of bleeding and gastric complications. Furthermore, if aspirin maintenance is interrupted for any reason, including sinus surgery, the process of desensitization may need to be repeated.

Surgical treatment

Similar to other forms of CRSwP, sinus surgery has the potential to improve outcomes by removing inflammatory polyps, evacuating eosinophilic mucus, and establishing wide apertures for the delivery of topical therapies postoperatively. This may entail extended surgery of the frontal, maxillary and sphenoid sinuses, as described in previous sections. Thorough surgery with complete removal of all polyps is recommended before the initiation of aspirin desensitization.

Treatment of Other Special Cases

Individuals with primary ciliary dyskinesia, when suspected or confirmed by testing, may benefit from a strategy similar to some cases of nonpolypoid CRS. In this condition, mucociliary clearance is inadequate and results in pooling of secretions predominantly within the maxillary and sphenoid sinuses, with subsequent superinfection and biofilm formation. Wide sphenoidotomy and maxillary antrostomy, possibly including modified medial maxillectomy, may be useful to maximize gravity-dependent drainage and facilitate postoperative topical irrigations, including steroids, surfactants, and topical antibiotics.[50]

Suspicion of a granulomatous disease may arise in the presence of sinonasal inflammation that progresses despite therapy with topical and systemic corticosteroids and primary sinus surgery. Such diseases as sarcoidosis, Wegener granulomatosis, and Churg-Strauss syndrome require submucosal biopsy for confirmation, which may require a surgical specimen. Cytotoxic medications may be indicated to control the systemic inflammation in these diseases, which require collaboration with a rheumatologist. Saline irrigations and topical corticosteroids may have a role, as does systemic antibiotic therapy to address secondary acute sinusitis. Sinus surgery may also be useful to remove obstructive soft tissue or bone that interferes with sinus drainage or ventilation.

SUMMARY

Refractory CRS is associated with unique challenges in diagnosis given the multifactorial nature, existence of unique subtypes, and limitations in available testing modalities. A broad, multidisciplinary approach is indicated with critical evaluation of patient, environmental, and disease factors. In many cases, evaluation of the patient throughout the disease process including after therapy serves a dual function of providing further characterization of the patient's disease while enabling recovery. The subtyping of CRS is progressively becoming more refined based on a deeper understanding of relevant pathophysiologic factors and distinct phenotypes. Treatment pathways will likely become more individualized over time in an attempt to address those issues relevant to the patient. To date, unique treatment principles apply to patients with refractory CRS based on presence versus absence of polyps, identification of specific pathogenic microorganisms, and disease subclassification.

REFERENCES

1. Fokkens WJ, Lund VJ, Mullol J, et al. European position paper on rhinosinusitis and nasal polyps 2012. Rhinol Suppl 2012;23:1–298.

2. Orlandi RR, Kingdom TT, Hwang PH. International consensus statement on allergy and rhinology: rhinosinusitis executive summary. Int Forum Allergy Rhinol 2016;6(Suppl 1):S3–21.

3. Hopkins C, Gillett S, Slack R, et al. Psychometric validity of the 22-item sinonasal outcome test. Clin Otolaryngol 2009;34:447–54.

4. DeConde AS, Mace JC, Bodner T, et al. SNOT-22 quality of life domains differentially predict treatment modality selection in chronic rhinosinusitis. Int Forum Allergy Rhinol 2014;4:972–9.

5. Lund VJ, Kennedy DW. Quantification for staging sinusitis. The Staging and Therapy Group. Ann Otol Rhinol Laryngol Suppl 1995;167:17–21.

6. Wright E, Agrawal S. Impact of perioperative systemic steroids on surgical outcomes in patients with chronic rhinosinusitis with polyposis: evaluation with the novel perioperative sinus endoscopy (POSE) scoring system. Laryngoscope 2007;117(Suppl 115):1–28.

7. Raithatha R, Anand VK, Mace JC, et al. Interrater agreement of nasal endoscopy for chronic rhinosinusitis. Int Forum Allergy Rhinol 2012;2:144–50.

8. McCoul ED, Smith TL, Mace JC, et al. Interrater agreement of nasal endoscopy in patients with a prior history of endoscopic sinus surgery. Int Forum Allergy Rhinol 2012;2:453–9.

9. Lund VJ, Mackay IS. Staging in rhinosinusitis. Rhinology 1993;107:183–4.

10. Marino MJ, Riley CA, Patel AS, et al. Paranasal sinus opacification-to-pneumatization ratio applied as a rapid and validated clinician assessment. Int Forum Allergy Rhinol 2016. [Epub ahead of print].

11. Snidvongs K, Lam M, Sacks R, et al. Structured histopathology profiling of chronic rhinosinusitis in routine practice. Int Forum Allergy Rhinol 2012;2:376–85.

12. Martinez-Devesa P, Patiar S. Oral steroids for nasal polyps. Cochrane Database Syst Rev 2011;(7):CD005232.

13. Schleimer RP. Glucocorticoids suppress inflammation but spare innate immune responses in airway epithelium. Proc Am Thorac Soc 2004;1:222–30.

14. Druilhe A, Létuvé S, Pretolani M. Glucocorticoid-induced apoptosis in human eosinophils: mechanisms of action. Apoptosis 2003;8:481–95.

15. Ohta K, Yamashita N. Apoptosis of eosinophils and lymphocytes in allergic inflammation. J Allergy Clin Immunol 1999;104:14–21.

16. Kalish L, Snidvongs K, Sivasubramaniam R, et al. Topical steroids for nasal polyps. Cochrane Database Syst Rev 2012;(12):CD006549.

17. Steinke JW, Payne SC, Tessier ME, et al. Pilot study of budesonide inhalant suspension irrigations for chronic eosinophilic sinusitis. J Allergy Clin Immunol 2009; 124:1352–4.

18. Pastacaldi C, Lewis P, Howarth P. Staphylococci and staphylococcal superantigens in asthma and rhinitis: a systematic review and meta-analysis. Allergy 2011;66:549–55.

19. Van Zele T, Gevaert P, Holtappels G, et al. Oral steroids and doxycycline: two different approaches to treat nasal polyps. J Allergy Clin Immunol 2010;125: 1069–76.e4.

20. Grammer LC. Doxycycline or oral corticosteroids for nasal polyps. J Allergy Clin Immunol Pract 2013;1:541–2.

21. Tanaka A, Ohashi Y, Kakinoki Y, et al. Immunotherapy suppresses both Th1 and Th2 responses by allergen stimulation, but suppression of the Th2 response is a more important mechanism related to the clinical efficacy of immunotherapy for perennial allergic rhinitis. Scand J Immunol 1998;48:201–11.

22. Gevaert P, Calus L, Van Zele T, et al. Omalizumab is effective in allergic and nonallergic patients with nasal polyps and asthma. J Allergy Clin Immunol 2013;131:110–6.
23. Tajiri T, Matsumoto H, Hiraumi H, et al. Efficacy of omalizumab in eosinophilic chronic rhinosinusitis patients with asthma. Ann Allergy Asthma Immunol 2013; 110:387–8.
24. Han JK, Marple BF, Smith TL, et al. Effect of steroid-releasing implants on postoperative medical and surgical interventions: an efficacy meta-analysis. Int Forum Allergy Rhinol 2012;2:271–9.
25. Han JK. Subclassification of chronic rhinosinusitis. Laryngoscope 2013;123: S15–27.
26. McCoul ED, Jourdy DN, Schaberg MR, et al. Methicillin-resistant *Staphylococcus aureus* sinusitis in nonhospitalized patients: a systematic review of prevalence and treatment outcomes. Laryngoscope 2012;122:2125–31.
27. Wallwork B, Coman W, Mackay-Sim A, et al. A double-blind, randomized, placebo-controlled trial of macrolide in the treatment of chronic rhinosinusitis. Laryngoscope 2006;116:189–93.
28. Videler WJ, Badia L, Harvey RJ, et al. Lack of efficacy of long-term, low-dose azithromycin in chronic rhinosinusitis: a randomized controlled trial. Allergy 2011;66: 1457–68.
29. Rudmik L, Soler ZM. Medical therapies for adult chronic sinusitis: a systematic review. JAMA 2015;314(9):926–39.
30. Rudmik L, Hoy M, Schlosser RJ, et al. Topical therapies in the management of chronic rhinosinusitis: an evidence-based review with recommendations. Int Forum Allergy Rhinol 2013;3:281–98.
31. Chiu AG, Palmer JN, Woodworth BA, et al. Baby shampoo nasal irrigations for the symptomatic post–functional endoscopic sinus surgery patient. Am J Rhinol 2008;22:34–7.
32. Goggin R, Jardeleza C, Wormald PJ, et al. Colloidal silver: a novel treatment for *Staphylococcus aureus* biofilms? Int Forum Allergy Rhinol 2014;4:171–5.
33. Biel MA, Sievert C, Usacheva M, et al. Antimicrobial photodynamic therapy treatment of chronic recurrent sinusitis biofilms. Int Forum Allergy Rhinol 2011;1:329–34.
34. Bhandarkar ND, Mace JC, Smith TL. The impact of osteitis on disease severity measures and quality of life outcomes in chronic rhinosinusitis. Int Forum Allergy Rhinol 2011;1:372–8.
35. Cho DY, Hwang PH. Results of endoscopic maxillary mega-antrostomy in recalcitrant maxillary sinusitis. Am J Rhinol 2008;22:658–62.
36. Costa ML, Psaltis AJ, Nayak JV, et al. Long-term outcomes of endoscopic maxillary mega-antrostomy for refractory chronic maxillary sinusitis. Int Forum Allergy Rhinol 2015;5:60–5.
37. Simmen D, Jones N. Manual of endoscopic sinus surgery and its extended applications. New York: Thieme Medical Publishers; 2005.
38. Turner JH, Vaezeafshar R, Hwang PH. Indications and outcomes for Draf IIB frontal sinus surgery. Am J Rhinol Allergy 2016;30:70–3.
39. Banhiran W, Sargi Z, Collins W, et al. Long-term effect of stenting after an endoscopic modified Lothrop procedure. Am J Rhinol 2006;20:595–9.
40. Smith TL, Singh A, Luong A, et al. Randomized controlled trial of a bioabsorbable steroid-releasing implant in the frontal sinus opening. Laryngoscope 2016. [Epub ahead of print].
41. Liang J, Higgins T, Ishman SL, et al. Medical management of chronic rhinosinusitis in cystic fibrosis: a systematic review. Laryngoscope 2014;124:1308–13.

42. Khalid AN, Mace J, Smith TL. Outcomes of sinus surgery in adults with cystic fibrosis. Otolaryngol Head Neck Surg 2009;141:358–63.

43. Liang J, Higgins TS, Ishman SL, et al. Surgical management of chronic rhinosinusitis in cystic fibrosis: a systematic review. Int Forum Allergy Rhinol 2013;3: 814–22.

44. Woodworth BA, Ahn C, Flume PA, et al. The delta F508 mutation in cystic fibrosis and impact on sinus development. Am J Rhinol 2007;21:122–7.

45. Holzmann D, Speich R, Kaufmann T, et al. Effects of sinus surgery in patients with cystic fibrosis after lung transplantation: a 10-year experience. Transplantation 2004;77:134–6.

46. Vital D, Hofer M, Benden C, et al. Impact of sinus surgery on pseudomonal airway colonization, bronchiolitis obliterans syndrome and survival in cystic fibrosis lung transplant recipients. Respiration 2013;86:25–31.

47. Leung MK, Rachakonda L, Weill D, et al. Effects of sinus surgery on lung transplantation outcomes in cystic fibrosis. Am J Rhinol 2008;22:192–6.

48. Dahlen B, Nizankowska E, Szczeklik A, et al. Benefits from adding the 5-lipoxygenase inhibitor zileuton to conventional therapy in aspirin-intolerant asthmatics. Am J Respir Crit Care Med 1998;157:1187–94.

49. Sweet JM, Stevenson DD, Simon RA, et al. Long-term effects of aspirin desensitization–treatment for aspirin-sensitive rhinosinusitis-asthma. J Allergy Clin Immunol 1990;85:59–65.

50. Mener DJ, Lin SY, Ishman SL, et al. Treatment and outcomes of chronic rhinosinusitis in children with primary ciliary dyskinesia: where is the evidence? A qualitative systematic review. Int Forum Allergy Rhinol 2013;3:986–91.

51. Bent JP 3rd, Kuhn FA. Diagnosis of allergic fungal sinusitis. Otolaryngol Head Neck Surg 1994;111:580–8.

Index

Note: Page numbers of article titles are in **boldface** type.

Otolaryngol Clin N Am 50 (2017) 199–204
http://dx.doi.org/10.1016/S0030-6665(16)30206-7
0030-6665/17

oto.theclinics.com

Moving?

Make sure your subscription moves with you!

To notify us of your new address, find your **Clinics Account Number** (located on your mailing label above your name), and contact customer service at:

Email: journalscustomerservice-usa@elsevier.com

800-654-2452 (subscribers in the U.S. & Canada)
314-447-8871 (subscribers outside of the U.S. & Canada)

Fax number: 314-447-8029

Elsevier Health Sciences Division
Subscription Customer Service
3251 Riverport Lane
Maryland Heights, MO 63043

*To ensure uninterrupted delivery of your subscription, please notify us at least 4 weeks in advance of move.

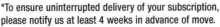

Printed and bound by CPI Group (UK) Ltd, Croydon, CR0 4YY

07/10/2024

01040500-0004